EXPLORING NEW FINDINGS ON AMYLOIDOSIS

Edited by **Ana-María Fernández-Escamilla**

Exploring New Findings on Amyloidosis
http://dx.doi.org/10.5772/61496
Edited by Ana-María Fernández-Escamilla

Contributors

Magda De Eguileor, Dmitry Kurouski, Hideo Tsukada, Ivana Sirangelo, Clara Iannuzzi, Gaetano Irace, Isabel Cardoso, Mobina Alemi, Luis Miguel Santos, James J. Driscoll, Tadashi Nakamura, Dae Sung Yoon, Wonseok Lee, Hyungbeen Lee, Gyudo Lee, Anna Novials, Joel Montane, Paisit Paueksakon, Jan Gettemans, Adriaan Verhelle, Oxana Galzitskaya, Olga Selivanova, Nikiat Dovidchenko, Kevan Hartshorn, Ruth Kandel, Mitchell White

Published by InTech

Janeza Trdine 9, 51000 Rijeka, Croatia

Publishing Process Manager Iva Simcic

Technical Editor SPi Global

Cover InTech Design team

First published September, 2016

Printed in Croatia

Additional hard copies can be obtained from orders@intechopen.com

Exploring New Findings on Amyloidosis, Edited by Ana-María Fernández-Escamilla

p. cm.

Print ISBN 978-953-51-2618-8

Online ISBN 978-953-51-2619-5

For EU product safety concerns:
IN TECH d.o.o., Prolaz Marije Krucifikse Kozulić 3, 51000 Rijeka, Croatia,
info@intechopen.com or visit our website at intechopen.com.

Meet the editor

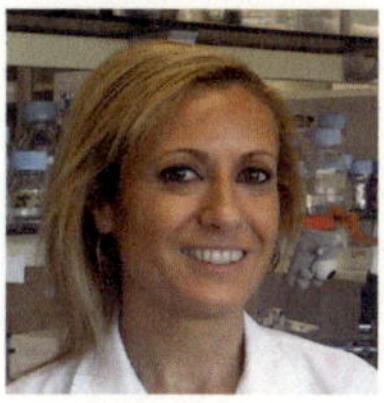

Ana-María Fernández-Escamilla is a senior researcher at Spanish National Research Council. In 2001, she received her PhD in Biophysical Chemistry at the University of Granada, Spain. She developed her career in prestigious Spanish and international research centers as European Molecular Biology Laboratory (Germany), funded by National and European competing grants. She participated in the development and testing of the computer algorithm "TANGO", designed to predict protein aggregation propensity. Currently, she develops as PI two R&D projects funded by public bodies and one biotech-company research contract. In 2014, she got positive assessment of research excellence by the Spanish National Evaluation and Foresight Agency. Her scientific research is focused on protein engineering combining theoretical and experimental approaches for biochemical, biophysical, and structural characterization of macromolecules.

Contents

Preface

Amyloid protein aggregates are involved in a number of "protein-misfolding diseases" of enormous social and economic impact for which there are still no effective therapies or strategies for their prevention or inhibition available. There is a heterogeneous group of amyloidogenic proteins associated with amyloid pathologies including amyloid-beta (Aβ) peptide linked to the most common type of dementia, Alzheimer's disease (AD); prion protein (PrP) related to spongiform encephalopathies; islet amyloid polypeptide (IAPP) connected to diabetes type II; transthyretin (TTR) linked to familial amyloidotic polyneuropathy (FAP) that often affects liver, nerves, heart, and kidneys; serum amyloid A protein (SAA) associated with AA amyloidosis that mostly affects kidneys; immunoglobulin light-chain (AL) amyloidosis that affects heart, kidneys, skin, nerves, and liver; and dialysis-related amyloidosis that develops when serum proteins in the blood (β2-microglobulin) are deposited in the joints and tendons.

One of the most recent biophysical definitions describes amyloids as elongated unbranched fibrils comprising a repeating intermolecular β-sheet motifs positioned perpendicular to the fibril axis. The resulting insoluble fibrillar structure is a highly ordered cross-beta structure that in the majority of the cases seems to be helically twisted. Amyloid-related diseases or amyloidosis are characterized by extracellular deposition of misfolded proteins in different organs, forming insoluble amyloid aggregates. Most of these protein aggregates lose their normal function and lead to cell damage, disruption of the tissue architecture, and organ dysfunction and death. Even though amyloid fibers have been extensively studied, current insights implicate prefibrillar intermediates rather than mature amyloid fibers in causing cell death.

Several events may trigger amyloid formation, such as protein mutations, unusual enzymatic cleavage patterns, and posttranslational modifications. However, not all amyloid fibers play a detrimental role in the host. An increasing number of studies show how amyloids also play an important role as beneficial (nontoxic) amyloid fibers termed "functional amyloids" (FAs). FAs are related to the formation of buds of insects, spider silk, coating fungal hyphae, bacterial host adhesion, bacterial biofilm formation, melanin synthesis, and human hemostatic system, whose molecular and functional mechanisms still remain undiscovered. Evidently, functional amylogenesis mechanisms require a strong regulation to avoid toxicity. In addition, I would like to highlight two recent studies. The first very interesting one by Camilla Betti (May 2016) describes the potential biotechnological application of induced target aggregation, a method based on expression of specific aggregation-prone peptides derived from the targeted proteins, as a very useful tool to knockdown protein functions in plants to produce favorable features in crops. The second study by Rubén Hervás et al. (Jan 2016) demonstrates that a functional amyloid (RNA-binding protein Orb2 of *Drosophila*) shares a wide group of features with toxic amyloids, including conversion to a structurally characteristic insoluble fibrous deposits via toxic oligomeric intermediates, which can be sequestered in vivo in hetero-oligomers by pathological amyloids. Furthermore, the toxic intermediates of this protein are extremely transient, corroborating the above-mentioned requirement for the strict regulation of the kinetic parameters during the amyloid formation process to differentiate this functional amyloid from pathological amyloids.

This book opens an exciting door to provide the latest information about the function and the mechanisms of the amyloid formation process from the structural, biophysical, biomedical, and nanotechnological perspective, combining the new findings on toxic and functional amyloids studies using the new technological advances in electron microscopy (EM), atomic force microscopy (AFM), and positron emission tomography (PET) among others, to fight against amyloid-based diseases.

When I was reviewing all the chapters, I decided to start the book with a clear and general perspective on amyloids. Chapter 1 by Isabel Cardoso, Luis Miguel Santos, and Mobina Alemi is written in a very accessible, comprehensive, and educational way that fulfills all the requirements for an introductory chapter. This chapter describes Alzheimer's disease (AD) as a form of localized amyloidosis that affects the central nervous system focusing on the neuroprotective role of transthyretin (TTR) and its amyloidogenic role in Familial Amyloid Polyneuropathy (FAP).

The next chapters deal with the progress in technique used to obtain structural and kinetic information on amyloid fibrils. Chapter 2 by Dmitry Kurouski aims to demonstrate the applicability of electron microscopy (EM) including transmission electron microscopy (TEM), scanning transmission electron microscopy (STEM), scanning electron microscopy (SEM), and cryo-SEM, and also atomic force microscopy (AFM) and vibrational circular dichroism (VCD) to advance the understanding of supramolecular architecture and the organization of amyloid fibrils and fibril polymorphism. Chapter 3 by Wonseok Lee, Hyungbeen Lee, Gyudo Lee, and Dae Sung Yoon describes the advances on alternative techniques, such as AFM and its extensions (dynamic liquid AFM; PeakForce quantitative nanomechanical mapping (QNM) and Kelvin probe force microscopy (KFPM)), as excellent methodologies to determine the biophysical properties of amyloid fibrils and the possible perspectives and future directions for the characterization of amyloid fibrils. Positron emission tomography (PET) imaging is an interesting technique for in vivo experiments. Chapter 4 by Hideo Tsukada describes PET as an excellent technique for the diagnosis of Alzheimer's disease using 18F-BCPP-EF—a novel PET probe for mitochondrial complex I (MC-I) activity—which could discriminate the neuronal-damaged areas with neuroinflammation, in young and aged monkeys demonstrating the normal aging effects on MC-I activity in the brain.

I consider crucial for the current research the combination of theoretical and experimental approaches to develop any scientific area. This methodology is described in Chapter 5 written by Oxana V. Galzitskaya, Nikita V. Dovidchenko, and Olga M. Selivanova who use theoretical and experimental approaches to describe possible kinetic models to elucidate the key features of amyloid nucleation and growth. Concretely, this chapter reviews the common features of the amyloid formation process by several proteins which have their own specific fibrillogenesis route determined by their amino acid sequence protein and strongly dependent on environmental conditions and seed addition.

As mentioned above, one of the possible triggers to induce amyloid aggregation is the post-translational modifications (PTMs) that affect protein structure and function. Chapter 6 by Clara Iannuzzi, Gaetano Irace, and Ivana Sirangelo is focused on one of the more frequent PTMs, protein glycation, and its determinant role on amyloid aggregation process and its implication on cellular cytotoxicity.

Currently, there are ample evidence that associate the inflammatory response to many neurodegenerative diseases, including Alzheimer's disease, Parkinson's disease, and multiple sclerosis. Chapter 7 by Ruth Kandel, Mitchell R. White, and Kevan L. Hartshorn shows how chronic inflammation in the brain is fundamental to AD pathogenesis which is precipitated through accumulation of amyloid-beta (Aβ) peptides. They suggest that the discovery of the neuroinflammation stimulus for Aβ production would allow early intervention to prevent development of AD.

The majority of the studies includes serious health connotations on amyloids due to clear relation with human pathologies but beyond of amyloid toxicity; each day the studies on amyloid functionality are getting force being "functional amyloids" a term well established. Chapter 8 by Magda de Eguileor, Rossana Girardello, Annalisa Grimaldi, Laura Pulze, and Gianluca Tettamanti describes "amyloidogenesis" as a widely distributed process in different cell types of evolutionary distant organisms that it has been integrated into additional physiological functions such as the reparation of body lesion.

The most prevalent amyloid pathologies are related to neurodegenerative diseases as Alzheimer's disease and Parkinson's disease, among others, but there are many amyloidoses which affect other organs: liver, nerves, heart, kidneys, joints, and tendons. Chapter 9 by Tadashi Nakamura is focused on "amyloid A (AA) amyloidosis", a complication of long-standing inflammatory diseases such as rheumatoid arthritis (RA). He also describes the new developments on its treatment, being currently under investigation, the novel therapies oriented to AA fibril formation and immunotherapy. These therapies will lead to improved prognosis in the near future. Another relevant amyloidogenic pathology is the "diabetes type II". Chapter 10 by Joel Montane and Anna Novials describes the capability of human islet amyloid polypeptide (hIAPP) to induce endoplasmic reticulum (ER) stress, resulting in an inflammatory processes and eventually apoptosis. Light-chain (AL) amyloidosis is the most common form of systemic amyloidosis (nonlocalized), affecting a wide range of organs, most commonly the kidneys. Chapter 11 by James J. Driscoll and Saulius Girnius shows the treatment advances and the novel therapeutic strategies against "AL amyloidosis" mainly focused on the development of proteasome inhibitors. Another frequent systemic amyloidosis or nonlocalized amyloidosis is the "amyloid nephropathy". Chapter 12 by Paisit Paueksakon discusses practical diagnostic approach and pathogenesis of amyloid nephropathy including discussion of treatment and prognosis. It also reviews several interesting techniques in typing of this amyloidosis as immunofluorescence, immunohistochemistry, and more recently laser microdissection and mass spectrometry.

From the new nanotechnology point of view, the amyloids are very interesting structures for nano-bio-technological applications, being this technology in turn very useful to obtain new insights on amyloidosis. Chapter 13 by Adriaan Verhelle and Jan Gettemans proposes the use of nanobodies (the heavy chain of heavy-chain antibodies) as possible inhibitors on the formation of the pathogenic gelsolin isoforms.

Finally, I would like to thank all authors for their significant contributions to the 13 chapters of this book and I greatly appreciate their work performed to orient this book not only to the experts in the field but also to those scientists, students and readers who, without any previous knowledge on the subject and in an easy way can get a general up-to-date overview on amyloids. I also thank InTech editorial team, especially Ms. Iva Simcic, for her efficient and professional help given to me. All of you have made my assignment as book editor enormously pleasant and educational as well. I am very grateful to Dr. J.C. Jiménez-López for suggesting me to be editor of this book. My warm thanks to my colleagues Joost Schymkowitz and Frederic Rousseau, well-known experts on amyloids, for reading this preface.

Ana-María Fernández-Escamilla, PhD
Environmental Protection Department,
Estación Experimental del Zaidín (EEZ),
Spanish National Research Council (CSIC),
Granada, Spain

Chapter 1

Modulating Role of TTR in Aβ Toxicity, from Health to Disease

Isabel Cardoso, Luis Miguel Santos and
Mobina Alemi

Additional information is available at the end of the chapter

http://dx.doi.org/10.5772/63194

Abstract

Amyloidosis is a generic term that refers to a wide spectrum of diseases that are characterized by the deposition of proteins in different organs, forming insoluble aggregates. Examples include islet amyloid polypeptide (IAPP) associated with diabetes type 2, prion protein (PrP) related with spongiform encephalopathies, (TTR) associated with familial amyloidotic polyneuropathy (FAP), and amyloid-beta (Aβ) peptide linked to Alzheimer's disease (AD), the most common form of dementia. Aβ peptide, thought to be the causative agent in AD, is generated upon sequential cleavage of the amyloid precursor protein (APP), by beta- and gamma-secretases, and it is believed that an imbalance between Aβ production and clearance results in its accumulation in the brain. TTR is a 55 kDa homotetrameric protein synthesized by the liver and choroid plexus of the brain and is involved in the transport of thyroid hormones and retinol. TTR protects against Aβ toxicity by binding the peptide, thus inhibiting its aggregation. Also, increased Aβ levels are found in both brain and plasma of AD mice with only one copy of the TTR gene, when compared to animals with two copies of the gene, suggesting a role for TTR in Aβ clearance. Growing evidence also suggests a wider role for TTR in central nervous system neuroprotection, including in the cases of ischemia, regeneration, and memory.

Keywords: Alzheimer's disease (AD), Aβ peptide, transthyretin (TTR), neuroprotection, blood–brain barrier (BBB)

1. Amyloidosis

1.1. Amyloidosis definition

Amyloidosis has long been used as a general term referring to a wide spectrum of protein-misfolding diseases [1], which are characterized by the extracellular deposition of those proteins in different organs, consequently forming insoluble aggregates called amyloid, a term popularized by Virchow in 1854 [2]. According to the Nomenclature Committee of the International Society of Amyloidosis (ISA), 31 identified proteins form extracellular amyloid fibrils in humans [3]. Amyloid fibrils are characterized by certain tinctorial properties, independently of the precursor protein forming the deposits, that for a long time were the only diagnosis available. These include apple-green birefringence under polarized light after staining with Congo red and yellow-green fluorescence after staining with thioflavin S and thioflavin T; thioflavin T has also been shown to interact with amyloid in suspension producing a specific fluorescent signal with a new excitation maximum at 450 nm. Ultrastructural studies by transmission electron microscopy (TEM) revealed that the amyloid material is fibrillary appearing as bundles of straight or coiled fibrils, non-branched, 7–10 nm wide and variable in length; in most cases, they seem to be helically twisted. Amyloid fibrils present a high content in β-pleated sheet as demonstrated by x-ray diffraction analysis and extensive antiparallel β-sheet strands with their axes running perpendicularly to the axis of the growing fibril (cross-β pattern).

Amyloid deposits are not entirely composed of the amyloid precursor protein. Several components have been found associated with all amyloid fibrils. These include serum amyloid P component (SAP), sulphonated glycosaminoglycans (GAGs), apoliproteins E and J, α1-antichymiotrypsin, several basement membrane components such as fibronectin, laminin and collagen type IV, complement proteins, and metal ions.

The extracellular deposition of fibrillary proteins leads to cell damage, organ dysfunction and death, and thus, these proteins are associated with a unique clinical syndrome, as seen in the case of the islet amyloid polypeptide (IAPP) associated with diabetes type 2 [4], prion protein (PrP) associated with the spongiform encephalopathies [5], transthyretin (TTR) associated with familial amyloidotic polyneuropathy [6] (FAP), and amyloid-beta (Aβ) peptide associated with Alzheimer's disease [7] (AD), among others.

Amyloid disorders are usually divided into two categories depending on the distribution of the amyloid deposits: localized and systemic amyloidosis. In localized amyloidosis, amyloid is restricted to a single tissue or organ, usually in the surroundings of the cells responsible for the synthesis of the precursor protein; in systemic amyloidosis, the amyloidogenic proteins are usually derived from circulating precursors that are either in excess, abnormal or both. Amyloidosis can also be hereditary or non-hereditary.

This chapter will focus in AD, a form of localized amyloidosis affecting the central nervous system, and the most common form of dementia. In particularly, we will discuss the neuroprotective role of TTR in AD, in addition to its amyloidogenic role in FAP, an example of systemic amyloidosis with a special involvement of the peripheral nerve.

2. Overview of AD

AD was firstly described by Alois Alzheimer in 1906 and is characterized by progressive loss of cognitive functions, ultimately leading to death [8]. This condition highly affects not only the life of patients but also the life of their caregivers. Pathologically, the disease is characterized by the presence of extraneuronal amyloid plaques consisting of aggregates of the Aβ peptide, and neurofibrillary tangles (NFTs) which are intracellular aggregates of abnormally hyperphosphorylated tau protein [9]. Aβ peptide is generated upon sequential cleavage of the amyloid precursor protein (APP), by beta- and gamma-secretases, and it is believed that an imbalance between Aβ production and clearance results in its accumulation in the brain.

2.1. From the first description to the confirmation

Alzheimer's disease was first described in the 1907's paper entitled "Uber eine eigenartige Erkankung der Hirnrinde," by Alois Alzheimer [10], in which he reported the behavior of a 51-year-old female patient (Auguste Deter) of the insane asylum of Frankfurt am Main. The patient presented several symptoms that caught Alzheimer's attention, apart from the central nervous system anatomical characteristics. Among others, time and space disorientation, rapid loss of memory, and mood swings were the most prominent symptoms [10]. In relation to pathological features, the observation of something that looked like "thick bundles" [10] of fibrils, later known as senile/amyloid plaques and NFTs [11], transformed AD into a unique condition, distinguishing it from the other neurological conditions known to date.

2.1.1. Symptoms and Diagnosis

Since 1907, clinicians have been trying their best to accurately identify AD-related symptoms and to divide and organize these symptoms in the simplest form. Burns et al. came out in 2002 with three different categories: (1) cognitive deficits that affect memory (amnesia and agnosia), speech (aphasia), and motor behavior; (2) psychiatric symptoms and behavioral disturbances, including depression, anxiety, delusions, and misidentification; (3) difficulties with the daily living activities, such as driving, using the telephone, dealing with money and, later in the disease, all the basic needs (feeding, dressing, toileting) [12–14]. As expected in such a complex condition, a huge symptomatic variation is found in AD patients, although a positive correlation between symptom severity and disease evolution is observed.

Although AD is seen as an elderly disease due to its higher prevalence in the older population (approximately 5.3 million people solely in the US, in 2015) [15], it is also the most frequent form of dementia under the age of 65, with up to 5% of all cases [16]. Of curiosity, every 67 s, one more person is diagnosed with AD, and, by 2050, one new case of AD is expected to develop every 33 s [15]. Due to this disease complexity, diagnosis guidelines had to be established, and for a long time, the main criteria adopted was the one decided at the 1984 consortium, by the National Institute of Neurological and Communicative Disorders and Stroke and the Alzheimer's Disease and Related Disorders Association (NINCDS–ADRDA). These criteria divided AD in three possible diagnosis scenarios, which were possible, probable, or definite AD [17]. More recently, some minor alterations have been proposed in order to comprise also the stages prior to the clinical observation of symptoms [18, 19], thus prompting three renewed stages: (1) preclinical Alzheimer's disease; (2) mild cognitive impairment (MCI) due to Alzheimer's disease; and (3) dementia due to Alzheimer's disease [20].

Despite all the attentions directed to the establishment of proper diagnostic criteria and guidelines available, the diagnosis of AD is still not an easy task. Actually, a recent meta-analysis showed that the sensitivity and specificity of the clinical diagnosis ranged from 53 to 99% and 55 to 99%, respectively [21]. Although alone it is considered a low value, when combined with other characterizing techniques (as neuroimaging and biomarkers—see Biomarkers section), it is possible to predict/diagnose AD with a high confidence.

Genetically, AD is usually divided in two forms: autosomal dominant familial AD (FAD; predominantly of early-onset—under the age of 65) and sporadic AD (also called and usually associated to the late-onset AD—more than 65 years) [22]. Although extensively used, it is important to point out that this classification is far too simplistic.

Despite all of the effort put into research, the primary event triggering AD remains yet a mystery. Nonetheless, for FAD, several mutations capable of triggering the disease have been identified, especially in three distinct genes: the amyloid precursor protein (APP) [23], the presenilin 1 (PSEN1), and the presenilin 2 (PSEN2) genes [24], in chromosomes 21q, 14q, and 1q, respectively. Although these three genes comprise approximately 55% of all mutations, they are only responsible for less than 1% of all cases of AD (http://www.molgen.vib-ua.be/ADMutations/). Contrary to FAD, sporadic AD does not exhibit autosomal-dominant inheritance but up to 60–80% of this form of AD is genetically determined [22].

2.2. The biochemical basis of AD

In spite of its multifactorial etiology, AD is characterized by two specific brain lesions, the amyloid plaques, and the NFTs, considered the hallmarks of AD. Also, associated with these abnormalities, it is often observed severe neural loss and reactive gliosis.

NFTs are filamentous inclusions (intracellular lesions), preferentially observed in pyramidal neurons, which are composed of filamentous aggregates of abnormally hyperphosphorylated microtubule-associated protein tau [25]. Even though NFTs are a hallmark of AD, they are also observed for other neurodegenerative disorders termed tauopathies (e.g., sporadic cortico-basal degeneration, palsy, and Pick's disease, progressive supranuclear palsy, Seattle family A, parkinsonism–dementia complex of Guam, and some frontotemporal dementias) [26, 27].

As for amyloid plaques, they can be distinguished in different plaques subtypes, depending on their composition, and being the neuritic and diffuse plaques the two major subtypes in AD. Neuritic plaques are constituted by the 40- and 42-amino acids (aa) Aβ peptides [28] (Aβ40 and Aβ42, respectively), surrounded by dystrophic neurites (axons and dendrites), microglia (monocyte- or macrophage-derived cells that reside in the brain), and reactive astrocytes [29]. Diffuse deposits are mainly composed of Aβ42 [28] and lack the neuritic and glial components [29], but evolve over time with formation of discrete niduses that eventually become neuritic amyloid plaques [30].

2.3. Amyloid-β precursor protein and Aβ formation

The amyloid-β precursor protein (APP) is a transmembrane receptor expressed ubiquitously in both neuronal cells and extra-neuronal tissues [31]. In humans, the APP gene is located in the chromosome 21, explaining partially the increased risk for Down syndrome patients to develop AD, and is composed of 18 exons [32]. Three major isoforms are expressed by alternative splicing: APP770 (full length), APP751 (lacking exon 8), and APP695 (lacking exon 7 and exon 8) [23, 31, 33]. APP belongs to a highly conserved family of type 1 transmembrane glycoproteins that extends also to invertebrate species, including the homologous: APL-1 (*Caenorhabditis elegans*), APPL (*Drosophila*), APLP1, and APLP2 (in mammals, besides APP) [34], and appa and appb (zebrafish) [35]. Following translation, APP is trafficked through the endoplasmic reticulum (ER), Golgi and trans-Golgi network (TGN), where it suffers specific endoproteolytic cleavages [33] that will originate several APP metabolites, among them the Aβ peptide. After reaching the membrane surface, APP can still undergo clathrin-mediated endocytosis and then be recycled to the surface again [36], during which Aβ can also be produced [37].

The 4 kDa Aβ peptide was first isolated and sequenced by Glenner and Wong, in 1984 [7] and can be found in the plasma and cerebrospinal fluid (CSF) of healthy humans and other mammals [38]. It was described as a 24 aa peptide but later, sequencing analysis revealed that the peptide could actually comprise 36–43 aa [39], being the two major species Aβ40 and Aβ42. In healthy individuals, these two forms make up about 90 and 10%, respectively, of the Aβ peptides that are normally produced by brain cells [40]. Despite the small difference in size and sequence of the various isoforms, they differ greatly in properties; for example, Aβ42 is more hydrophobic, thus, more prone to aggregation (compared to the less hydrophobic Aβ40). In fact, it readily aggregates in vitro, being considered the more amyloidogenic and hence pathogenic species [41].

2.3.1. Towards amyloid or not?

APP processing can originate different metabolites that bear very different physiological functions, depending on the proteolysis pathway adopted: the amyloidogenic or non-amyloidogenic pathway (**Figure 1**). In the non-amyloidogenic pathway, APP is firstly cleaved by the α-secretase, a zinc metalloproteinase of the ADAM family [42], followed by the action of γ-secretase. The latter is a high molecular weight complex of four proteins: presenilin 1 or 2 (PSEN1, PSEN2), nicastrin (NCT) [43, 44], anterior pharynx-defective 1 (APH1), and presenilin enhancer 2 (PEN2) [45]. The cleavage by the α-secretase (at Lys687 of APP770) [46], within the Aβ domain, abrogates the production of Aβ, resulting in the release of a large soluble ectodomain of APP (sAPPα, ~100 kDa), leaving behind a 83-residue carboxi-terminal fragment (CTFα, of ~10 kDa) [47]. Then, γ-secretase cuts the CTFα, liberating the extracellular p3 peptide and the 50 aa APP intracellular domain (AICD, of ~6 kDa) [48].

On the other hand, as suggested by its name, the amyloidogenic pathway gives rise to the amyloidogenic Aβ peptide, and similar to the previous pathway, it consists of two sequential cleavages, first by the β-secretase (beta-site APP–cleaving enzyme 1–BACE-1), and then by γ-secretase. The first protease cleaves APP at Met671 [49], releasing the large soluble ectodomain sAPPβ [33]. The remaining 99 aa CTFβ (of ~12 kDa) [50] is then cleaved by the γ-secretase, in the membrane, and originates, as said above, the Aβ peptide and the AICD [48]. This process generates different Aβ species, with variable hydrophobic C-termini (related to the γ-secretase cleaving site), that present different propensity to oligomerize [51] and, consequently, to form the amyloid plaques. Noteworthy, AD-linked mutations in the PSEN1 and PSEN2 proteins, particularly important in the case of FAD, influence γ-secretase-mediated processing of APP, and selectively enhance Aβ42 production compared to Aβ40 [52].

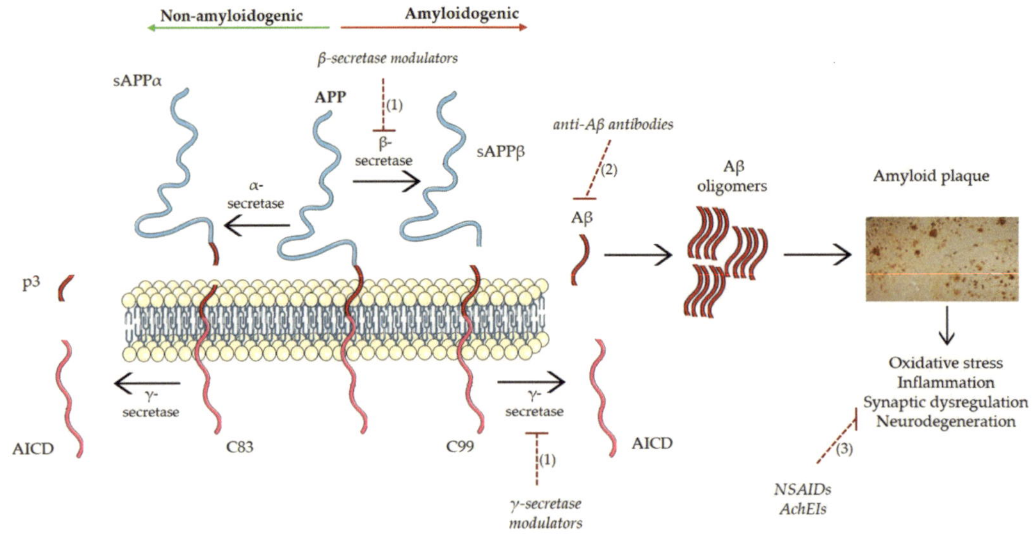

Figure 1. The amyloidogenic and non-amyloidogenic pathways of APP. In the non-amyloidogenic pathway, APP is cleaved by the α-secretase releasing the sAPPα neuroprotective N-terminal fragment, which contains part of the Aβ sequence. The 83 aa APP fragment (C83) then suffers the action of the γ-secretase, liberating the p3 peptide and the AICD fragment. The amyloidogenic pathway involves the sequential cleavage of APP by the β-secretase which releases the soluble ectodomain sAPPβ. The remaining C99 fragment of APP is then cleaved by the γ-secretase, resulting in the formation of the Aβ peptide. Due to its high propensity to aggregate, Aβ peptide oligomerizes, accumulates and forms amyloid senile plaques, in turn leading to the described alterations of AD. Current therapeutic approaches in AD include: (1) inhibition of β- and γ-secretases, (2) improving Aβ clearance, and (3) amelioration of inflammation and synaptic dysregulation.

Although tightly related to AD onset, APP processing is a normal metabolic event and Aβ is a normal product of cellular metabolism throughout life, circulating as a soluble peptide in biological fluids [53]. Plus, Aβ deposition can also be found, together with NFTs, in the brain of non-demented elderly people [54].

2.4. Alzheimer's disease hypotheses

AD is one of the human diseases with the highest number of hypothesis formulated trying to explain its pathogenesis, with very different and plausible molecular mechanism to back them up. Within the list, the amyloid cascade hypothesis stands out, together with the so-called "tau and tangle" hypothesis, strengthened by the fact that they are based in the two hallmarks of AD.

2.4.1. *Amyloid cascade hypothesis*

Since its formalization, in 1992 by Hardy and Higgins, the amyloid cascade hypothesis has had a prominent role in explaining the etiology and pathogenesis of AD. They suggested that amyloid deposition was the primary influence driving AD pathogenesis [55], due to two key observations: the detection of Aβ as the main constituent of amyloid plaques, and the discovery of mutations in the APP, PSEN1 and PSEN2 genes associated with FAD [56]. This hypothesis stated that a dysregulation in APP processing or Aβ clearance would provoke an increase in the Aβ42/Aβ40 ratio, which would promote aggregation, accumulation, and plaque formation. In turn, this would be responsible for the subsequent pathology (including tau aggregation, phosphorylation, neuronal attrition, and clinical dementia) [57]. Due to its inability to entirely explain AD pathogenesis, especially by the lack of correlation between plaque burden and clinical manifestations [58], this hypothesis has been upgraded over the past few years. Scientists started to divert their attention from the effects of the amyloid deposits, to study the other forms (monomers, oligomers, and protofibrils—usually shorter and thinner then mature fibrils) [59] of Aβ peptide-induced neurotoxicity. Some studies suggest that Aβ toxicity functions in a plaque-independent manner, indicating that oligomeric intermediates present higher toxicity to the cells [60] and that activation of signaling pathways due to intraneuronal accumulation of Aβ oligomers is responsible for tau hyperphosphorylation and subsequent deposition [61]. Several explanations have been proposed, with some defending that oligomeric toxicity is related to a greater capacity for diffusion and a larger collective surface area for interacting with neuronal and glial cells [60], while other proposed that it is not related to a specific prefibrillar aggregate (dimer, trimer, and so on) but rather to the propensity that each species has to grow and undergo fibril formation [62].

A more consensual vision about Aβ is that it possesses a dual role: On one hand, it can be a neurotrophic agent or a neuroprotector against excitotoxicity (by activating the phosphatidylinositol-3-kinase (PI-3K) pathway); on the other hand, an inducer of neuronal degeneration (at high concentrations) in mature neurons [63].

Other interesting and amyloid cascade-opposite hypotheses have been proposed, stating that Aβ should not be seen as the initiating factor for neurodegeneration in AD, but instead, its deposition is nothing more than a protective mechanism to neuronal insult, in which Aβ binds and removes harmful substances by blocking them in plaques [64, 65].

2.4.2. *Tau hypothesis*

"Tauists" defend a collection of ideas that maintain the primacy of NFTs formation as the AD-causing event, which Mudher and Lovestone designated as the "tau and tangle hypothesis" [57]. It started to emerge due to solid evidence that amyloid plaques do not account for the complex pathophysiology of AD [66], opposed to the observed highly positive correlation between NFTs and cognitive deficits [67]. It argues that in AD the normal role of tau (microtubules stabilization) is impaired and that NFTs accumulate and occupy much of the neuron, resulting in neuronal death. This was supported by the visualization of the extracellular tangles in the shape of neurons, abundant in the late stages of disease [57]. Also, the discovery of mutations within the tau gene that cause fronto-temporal dementia and parkinsonism linked to chromosome 17 (FTDP-17), demonstrating that tau dysfunction, in the absence of amyloid pathology, was enough to cause neuronal loss and clinical dementia [68], further strengthened this hypothesis. However, tau mutations do not originate amyloid plaques, whereas APP and presenilin gene mutations give rise to amyloid and tau depositions, strongly evidencing that amyloid pathology is upstream of tau pathology [57]. More recently, a more embracing tau hypothesis was proposed, in which a series of damage signals (Aβ oligomers, oxygen-free radicals, iron overload, cholesterol levels in neuronal rafts, low-density lipoprotein (LDL) species and homocysteine, among other) trigger, by innate immunity, the activation of microglial cells with the consequent release of pro-inflammatory cytokines that modify neuronal behavior through anomalous signaling cascades, which finally, promote tau hyper-phosphorylation [66]. In turn, tau hyperphosphorylation will contribute to further activation of microglial cells and stimulation of the deleterious cycle, which will lead to progressive neuronal degeneration [66]. The degree of tau phosphorylation in the AD brain is reasonably well correlated with the severity of AD symptoms; however, fetal tau, a much more phosphorylated form of tau than adult tau, does not induce AD-like pathology [69]. In summary, there is no direct evidence for the neurotoxicity of hyperphosphorylated tau (as in the case of Aβ toxicity).

2.4.3. *"Other" hypothesis*

2.4.3.1. *GSK-3 hypothesis*

Glycogen synthase kinase-3 (GSK-3), a multi-tasking kinase with major roles in brain signaling, has been recently proposed as a central player in AD pathology. This was supported by observing that the deregulation of this protein is responsible for many of the pathological hallmarks of the disease, in both sporadic and familial AD cases [70]. It was suggested that the hyperactivity of GSK-3β, the most abundant of two isoforms (GSK-3α and GSK-3β) expressed in neurons, is intimately involved with cognitive impairment [71], Aβ production [72], tau hyperphosphorylation [73], acetylcholine synthesis [74], neuronal death [75], and neuroinflammation [76] in AD. Furthermore, regarding Aβ interaction, it was observed that Aβ also regulates GSK-3β activity [77, 78] making it difficult to establish which event is located upstream. Thus, this hypothesis is seen as an integration and extension of the amyloid cascade hypothesis, still conferring to Aβ a central role in AD pathology. Although GSK-3 modulation appears to be an excellent therapeutic approach, no effective result has been observed in trials, perhaps due to its activity in multiple targets.

2.4.3.2. *Oxidative stress/mitochondrial hypothesis*

The brain is especially vulnerable to free radical damage as a result of its high oxygen consumption rate, abundant fatty acids content, and the relative low levels of antioxidant enzymes

http://dx.doi.org/10.5772/63194

[79]. The most appealing feature of the oxidative stress hypothesis is its slow and cumulative damaging nature that could, over time, account for the late life onset and slowly progressive nature of AD, and neurodegeneration in general [80]. Also supporting this hypothesis is the suggested unbalanced levels of heavy metals in the brain, among others, iron (Fe), copper (Cu), aluminum, and mercury, which function as catalysts for oxygen free radical generation [80]. There has been high controversy in the measurement of these elements, especially Fe, but most studies reveal an apparent unbalance in AD brains compared to controls. In a recent study, Fe was found significantly increased in patients with severe AD [81] (as previously reported [82]). Nonetheless, some consider that this "accepted" elevation, even if significant in some studies of AD pathology, does not account for brain degeneration, and so, presents itself as a misleading therapeutic target with considerable risks for patients (reviewed in [83]). As for Cu, it has been shown to be decreased in AD brains [81], which at first goes against the oxidation hypothesis. More recently, and also in the presence of some contradictory results [84], copper was found to bind strongly to Aβ aggregates, inhibiting in vitro amyloid fibril formation [85]. In addition, and when bound to the aggregates, copper exhibited a redox role, by degrading hydrogen peroxide [86]. Protein and DNA oxidation (in particular mitochondrial DNA), and lipid peroxidation (which affects the phospholipid-rich membrane) were also found to be increased in AD brains [80].

Another hypothesis intimately related to the brain redox status is the mitochondrial cascade hypothesis [87]. Mitochondria are considered the cell "powerhouses"; however, when in a non-physiological energy production, they can provoke severe damage by increasing the reactive oxygen species (ROS). Curiously, mitochondria are the first target of ROS, suffering DNA oxidation, which may lead to a further increase of ROS production, generating a vicious cycle [88]. The authors of this hypothesis state that sporadic and autosomal dominant AD are not etiologically homogeneous and that mitochondrial dysfunction works as a link for both. Very briefly, in autosomal dominant forms, Aβ-induced mitochondrial dysfunction leads to the other AD-characteristic histopathologies, while in sporadic AD, mitochondrial malfunction induces the AD pathologies, including processing of APP to Aβ [89].

2.4.3.3. The cholinergic hypothesis

The cholinergic hypothesis was proposed after the observation of a decrease of choline acetyltransferase (ChAT) in AD patients [90]. It states that the loss of cholinergic cells in the septal nuclei and basal forebrain (described in patients with advanced AD [91]) compromises the innervation of the cerebral cortex and related structures, which play an important role in cognitive functions, especially memory [92]. More recent studies have suggested a bidirectional pathway linking Aβ toxicity in cholinergic dysfunction and the interaction of cholinergic regulatory mechanisms in the processing of APP [93]. Discrediting this hypothesis, later studies showed that the cholinergic degeneration [94] and the decrease in ChAT enzyme activity [95] are not observable in the early stages of disease. This was accompanied by the fact that treatment with acetylcholinesterase inhibitors does not offer long term cure, although it has shown consistent, despite modest, benefits in symptoms improvement [96]. Nonetheless, some studies point out that compensatory mechanisms could overcome the cholinergic defects, disguising its effects in early stages of AD or mild cognitive impairment [97].

2.4.3.4. Calcium hypothesis

The calcium hypothesis was first introduced by Khachaturian in 1982, stating that cellular mechanisms which maintain the homeostasis of cytosolic Ca^{2+} play a key role in brain aging and that sustained changes in Ca^{2+} homeostasis could provide the final common pathway for age-associated brain changes [98], or in this case, be the proximal cause of neurodegeneration in AD. Out of curiosity, this proposal was purely speculative at the time, only sustained on circumstantial evidence from a handful of studies [98]. It was observed that the persistent elevation of the levels of Ca^{2+} leads to the constant elimination of newly acquired memories, due to a stimulation of long-term depression mechanisms [99]. In fact, calcium signaling dysfunctions occur during the initial phases of the disease, and even before the development of pronounced symptoms [100]. However, whether it is calcium dyshomeostasis that provokes Aβ production and accumulation [101], or vice-versa [102], remains to be elucidated. Either way, in addition to the Aβ unbalance, increased levels of Ca^{2+} promoted protein tau hyper-phosphorylation [103]. It was also suggested that amyloid oligomers induce membrane permeabilization, leading to increased intracellular Ca^{2+} concentration [104]. Nevertheless, there is some disagreement as to the mechanism by which amyloid oligomers increase intracellular calcium.

2.5. Biomarkers and risk factor

Despite of the extensive Knowledge on the causative gene mutations responsible for familial AD, the sporadic (non-genetic) form of this disease, which results from the diverse interactions between genetic and environmental factors, is still lacking characterization. Thus, researchers are continuously looking for specific molecules that should be altered exclusively in AD, and preferentially in the asymptomatic period. This, combined with the meticulous description of the patient risk factors, may give the opportunity for an early action and increase the success rate of therapeutics.

2.5.1. Biomarkers

By definition, and according to the International Programme on Chemical Safety, biomarker is "any substance, structure, or process that can be measured in the body or its products and influence or predict the incidence of outcome or disease" [105]. The search for early AD biomarkers has been highly targeted over the last years, as investigators believe that the generation of an effective treatment for AD is only possible if the disease is detected at very early stages. Thus, the discovery of biomarkers is of extreme importance for the early diagnosis of AD and even for predicting the conversion of MCI into AD patients.

The search for solid AD biomarkers started with those who seem to be altered in this condition when compared to normality. Several studies showed that the combination of CSF total- and phospho-tau, and CSF and plasma Aβ42 is able to predict with increased sensitivity and specificity the development of AD in patients with MCI [21, 106, 107], in addition to the already established role of the ApoE-ε4 isoform [108] (major susceptibility gene—see Section 2.5.2. Risk Factors). Studies in FAD-causing mutations carriers showed increased levels of CSF total-tau and plasma Aβ42, although having reduced CSF Aβ42 levels, at least 10 years before the symptoms establishment [106]. Also, the ratio of Aβ42/Aβ40 in CSF and plasma was found decreased, respectively, for non-demented mutation carriers [109] and cognitively normal elders (which evolved to MCI or AD) [110]. Other CSF biomarkers, such as BACE-1 [111] and sAPPα/β [112], are also suggested; however, independent studies were not consistent [106], possibly due to technical difficulties in the biomarkers quantification [113]. Our group has also proposed TTR as a biomarker in plasma, demonstrating a negative correlation with AD severity [114], which supported prior observations for CSF levels. In that study, the authors also considered TTR a selective biomarker for AD [115]. Other studies contradict this idea suggesting that TTR potential as biomarker raises some doubt since its levels appear to fluctuate substantially within a single individual over a 2-week interval [116].

In addition to the so-called fluid biomarkers, physicians have at their disposal powerful imaging technology. With the improvement in PET (positron emission tomography) and MRI (magnetic resonance imaging) spectroscopy resolution, neuroimaging has been gaining importance and increasing the confidence in AD diagnosis. Due to the possibility of using specific tracers, such as a derivate of thioflavin T that crosses the blood–brain barrier (BBB) and binds selectively to Aβ (C11-labeled Pittsburgh Compound B–PiB), it is possible to identify amyloid deposition in the brain in vivo [117]. In 2004, Klunk and colleagues performed the first study of brain amyloid imaging (BAI) using the PiB compound, in which they showed a robust relationship between amyloid deposition and PiB retention [118]. The combination of increased BAI signal, low CSF Aβ42, and high CSF p-tau in a subject with dementia is seen as a "definite" diagnosis of AD. Furthermore, BAI and CSF profiles can be used to predict patients with MCI who will progress to frank dementia with high degree of confidence [119]. Despite the value of this compound, the resulting data should be subjected to careful analysis since healthy subjects also present amyloid deposition, hindering the differentiation between symptomatic AD and asymptomatic controls with amyloid plaques [120]. MRI (structural evidence) is also a common technique often used, alone or in combination with CSF tau and Aβ42, to predict development of AD [121]. Curiously, a recent study showed that the MRI together with PiB-PET makes the best combination of biomarkers, thus showing the best AD predictive value [119].

2.5.2. Risk factors

2.5.2.1. Environmental factors

As Stephen King wrote in The Gunslinger: "Time's the thief of memory," and so, the most worldwide accepted (and intuitive) risk factor is aging. In every species, age brings a slowing of brain function [122], thus preventing the brain to properly respond/recover from insults. The increasing of life expectancy, in addition to the increasing of population (attributed to the postwar "baby boom"), turned aging in a major risk factor. Also gender appears to play a role in disease development, since data show that women are more prone to this disease than men. Although women present higher life expectancy, also in younger study groups (60–80 years), where differences in death rate are insignificant, women present higher incidence of cases [123]. The specific mechanism is unknown; however, several factors have been proposed to influence, such as: age-related sex hormone reduction, risks of other diseases (diabetes, depression, cardiovascular disease), and differences in brain anatomy and metabolism [124].

The cardiovascular risk factors, which appear sometimes as a distinct group of factors, include diabetes mellitus [125], overweight [126], hypertension [127], and high cholesterol levels [128]. Individually or in cooperation, these factors increase the predisposition for cognitive decline. The midlife control of the above cardiovascular factors has been associated with a reduction in white matter lesions in late life [127]. As for cholesterol, results appear to be inconsistent; however, lipid-lowering treatments present benefits against white matter lesions [126].

Contrasting with the previous risk factors, wine consumption, coffee consumption, the use of non-steroidal anti-inflammatory drugs (NSAIDs), and physical activity are associated with reduced risks, thus showing some protective effects [129].

2.5.2.2. Genetic factors

ApoE exists as three isoforms ε2, ε3 and ε4, with ε3 having the highest prevalence. As Corder and colleagues stated, in 1993, ApoE plays an important role in AD, with the risk of developing disease increased in carriers of the ApoE-ε4 allele, such that a double dose of this allele was nearly enough to cause AD by the age of 80 [130]. Despite the broad molecular evidence about ApoE role in AD, its genetic variation is also present in other kinds of neurological disorders, including Parkinson's disease and multiple sclerosis [22]. In 2009, three novel AD genes were identified, presenting high degree of association: CLU (clusterin or apolipoprotein J), CR1 (complement component (3b/4b) receptor 1), and PICALM (phosphatidylinositol-binding clathrin assembly protein). Down's syndrome (or trisomy 21) is also considered a genetic risk factor. This condition is the result of a third copy of the chromosome 21, which coincides with the location of the APP gene [131], giving rise to an increased accumulation of Aβ.

2.6. Drugs and treatments

Due to the complexity of AD, a vast number of targets and pathways may be chosen to intervene. Cholinergic degradation inhibitors, immunotherapy, secretase inhibitors, anti-inflammatory drugs, and tau- and Aβ-deposition interfering drugs (**Figure 1**) are but a few examples of the many classes of drugs that are being tested at the moment.

The first drugs developed for AD, acetylcholinesterase inhibitors (AchEI), aimed at increasing acetylcholine levels (see "Cholinergic hypothesis"). Currently, FDA has five drugs approved for the "treatment" of AD in the initial stages: 4 AchEI (Donepezil, Rivastigmine, Galantamine, and Tacrine) and 1 NMDA receptor antagonist (Memantine) (http://www.alzforum.org). As referred above, they treat and ameliorate the symptoms, but do not cure.

In 2010, Rinne and colleagues showed for the first time target engagement from a disease-modifying drug in humans, using the monoclonal anti-Aβ antibody bapineuzumab [132, 133]. This study showed a reduction of fibrillar amyloid in the brain of AD individuals, but did not improve cognition and stopped at phase 3 [133]. Crenezumab, another anti-Aβ, was selected for pre-symptomatic treatment trials of Colombian mutant PSEN1 kindred [133], however, showed extensive cross-reaction with non-Aβ related proteins [134]. Intravenous immunoglobulins (IVIG) have also been proposed as a potential treatment, based on the hypothesis That IVIG contain naturally occurring antibodies that specifically promote clearance of Aβ peptides from the brain [135].

β- and γ-secretase modulators [133], Aβ and tau deposition modulators (e.g., scylloinositol and methylene blue, respectively [39]), and molecules addressing oxidative damage (resveratrol) are also potential drugs under study. Recently, deep brain stimulation (DBS) performed by the group of Dr Lozano in AD patients showed promising results, with improvements and/or slowing in the rate of cognitive decline [136], increased hippocampus volume and glucose metabolism [137]. The authors propose that DBS is able to influence the structure of the brain and that hippocampal atrophy can potentially be slowed, suggesting restorative properties to DBS [137].

A general recommended therapy is a good diet and a healthy lifestyle, in order to control cardiovascular risk factors, decreasing cerebrovascular events. No effective treatment has been found, thus increasing the interest for the early diagnose of AD, to allow a more effective and early stage intervention.

3. Blood–brain barrier and Alzheimer's disease

The BBB is a profoundly specialized brain endothelial structure of the differentiated neurovascular system. These specialized endothelial cells interacting with astrocytes, microglia, and pericytes, confine components of the circulating blood from neurons. Furthermore, the BBB controls the chemical composition of the neuronal environment which is required for the functioning of neuronal circuits, synaptic transmission, synaptic remodeling, angiogenesis, and neurogenesis. BBB malfunction, through the disruption of the tight junctions (TJs) and alteration of the transport of molecules between blood and brain, brain hypoperfusion, and inflammatory responses, may begin or contribute to the process of different diseases such as AD, Parkinson's disease, amyotrophic lateral sclerosis, multiple sclerosis. These data support developments of new therapeutic strategies for the neurodegenerative disorders focused at the BBB [138].

3.1. The blood–brain barrier: the earliest findings

In 1885, when scientist Paul Ehrlich injected trypan blue dye into the bloodstream of mice, he noted that the stain colored all of the animal organs, except the brain [139]. In 1913, one of the Ehrlich's students, Edwin Goldmann, performed a follow-up experiment by injecting the same dye into the brain of mice. He observed that injection of trypan blue directly into the CSF stained all cell types in the brain but failed to penetrate into the periphery [140]. Although aiming at finding new compounds that could attack disease-causing microbes, these experiments suggested a physical barrier between the brain and the blood, becoming the stepping stones on BBB research. Lewandowsky was the first to use the term blood–brain barrier while studying the limited permeation of potassium ferrocyanate into the brain [141]. However, it took until the 1960s for the specific anatomy of the network of brain–blood vessels comprising the BBB to be glimpsed [142]. Using electron microscopy, in 1967, Reese and Karnovsky showed that the BBB is localized at the level of TJs between adjacent brain endothelial cells [143, 144].

It is now known that the brain of mammals is separated from the blood by the BBB, localized to the brain capillaries and pia-subarachnoid membranes, and by the blood-CSF barrier, confined to the choroid plexus [145]. At the junctional complex formed by the TJs and adherens junctions (AJs), brain endothelial cells are connected to each other [142]. Transcellular transport at the BBB occurs through several mechanisms including passive and active transport through different receptors and transporters. Interestingly, endothelial cells, pericytes, and astrocytes present at the BBB also express several enzymes such as cholinesterase, aminopeptidases and endopeptidases that alter endogenous and exogenous molecules, which can negatively influence neuronal function. This produces a metabolic barrier which protects the central nervous system (CNS) [146].

3.2. The neurovascular unit at the BBB; endothelial cells, pericytes, and glial cells

3.2.1. Endothelial cells and pericytes

A cerebral capillary lumen is enclosed by a single endothelial cell. Anatomically, the BBB endothelial cells are distinguished from those at the periphery by enhanced mitochondrial content [147], loss of fenestrations [148], least pinocytotic activity [149], and the presence of TJs [150]. The BBB tightly sealed monolayer of endothelial cells usually prevents the free exchange of solutes between blood and brain [151] except for the lipid-soluble molecules smaller than 400 Da with less than nine hydrogen bonds, which can cross the BBB without any support, via lipid-mediated diffusion [146].

As for pericytes (granular or filamentous), they are connected to the abluminal membrane of the endothelial cells [152]. Pericytes and endothelial cells are ensheathed by the basal lamina, composed of collagen type IV and other extracellular matrix proteins [153]. However, there is not much known about the involvement of pericytes at the BBB, but the addition of pericytes to co-cultures of endothelial cells and astrocytes has been shown to stabilize capillary-like structures [154]. In conditions associated with increased BBB permeability such as hypoxia or traumatic brain injury, pericytes have also been shown to migrate away from brain microvessels [155, 156]. Moreover, pericyte-derived angiopoietin provokes expression of TJs such as occludin in endothelial cells [157], confirming that pericytes are involved in the maintenance of the barrier properties in the cerebral endothelium [142].

3.2.2. Glial cells

Astrocytes are another cell type present in the neurovascular unit. These cells are usually located between neurons, pericytes, and capillary endothelium, and communicate with these cells via their several foot processes [138]. It is long believed that astrocytes are crucial in the development of the BBB properties [158]. It has been shown that co-culture of brain endothelial cells with astrocytes can enhance TJs of the brain endothelium [159]. Furthermore, endothelial cultures incubated with astrocyte-conditioned media have shown to improve BBB characteristics in vitro by de novo protein synthesis of γGTP in cerebral microvessel endothelial cells, which indicate that the glial cells may induce the cerebral capillary endothelial cells to express differentiated properties which allow the endothelium to function as the blood–brain barrier [160]. Also, astrocytes have been shown to regulate cerebral microvascular permeability [161], via dynamic calcium signaling between astrocytes and the endothelium [162]. This has been explained by Zonta et al., whereby an increase in neuron-induced astrocyte calcium promotes secretion of vasodilatory substances from perivascular astrocyte endfeet, resulting in improved local blood flow [163]. This work constituted a breakthrough in the knowledge of both astrocyte function and regulation of the activity-dependent cerebral blood flow [164].

Finally, another glial cell type present in the BBB is microglia which migrates from the yolk sac into the CNS parenchyma during embryogenesis [165]. Microglia performs critical functions in innate and adaptive brain immune responses. Microglia, when activated, transforms from “ramified” to an "ameboid" and ultimately to a “phagocytic” form. This evolution is correlated with alterations in expression of surface antigens and cytokines release [138]. Studies have shown that perivascular microglial cells are derived from bone marrow [166].

In vivo studies demonstrated that resident microglia cells in the brain parenchyma also communicate with CNS microvessels. This may suggest that microglia plays an important role in regulating BBB features during embryogenesis and diseases [167], besides an indisputable function in CNS development and homeostasis [168]. Furthermore, it has been shown that during embryonic stages of CNS vascularization, stabilization, and fusion of brain endothelial cells are mediated by resident microglial cells [167]. Also, interestingly, it has been shown that specific depletion of microglia results in reduced vessel density in a mouse model of choroidal neo-vascularization [169]. There are studies which suggest that microglial activation may be related to BBB disruption [170] apparently by producing ROS, through NADPH oxidase, which in turn impairs BBB function. Furthermore, TNF-α released from activated microglia has shown to affect BBB integrity, as permeability of endothelial cells co-cultured with microglia, was increased when microglial cells were activated by LPS and it was blocked by a neutralizing antibody against TNF-α, indicating that TNF-α contributes to BBB dysfunction [171]. The post-traumatic inflammatory response is shown to be associated with expression of cytokines such as IL-1β or metalloproteinases particularly MMP2, 3 and 5 produced mainly by microglia at the lesion site. It has also been demonstrated that these proteins can cause disruption of the basal lamina and/or redistribution and degradation of the TJs complexes [172, 173] resulting in BBB breakdown and neurological disorders after traumatic injury [174].

3.3. Junctional complexes and cytoskeleton linked proteins at the BBB

The presence of junctional complexes is one of the main characteristics of inter-endothelial space of the cerebral microvasculature which include TJs, AJs, and possibly gap junctions. Both TJs and AJs restrict permeability across the endothelium, whereas gap junctions (if present) mediate intercellular communication [175].

3.3.1. Tight junction proteins

Occludin, the first integral membrane protein within the TJ family identified [176], is a 60–65 kDa protein with four transmembrane domains which is highly expressed in the cerebral endothelium [177, 178], whereas it is much less present in non-neural endothelial cells [179]. A construct with a deletion in the N-terminal of occludin showed a considerable effect on the TJ integrity [180]. Deletion of occludin in mice has been shown to cause a complex phenotype and postnatal growth retardation [181]. However, occludin functions are not limited to its role as a TJ protein. For instance, there are studies demonstrating that occludin can regulate epithelial cell differentiation [182] and control cell apoptosis in mouse hepatocytes [183]. Also, it has been shown, in a mouse model of multiple sclerosis, that occludin dephosphorylation leads to noticeable signs of disease which occur just prior to apparent changes in the BBB permeability [184]. In cerebral ischemia, occludin and other TJs were shown to be vulnerable to attack by matrix metalloproteinases [185].

The claudin family, 20–24 kDa proteins, includes more than 20 members that build TJ strands through homophilic interactions [186]. Claudin 3, 5, and 12 play important roles at the BBB [187, 188]. Each claudin regulates the diffusion of a group of molecules of a certain size. For instance, mice neonates with deletion of claudin-5 die due to a size-selective loosening of the BBB for molecules smaller than 800 Da [188]. It is speculated that claudins determine the primary "seal" of the TJ and occludin functions as an additional support structure [142]. It has been demonstrated that overexpression of claudin species can induce development of TJ-like strands, while expression of occludin does not lead to the formation of TJ; rather, occludin only localizes to TJ in cells that have already been transfected with claudins [189].

In addition to the claudin/occluding proteins, junctional adhesion molecules (JAMs) perform an important role in the organization of TJ assembly as it has been reported that these proteins can reduce cell permeability and enhance resistance to macromolecules [190]. JAM-1, a 40-kDa member of the IgG superfamily composed of a single membrane-spanning chain with a large extracellular domain [191], is postulated to mediate the attachment of neighboring cell membranes via homophilic interactions [192]. However, there is not much known about JAMs exact function in the mature BBB, but in the rat cortical cold injury model, a characterized in vivo model of BBB breakdown it has been shown that endothelial JAM-1 is significantly reduced which strengthens the idea that JAM-1 contributes to TJs integrity [193].

3.3.2. Adherens junction proteins

The first component of AJs is the vascular endothelial (VE)-cadherin, an endothelial-specific integral membrane protein which is linked to the cytoskeleton via catenins [175] and mediates cell-cell adhesion via homophilic interactions between the extracellular domains of proteins expressed in adjacent cells [194]. In vitro and in vivo studies have shown that VE-cadherin is required for the cells to regulate vessel maintenance, that is, for the correct organization of the new vessels and for the endothelial integrity in the quiescent vessels [195]. Various mechanisms have been suggested for how VE-cadherin regulates endothelial functions; such as direct activation of signaling molecules with a role in survival and organization of the actin cytoskeleton and regulation of gene transcription cofactors and formation of complexes with growth factor receptors [138].

Even though AJs are required at the BBB to decrease the endothelial permeability [196], it is principally the TJs that present the low paracellular permeability and high electrical resistance [142, 197].

Another component of AJs is Platelet endothelial cell adhesion molecule 1 (PECAM-1), an integral membrane protein of the Ig superfamily with six extracellular domains, a short transmembrane, and a large cytoplasmic domain which is highly expressed in blood and vascular cells especially endothelial cells [198]. PECAM-1 plays a major role in the migration of leukocytes across endothelium [138] and contributes to the steady-state barrier function of endothelial cells. It also functions as a mechano-sensor and stimulates reconstruction of the barrier integrity following perturbations, including the BBB [199, 200]; all physiologic processes that rely on the junctional integrity and signaling [198].

3.3.3. Associated proteins

There are various proteins in the cytoplasm that associate with the transmembrane components of the TJ [142]. Multi-domain scaffolding proteins of membrane-associated guanylate kinase-like homolog family, including zonulae occludentes (ZO) proteins, such as ZO-1 and ZO-2, are characterized for their contributing to the cytoskeletal anchorage for the transmembrane TJ proteins, binding to the claudins, occludin, and actin [201, 202] and controlling the correct distribution of claudins [203].

ZO-1, a 220-kDa protein, is one of the first and best-studied proteins in TJs [204]. It is expressed in epithelial and endothelial cells and even other cells which do not have TJs [205]. It has also been observed to be associated with AJs [206] and gap junction proteins [207]. ZO-1 is located just below the TJ membrane contact points and has been found to be important for both function and stability of TJs. ZO-1 dissociation from the junctional complex is shown to be correlated with increased permeability in the BBB in vitro model [208]. ZO-2, a 160-kDa protein with a high sequence homology to ZO-1 [209], interestingly, has been demonstrated to function redundantly with ZO-1, replacing it and promoting the formation of TJ in the cells lacking ZO-1 [210].

Another component present in the junctional complexes is actin. Although actin has been basically considered structural in function, it is now obvious that the anchorage of AJs and TJs to the actin cytoskeleton is critical for both barrier stability and also for the regulation of cell polarity, cellular movement, fluid sensing, and cell-contact inhibition [211]. Studies using mice lacking the actin-binding protein dystrophin have demonstrated increased brain vascular permeability due to disorganized α-actin cytoskeleton in endothelial cells and astrocytes [212]. These findings demonstrate that properly arranged actin filaments and their binding to the TJ and/or AJ proteins are critical for normal barrier function. Studies have also shown that HIV-1 gp120 and alcohol are able to alter the cytoskeleton and induce stress fiber actin formation, causing increased permeability of the human BBB endothelium [213]. It has been suggested that alcohol-mediated changes in the brain endothelial cells (BEC) monolayers may increase diffusion of plasma components and viral penetration across the BBB, and therefore, especially at levels attained in heavy drinkers, accelerate HIV-1 penetration into the brain [138].

3.4. Transport at the BBB

Transcellular transport at the BBB happens through several mechanisms. Small lipophilic molecules can access the brain by passive diffusion. Brain CSF bulk flow mediates transport of molecules with different sizes into the CSF at a slow rate [214]. For potentially toxic molecules and metabolic waste products, the CSF works as a sink. These molecules are then eliminated from the CSF back into the blood by active transport or facilitated diffusion across the choroid plexus epithelium, or by vacuolar transport across the epithelial arachnoid granulations [138]. Efflux pumps return many undesired molecules back to the blood to regulate passive transport into the brain [215]. The flow of the plasma oxygen and carbon dioxide across the BBB is diffusive. Therefore, oxygen supply and carbon dioxide elimination are blood-flow dependent, so the gas transport is sufficient as long as cerebral blood flow is within physiological limits [216].

Small polar molecules, such as glucose, amino acids and nucleosides, can pass the BBB by carrier-mediated transport. These carriers can be multi-ligands or specific to only one molecule, such as GLUT1 glucose transporter, the L1 large neutral amino acid transporter, and the CNT2 adenosine transporter which have been cloned from BBB-specific cDNA libraries [146]. The direction of the concentration gradient is usually from blood to brain, regulated by brain demands and the concentration of metabolites in plasma [138]. Ion transporters such as the sodium pump localized on the abluminal membrane are important to sustain the high-concentration gradient for sodium at the BBB, so that sodium-dependent transport can happen. Also, sodium–hydrogen exchanger expressed at the luminal membrane and chloride–bicarbonate exchanger expressed at both sides [217] play significant roles in regulating intracellular pH in the endothelium.

Moreover, large solutes, such as proteins and peptides, are transported across the BBB by receptor-mediated or adsorption-mediated endocytic transport [218, 219]. Analysis of the rat BBB transcriptome has shown that 10–15% of all proteins in the neurovascular unit are transporters which emphasize the critical role of these molecules at the BBB [215, 220]. As a consequence of this controlled transport, the concentration of amino acids and proteins can suffer considerable variations, whereas relatively small differences exist in the concentration of ions between blood and CSF [221].

In the BBB, the ABC transporters for efflux are permeability glycoprotein (P-gp, multidrug resistance protein, ABCB1), the multidrug resistance-associated proteins and breast cancer resistance protein [222, 223] whose major role is to operate as active efflux pumps, transporting a diverse range of lipid-soluble compounds out of the brain capillary endothelium and the CNS, eliminating potentially neurotoxic endogenous or xenobiotic molecules [216, 224]. P-gp is expressed at the luminal and abluminal membrane, as well as in pericytes and astrocytes [225], and is distributed along the nuclear envelope, in caveolae, cytoplasmic vesicles, Golgi complex, and rough ER [138]. The endothelial cells at the BBB also express several transporters for hormones, some cytokines, and chemokines [226]. Large proteins, such as transferrin, LDL, leptin, immunoglobulin G (IgG), insulin, and insulin-like growth factor also use receptor-mediated transport systems to pass through the BBB [146].

Internalization of ligands and receptors from the plasma membrane is cholesterol sensitive [227] and comprises endocytosis of caveolae, vesicles enriched in caveolin-1 [228]. The caveolar membranes carry several receptors including those for insulin, albumin, receptor for advance glycation endproducts (RAGE), LDL, HDL [229] and are also closely associated with P-gp. Moreover, caveolin-1 can affect the levels of TJs in endothelial cells of the BBB [230]. Interestingly, study of the ultrastructure of the BBB in young and aged mice during ischemia has demonstrated that permeability is associated with a remarkable increase in endothelial caveolae and vacuoles although TJs were generally intact [231].

3.5. Aβ clearance at the BBB

Increase in either total Aβ levels or the relative concentration of both Aβ40 and Aβ42 (where the former is more concentrated in cerebrovascular plaques and the latter in neuritic plaques) have been implicated in the pathogenesis of both familial and sporadic AD.

There are several identified pathways for the removal of the Aβ from the brain. Aβ peptides mainly produced in neurons are degraded by peptidases. Through efflux transporters located in cerebral vessels, Aβ flows out from brain parenchyma into the plasma. Aβ is also removed through perivascular pathways into the cervical lymph nodes as Aβ within ISF diffuses in the extracellular spaces of the brain parenchyma entering basement membranes of capillaries, passing into the tunica media of arteries, and draining out of the brain. Aβ can also be taken up by different cells in the brain [232]. A few AD cases are familial AD, associated with genetic mutations which promote an increase in the production of Aβ [233]. On the other hand, the cause of the sporadic AD, the majority of the AD cases, is considered to be the impaired clearance of Aβ from the brain [234, 235]. In this viewpoint, AD is associated with cerebrovascular disorder, which drives the accumulation of Aβ at the blood vessels (cerebral amyloid angiapothy, CAA) and in the brain parenchyma, extracellularly [138, 236], and intraneuronal lesions—NTFs [237].

In the healthy brain, Aβ concentration is accurately regulated by its rate of production, its enzymatic degradation [238], its rapid clearance across the BBB through LRP1 [239, 240], and influx back into the brain by RAGE [241]. These receptors are multi-ligand cell surface receptors that, in addition to Aβ, mediate the clearance of a large number of proteins. P-gp, belonging to the superfamily of ATP-binding cassette (ABC) transporters, is also involved in effluxing Aβ out of the brain. While LRP1 and P-gp appear to mediate the efflux of Aβ from the brain to the periphery, RAGE has been strongly implicated in Aβ influx back into the CNS. With increasing age and also in AD pathology, the expression of the Aβ efflux transporters is decreased and the Aβ influx transporter expression is increased at the BBB, adding to the amyloid burden in the brain and its gradual neurotoxic oligomerization [242]. Thus, continuous Aβ elimination by transport across the BBB and/or metabolism is essential to prevent its potentially neurotoxic accumulations in the brain [234]. Studies have demonstrated several transport proteins such as α2-macroglobulin, TTR, apolipoprotein E (apoE), and apolipoprotein J (apoJ), which bind to Aβ and control its clearance, metabolism, and aggregation [243]. It has been shown that apoJ can increase the BBB clearance of Aβ42 [244], while apoE disrupts the clearance of free Aβ across the mouse BBB, in an isoform-specific manner (apoE4>apoE3 or apoE2), by driving Aβ transport from LRP1 to VLDLR which internalizes Aβ-apoE complex at a slower rate than LRP1 [245]. Another transport pathway is the bulk flow of the ISF into the CSF through the perivascular Virchow-Robin arterial spaces, which is followed by drainage into the plasma across the arachnoid villi [243].

3.5.1. Aβ transport by LRP1

LRP1, the major efflux transporter for Aβ across the BBB [239] and a member of the LDL receptor family, acts as both a multifunctional scavenger and a signaling receptor. LRP1 is synthesized as a precursor molecule (600 kDa) in the ER. Then in the Golgi network, a cleavage generates an 85 kDa transmembrane beta-subunit (containing two intracellular NPxY motifs) that remains non-covalently connected to the extracellular 515 kDa alpha-subunit (containing 4 ligand-binding domains for more than 30 ligands) [246].

Transcytosis of Aβ across the BBB starts with its binding to LRP1 at the abluminal side of the cerebral endothelium [239, 240]. However, this has been controversial due to the studies that failed to demonstrate a role for LRP-mediated transcytosis, but rather showed a role for LRP receptors in endocytosis and degradation of Aβ [247]. Anyway, the significant function of LRP1 in AD is not only portrayed by LRP1-mediated endocytosis of Aβ but also by data showing that the cytoplasmic domain of LRP1 has been involved in APP processing [248]. Cleavage of the extracellular domain of LRP1 by beta-secretase (BACE1) releases soluble LRP1 (sLRP1) in plasma [249]. Reduced expression of LRP1 has been described during aging in animal models and in AD individuals [240, 249]. In astrocytes, LRP1 also mediates degradation of amyloid deposits via apoE [250].

3.5.2. Aβ transport by RAGE

RAGE, a multiligand receptor in the immunoglobulin superfamily, which can bind to various ligands including Aβ and advanced glycation end products (AGE proteins) [251], is the most influential influx transporter for Aβ across the BBB [241]. Interestingly, and unlike many receptors (including LRP1), RAGE expression is triggered by the accumulation of RAGE ligands, meaning that the levels of RAGE expression are determined by the levels of its ligands. In the healthy brain, RAGE is expressed at minimal levels at the BBB, except at the endothelium of bigger microvessels of the brain. However, when RAGE ligands increase in the AD brain, RAGE expression rises in the affected cerebral vessels, neurons or microglia [251]. This mechanism worsens the cellular dysfunction due to RAGE-Aβ interactions. Circulating Aβ can enter the brain by a special receptor-mediated transport mechanism that is dependent on

RAGE expression on the luminal surface of brain vessels [252]. Following Aβ binding to RAGE at the luminal membrane of the BBB, transcytosis of circulating Aβ across the BBB into the brain parenchyma and its binding to neurons occurs. Moreover, activation of NF-kB in the endothelial cell leads to proinflammatory cytokines secretion and cerebral blood flow suppression [241]. Aβ-RAGE interaction not only generates oxidative damage to RAGE-expressing neurons, which results in neuronal degeneration, but also activates microglial cells, indirectly leading to inflammation [251]. Therefore, repression of Aβ-RAGE interaction in the BBB can inhibit Aβ influx, oxidant stress, and cytokine production. The inhibitors of Aβ/RAGE interaction have been shown to improve the BBB function and the cerebral blood flow responses to the brain activation, and to reduce neuroinflammation. Some RAGE/Aβ blockers are currently being tested in AD patients [138]. While RAGE is involved in the influx of Aβ into the brain, the soluble isoform of RAGE (sRAGE) has been detected in the plasma. It seems that sRAGE competes with cell-surface RAGE for ligand binding, thus increasing the elimination of circulating Aβ [145].

3.6. BBB dysfunction in AD

Failure in the BBB function is an outstanding event in the development and progression of several CNS diseases including multiple sclerosis [253], ischemia [254], Parkinson's disease, and AD [255]. While in some of the diseases increased BBB permeability is an outcome and consequence of the pathology (such as ischemic stroke), in other cases, BBB failure may be a causative event for the disease (such as multiple sclerosis). Furthermore, BBB dysfunction can be mild with temporary opening of TJs, or it can be a chronic breakdown [256], with changes in transporters and enzymes happening at the same time [216].

Although cerebrovascular abnormalities have been noted in AD, the starting point between BBB failure and AD pathology is not clear yet [142, 257]. Nevertheless, BBB homeostasis is altered in the initial stages of AD leading to the production of proinflammatory cytokines and suppressors of the cerebral blood flow by endothelial cells; then, amyloid deposits are observed in cerebral capillaries and vessels in the later stages of AD [258]. A large number of alterations in the structure and function of the BBB were shown to occur in AD. For instance: decreased LRP1 expression in human brain microvasculature [239], increased LRP1 oxidative damage [259], impaired microvascular P-gp [260], increased expression of RAGE in the cerebral vessels, neurons and microglia [251]. Moreover, it has been shown to occur: decreased glucose consumption by the brain, thus predicting a decay in cognitive function [261], which has been described by the reduction in the GLUT-1 transporters expression (protein levels) in AD hippocampus microvessels [262] but not a decrease in GLUT-1 mRNA levels [263]. Other alterations have been described, such as: decreased endothelial mitochondrial density, increased endothelial vacuolization, accumulation of collagen and perlecans in the basement capillary membrane [264], and increased pinocytotic vesicles [265].Also, it has been reported a reduced number and smaller diameter of capillaries in CNS implying the diminished overall surface for LRP1-mediated transcytosis of Aβ across the BBB, and also a decreased length of brain capillaries [266] which lowers transport of energy substrates and nutrients across the BBB, and reduces the clearance of neurotoxins from the brain [138]; Overexpression and accumulation of occludin in frontal cortex and basal ganglia of AD brains [267] have also been described as well as lower expression of genes such as the homeobox gene MEOX2 (or GAX), a regulator of vascular differentiation [268]. Finally, activated microglia [269] and astrocytes, the resident brain immune cells present in neurovascular unit of the BBB, have been observed surrounding Aβ plaques in AD brains, releasing inflammatory cytokines, such as IL-1 and IL-6, TNF-α, and transforming growth factor-β [174].

4. Periphery and Alzheimer's disease

4.1. Aβ levels at the periphery

Although studies in rodents have shown an increase in plasma Aβ levels, data in human AD patients have been contradictory; while some demonstrate increased levels of circulating Aβ [270], others report decreased [271] or unchanged [272] levels. Nevertheless, the significant role of circulating Aβ in AD pathology cannot be neglected. Interestingly, Aβ is also produced outside the brain in considerable amounts by the platelets, skeletal muscle, vascular walls, kidney, heart, liver, and by other non-neural tissues [273–275]. These pools may also provide a dynamic exchange of Aβ between the brain and periphery. However, Aβ peptides in the periphery cannot form filamentous structures, probably due to the presence of multiple circulating molecules that bind Aβ and thereby change its free-plasma levels [276].

4.1.1. Plasma proteins involved in peripheral sink and clearance of Aβ

Continuous removal of Aβ, not only from the brain but also from blood and from the entire organism, is essential for preventing its accumulation in the brain. Aβ in the plasma is bound to a number of proteins such as albumin [277], apoE and apoJ [278], TTR and a soluble form of LRP1 (sLRP1). In healthy human plasma, sLRP1 is a major endogenous brain Aβ sinker that sequesters 70–90% of plasma Aβ. sLRP1 has been demonstrated to bind the majority of circulating Aβ preventing RAGE-dependent influx of Aβ back to the brain, while improving its systemic clearance [279]. These data confirm the peripheral sink hypothesis, which imply systemic clearance of Aβ via binding proteins in serum and preventing its uptake through RAGE. Accordingly, this explains how some therapeutics, such as peripheral administration of sLRP1 or antibodies against Aβ [280], decrease Aβ levels in the brain. Moreover, AD patients show decreased plasma sLRP1 levels and increased oxidative damage to sLRP1, reducing its binding capacity for Aβ. This, in turn, increases the free Aβ fraction in plasma [279], that is, accessible for RAGE-dependent influx back to the brain [281].

Higher sRAGE levels are linked to reduced risk of developing several disorders such as cardiovascular disease and AD. Levels of sRAGE are decreased in AD and in vascular dementia, which may confer a target for therapeutic purposes [282]. It has been demonstrated that systemic administration of a truncated form of RAGE decreases Aβ load in a transgenic mouse model [241]. Moreover, sRAGE has an inverse relationship with cholesterol, presenting another modulatory impact on Aβ metabolism due to the role of cholesterol as a mediator of inflammation and APP processing [145].

4.1.2. Alterations in other plasma proteins in AD

Few proteins are synthesized solely by the brain or are present in higher concentrations in CSF compared with the blood. In conditions of the BBB failure, these CSF markers can appear or be increased in the plasma [283]. Hence, estimating levels of CSF proteins in the plasma may be a reliable method to control BBB integrity. For instance, S-100 is primarily produced in the brain by astrocytes and when the BBB is disturbed it is quickly released from the brain and appears in the blood [284].

4.2. Liver and Aβ elimination

At the periphery, the liver play important roles not only in the storage and in the release of nutrients and proteins but also in the neutralization and elimination of a variety of toxic substances such as Aβ from the plasma.

The receptor for LDL (LDLr), LRP1, and megalin/LRP2 play important roles in endocytosis of lipoproteins and systemic lipid homeostasis. Moreover, LRP1 mediates the clearance of a multitude of extracellular ligands such as Aβ and regulates diverse signaling processes such as growth factor signaling, inflammatory signaling pathways, apoptosis, and phagocytosis in liver.

In the liver, LRP1, which can be blocked by the receptor-associated protein (RAP), has been shown to be the predominant transporter that mediates systemic clearance of Aβ [285]. LRP1 localized to hepatic cells binds to and systemically clears circulating Aβ. Reduced hepatic LRP1 levels are associated with decreased peripheral Aβ clearance in aged rats. In aged squirrel monkeys, systemic clearance of Aβ is also reduced and associated with increased Aβ levels in the brain. In addition to the liver, sLRP1-Aβ complexes and free Aβ are removed through the kidneys [279]. Liver was also demonstrated to be the major source of Aβ and to be able to regulate brain Aβ levels [286].

The half-life of circulating Aβ is short, in the range of minutes [287, 288]. This also suggests that rapid systemic clearance of Aβ prevents reuptake by RAGE after efflux.

It has been shown that some proteins such as insulin [289] and TTR [290] increase LRP1 levels in hepatic plasma membrane, and in turn enhance peripheral Aβ clearance. Insulin-degrading enzyme, a zinc metalloendopeptidase that hydrolyzes numerous peptides, including Aβ [238], insulin [291] and the AICD, has been purified from several mammalian tissues including liver, brain and blood cells [292]. Furthermore, experiments in rats demonstrated that after 3.5 min post-infusion of radiolabelled Aβ into the lateral ventricle, 40% of the injected radioactivity was already in the blood and urine, and internalized by the liver and the kidneys, indicating not only a quick clearance mechanism but also the involvement of systemic organs in the elimination and catabolism of Aβ [293]. Therefore, the capacity of the liver to internalize, catabolize, and eliminate large doses of Aβ, may explain not only the low plasma Aβ levels but also its small variation noted with age and disease stages.

In some cases, both parenchymal and non-parenchymal liver cells take up proteins, whereas in other cases this is done mostly by hepatocytes, as happens for TTR, apoA-I, SAP and Aβ. In vivo and in vitro experiments showed that hepatocytes are the main cells involved in Aβ uptake (about 90%) and in its catabolism [288].

5. Transthyretin

Transthyretin (TTR), formerly called prealbumin due to its electrophoretic characteristics, located just in front of the albumin band, is a plasma protein secreted mainly by the liver and choroid plexus (CP) [294]. The name "transthyretin" discloses its dual physiological role as a carrier for thyroid hormones [295] and retinol, the latter through the binding to retinol-binding protein (RBP) [296]. TTR was first described in the CSF [297] and shortly after in the plasma [298].

Although the involvement of TTR in the transport of thyroid hormones and RBP, as well as in FAP, is very well established, its involvement in neuroprotection is part of a very recent knowledge and constantly evolving.

5.1. TTR gene structure and expression

TTR is codified by a single copy gene localized in the long arm of chromosome 18 [299]. The entire nucleotide sequence including the 5′ (transcription initiating site) and the 3′ (untranslated region) flanking regions was determined [300, 301] and attributed to the region 18q11.2–q12.1 [302]. The full gene is 7.6 kilobase (kb) long comprising 4 exons and 3 introns [300, 301]. Exon 1 contains 95 basepairs (bp), including 26 bp 5′ untranslated, and codes for a 20 aa residue leader peptide and aa 1–3 of the mature protein; exon 2 (131 bp), 3 (136 bp), and 4 (253 bp) hold the coding sequences for aa residues 4–47, 48–92 and 93–127, respectively. The introns (A, B and C) are 934, 2090 and 3308 bp long, respectively. Introns A and C contain two open reading frames (orf) of unknown significance [301].

The TTR mRNA spans ~0.7 kb and contains a 5′-untranslated region (26–27 nucleotides), a coding region (441 nucleotides), and a 3′-untranslated region (145–148 nucleotides) preceding the poly(A) tail [294, 303]. Human [299], rat [304, 305] and mouse [306] coding regions exhibit a considerable degree of homology (~85%), suggesting a phylogenetically preserved modulating role in gene expression.

TTR is predominantly synthesized by the liver where more than 90% of the protein is produced. The remaining is produced by the CP and the retina. TTR is detected in the fetal blood very early during development, as soon as eight weeks after conception [307]. TTR plasma concentration is age dependent, and in healthy newborns, it is about half of that in adults [308, 309]. TTR values vary from 20 to 40 mg/dL. In spite of the low TTR levels in CSF (~2 mg/dL), the CP is presented as the major site of TTR expression, expressed as a ratio of TTR/mass of tissue, corresponding to a ~30-fold higher than that found in plasma [310]. TTR represents 20% of the total CSF proteins [310].

With respect to the regulation of TTR expression, several studies showed that liver and CP TTR expression are increased in response to sex hormones, as demonstrated in mice [311,

312]. In rats, hydrocortisone and psychosocial stress are also inducers of TTR in the CP [313]. Others studies indicate that TTR can be expressed by brain cells, for instance in response to the heat shock factor 1 (HSF1) and to the AICD fragment of APP, as we will discuss further ahead in the context of TTR protection in AD.

5.2. TTR protein structure

The TTR mRNA codifies for the TTR-monomer; the polypeptide of 147 aa residues whose N-terminal region is a hydrophobic signal peptide of 20 aa residues. The TTR monomer is subjected to a cleaving process, during its migration through the ER, giving rise to the native TTR monomer after breaking of the signal peptide [294]. Assembly of four identical subunits (13,745 Da) occurs yielding the mature tetrameric protein, with a molecular mass of 54,980 Da [314].

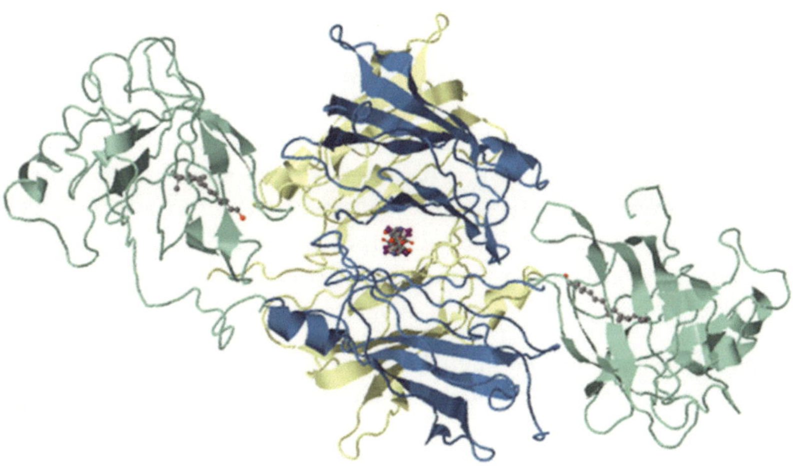

Figure 2. The human TTR tetrameric structure complexed with two molecules of RBP (light green), which in turn is bound to retinol, and with T4 (binding in the central channel).

The tridimensional structure of TTR was made available at 1.8 Å resolution by X-ray diffraction studies on the crystallized protein [315]. Each monomer contains two β-sheets formed by strands DAGH and CBEF. All, except strands A and G, display an antiparallel orientation, and are arranged in a topology similar to the classic Greek key barrel. The strands are 7–8 residues long, except strand D, which, is only 3 residues in length. Only about 5% of the aa residues are located in one segment of α-helix comprising residues 75–83, at the end of strand E. Two monomers associate forming the dimer by interactions between chains F and H of each monomer. Fixing the chains of one monomer as A–H and the ones of the other monomer as A′–H′, the arrangement within a dimer is DAGHH′G′A′D′ and CBEFF′E′B′C′. The tetramer consists of two dimers with connecting edges occurring between the AB loop of one dimer with the H strand of the other dimer (**Figure 2**). The quaternary structure of TTR has the shape of a globular protein with an overall size of 70 Å × 55 Å × 50 Å [315]. The two dimers are slightly rotated in relation to each other along the y axis.

5.3. Physiology and Metabolism

5.3.1. Transport of thyroxine (T_4)

Thyroid hormones are transported in blood circulation and delivered to the target tissues, with an incredible high amount of the hormones (99%) bound to serum proteins. In human plasma, TTR, thyroxine-binding protein (TBG) and albumin are responsible for the delivery of T_4 into the target tissues. Although TBG is much less concentrated in the plasma than TTR, it presents the highest affinity constant for T_4 (Ka = 1×10^{10} M^{-1}) and transports about 70% of the plasma T_4. TTR has an intermediate affinity for T_4 (Ka = 7×10^7 M^{-1}) and transports about 15% of the hormone, and finally, albumin presents the lowest binding affinity (Ka = 7×10^5 M^{-1}) [316].

The four monomers of the TTR tetramer, demarcate an open channel through the molecule where two binding sites for thyroid hormones are located (**Figure 2**). These two binding sites present negative cooperativity [317] implying that when the first thyroid hormone molecule occupies the first site, the affinity for the second molecule is highly reduced.

T_4 transport into the brain is of particular interest and has raised much controversy [318]. Although TTR is the major T_4-binding protein in the CSF, studies done in *ttr* knock-out mice ($TTR^{-/-}$) [319] revealed that TTR is not essential for thyroxine to reach the brain and other tissues [320]. In addition, measurement of several parameters of thyroid hormone function indicates that these mice are euthyroid despite strongly reduced total T_4 plasma levels [321]. No other protein was found to replace TTR in the transport of T_4 in the CSF, and T_4 levels were normal in the cortex, cerebellum, and hippocampus while strongly reduced in the CP of the $TTR^{-/-}$ mice [322].

Therefore, it was suggested that TTR might be a reservoir for T_4 both in the plasma and in the CP and CSF, which might become important under conditions of increased hormone demand.

5.3.2. Transport of vitamin A

TTR is also responsible for retinol transport through binding to retinol-binding protein (RBP, **Figure 2**). RBP is a 21 kDa monomeric protein comprising 182 aa residues [323]. The conformational structure of RBP bound to retinol was determined by x-ray crystallography [324]. In most instances, RBP is transported in the bloodstream in the form of a saturated holo-RBP protein equimolarly attached to TTR [325]. Although TTR has four binding sites for RBP [326, 327], under physiological conditions only one RBP molecule is bound to TTR due to the RBP limiting concentration.

5.3.3. TTR metabolism

The biological half-life of TTR is about 2–3 days in humans [328, 329], 22–23 h in monkeys [330] and 10–13 h in rats [331]. The major sites of TTR degradation in the rat are liver (36–38%), followed by the muscle (12–15%) and skin (8–10%) [332].

The normal physiology of TTR is not completely understood, in particular, its cellular uptake. Nevertheless, several observations suggest that TTR internalization is receptor-mediated, both in human hepatoma cells (HepG2) [333] and in chicken oocytes [334]. Megalin, a receptor implicated in the renal re-uptake of plasma proteins carriers of lipophilic compounds, was shown to play a role in renal uptake of TTR [335]. Furthermore, different TTR mutations presented different levels of cell association and degradation, suggesting that the structure of TTR is important for megalin recognition. TTR internalization was further explored by studying TTR uptake using hepatomas and primary hepatocytes [336]. This work showed direct evidence for TTR internalization by a specific receptor, forming a ~90 kDa complex. TTR internalization was inhibited by RBP (70% decrease) and T_4 (20% decrease) and TTR mutants revealed differences in uptake, indicating again that the recognition by receptor is structure dependent. Internalization was also inhibited by lipoproteins and RAP, a ligand for all members of the low-density lipoprotein receptor family (LDLr). All together, these results suggest a common pathway for TTR and lipoprotein metabolism and the existence of a RAP-sensitive receptor for TTR internalization. TTR is also internalized by several other cells types in cell culture, such as astrocytoma cells [337], cardiomiocytes [338, 339], neurons [340, 341], endothelial cells and others. More recently, TTR was also shown to be uptaken by sensory neurons, an event also mediated by megalin [340].

5.3.4. Proteolytic activity

TTR was also found to act as a cryptic protease and the first substrate described was apoA-I [342, 343]. TTR is also able to cleave lipidated apoA-I (mainly in the lipid poor pre β-HDL subpopulation) which can be relevant in the lipoprotein metabolism [343]. Moreover, apoA-I cleaved by TTR presents less ability to promote cholesterol efflux [343] and shows increased amyloidogenecity and propensity to form aggregates. Liz et al. also described that TTR was able to cleave amidated neuropeptide Y (NPY) and that its proteolytic activity affects axonal growth, leading to the conclusion that TTR has natural substrates in the nervous system [344]. Newly, the same authors described TTR as a metallopeptidase [345], and this result was supported by another study that showed the involvement of a carboxylate and an ammonium group, possibly from a lysine side chain, in the TTR hydrolytic activity [346]. Costa et al. showed for the first time that TTR can cleave Aβ peptide in vitro [347] and implications in Aβ clearance in AD will be addressed further ahead.

5.4. TTR as a cause of disease

TTR is associated with the most prevalent type of hereditary systemic amyloidosis. The pathologic conditions include FAP and familial amyloidotic cardiomyopathy (FAC). A non-hereditary condition is also related to TTR, the systemic senile amyloidosis (SSA), and affects about 25% of people over 80 years of age. In SAA, the deposits occur in the heart and are composed of wild-type (WT) TTR.

FAP is related to a peculiar form of hereditary autosomal dominant polyneuropathy. Corino de Andrade first described the disease in 1952 [6] in the Portuguese population mainly from the northern part of the country. Characterized by systemic deposition of amyloid and with a special involvement of the peripheral nerves, the age of onset of the disease is usually between 20 and 35 years of age, with a fast progression to death within 10–15 years.

Clinically, FAP is characterized by early impairment of temperature and pain sensation in the feet, and autonomic dysfunction leading to paresis, malabsorption, and emaciation. Painless injury to the feet complicated by ulcers, cellulitis, osteomyelitis, and Charcots joints may also occur [348]. Motor involvement occurs with disease development causing wasting and weakness, and there is a progressive loss of reflexes. The amyloid deposits can occur in any part of the peripheral nervous system, including the nerve trunks, plexus, and sensory and autonomic ganglia. The other organ frequently involved in FAP, which is the heart. Clinically, the cardiomyopathy may present as an arrhythmia, heart block, or heat failure.

The first report relating immunologically TTR as the main protein in FAP fibrils was in 1978 by Costa and colleagues [349]. In 1984, the Val30Met mutation was identified in the protein isolated from Portuguese FAP patients. This variant was shown to be a biochemical marker for FAP [350] that resulted from a point mutation in the exon 2 of the TTR gene [351]. Since the identification of the Val30Met variant, many others aa substitutions were identified in the TTR protein and now over 100 mutations are described (http://amyloidosismutations.com/mut-attr.php); these variants are associated with different clinical phenotypes and a considerable number of non-pathogenic TTR mutations have been identified, including a T119M variant described to be protective.

TTR tetramer dissociation is believed to be on the basis of a series of events leading to TTR amyloid formation. In fact, the amyloidogenic potential of the TTR variants relates inversely with its tetrameric stability, and it is thought that upon dissociation of the tetramer, non-native TTR monomers are formed which can assemble, forming amyloidogenic intermediate species, such as oligomers and aggregates. Similarly to other amyloidogenic proteins, it is now believed that cellular toxicity is derived from the initial intermediate species occurring in the initial stages of FAP [352]. TTR stabilization has been proposed as a key step for the inhibition of TTR fibril formation and has been the basis for FAP therapeutic strategies. Such stabilization can be achieved through the use of small compounds sharing molecular structural similarities with T_4 and binding in the T_4 central-binding channel. Most of such compounds belong to the class of NSAIDs as it is the case of diflunisal and tafamidis, currently being administrated to FAP patients. For instance, in FAP patients, diflunisal was shown to stabilize TTR, increasing its serum concentration [353], and to reduce the rate of progression of neurological impairment and to preserve quality of life [354].

6. TTR and neuroprotection

Several lines of evidence indicate that TTR possesses neuroprotective properties in multiple contexts. Studies with $TTR^{-/-}$ mice revealed that these animals show reduced signs of depressive-like behavior, probably due to the modulation of noradrenergic system by the increase of noradrenaline in the limbic forebrain [355]. Additionally, increased levels of NPY, known as an antidepressant neurotransmitter [356], were reported in dorsal root ganglia (DRG), sciatic nerve, spinal cord, hippocampus, cortex, and CSF of $TTR^{-/-}$ mice [357], supporting the importance of TTR in the modulation of depressive behavior. Furthermore,

Sousa and co-workers also described that $TTR^{-/-}$ mice present memory impairment compared with wild-type ($TTR^{+/+}$) animals, indicating that the absence of TTR accelerates cognitive deficits usually associated with aging [358].

In addition, TTR was associated with nerve regeneration. Fleming et al. revealed, for the first time, that TTR acts as an enhancer of nerve regeneration, following the observation that $TTR^{-/-}$ mice have decreased ability to regenerate from a sciatic crushed nerve [359]. Later, the same authors showed that the absence of TTR leads to impaired retrograde transport and decreased axonal growth, and also that the effect of TTR in neurite outgrowth and nerve regeneration is mediated by megalin-dependent internalization [340].

It was also established a relationship between TTR and ischemia, one of the major causes of brain injuries in world. Santos and co-workers proposed that in a compromised heat-shock response, CSF TTR contributes to control neuronal cell death, edema, and inflammation, influencing the survival endangered neurons [360].

More recently, a new neuroprotective role in the CNS was attributed to TTR, as a transcription inducer of insulin-like growth factor receptor I (IGF-IR), known as a protective receptor against apoptosis [361]. Vieira and colleagues described, for the first time, that TTR induces increased levels of IGF-IR, showing that TTR triggers IGF-IR nuclear translocation in cultured neurons [341].

6.1. TTR protection in Alzheimer's Disease

There are several reports suggesting a relevant protective role of TTR in AD. However, the precise mechanism(s) is not entirely understood.

In 1993, Wisniewski described that Aβ40 fibril formation was inhibited upon incubation with human CSF [362], which was explained by the sequestration of Aβ by extracellular proteins circulating in CSF such as apoE and apoJ [362–364]. The earliest description of TTR protection in AD was presented by Schwarzman and colleagues in 1994 when they observed that, in CSF and contrarily to the expectations, apoE was not the major protein binding to Aβ, but TTR [365], proposing the sequestration hypothesis as a possible explanation for the peptide aggregation and consequent progression of AD. This hypothesis suggested that certain extracellular proteins sequester normally produced Aβ, thereby preventing amyloid formation and its toxicity. Amyloid formation would occur when sequestration failed [365, 366], which could be related either with an Aβ overproduction, a reduction in the levels of the sequestering proteins, inability of those proteins to interact with the peptide, deficient clearance mechanisms, or a combination of all the events above stated.

Supporting a protective role for TTR in AD are its decreased levels observed both in the CSF [367] and in the plasma [114, 368] of AD patients as compared to age-matched subjects. Serot and coworkers suggested that the decrease in TTR levels in the CSF of AD brains was possibly related with an epithelial atrophy in the CP [367]. Interestingly, very recently, studies in an AD transgenic mouse model reported CP dysfunction and revealed a specific increase only of the Aβ42 isoform in epithelial cytosol and in stroma surrounding choroidal capillaries, accompanied by a thickening of the epithelial basal membrane, greater collagen-IV deposition around capillaries in CP that probably restrain solute exchanges, and attenuated expression of epithelial aquaporin-1 and TTR protein compared to non-transgenic mice [369].

Modulation of Aβ aggregation and toxicity was also investigated in brain vascular smooth muscle cells, isolated from dogs and AD patients, containing intracytoplasmatic granules of Aβ produced in the presence of apoE. In this model, TTR was able to rescue the cells from this accumulation and the positive thioflavin S staining, initially observed, was no longer detected [370].

Although not fully consensual, several authors reported the presence of TTR in amyloid plaques both in AD patients [371–373] and in AD transgenic models [372], strengthening a role for TTR in Aβ deposition and in AD. TTR was also identified as a survival gene, and its differential overexpression in mice hippocampus was suggested to be responsible for the lack of neurodegeneration observed in the Tg2576 transgenic mice overexpressing the mutant form of human amyloid precursor protein with the Swedish mutation (APP_{Sw}) [374]. Up-regulation of TTR and other survival genes was induced by the sAPPα, a neuroprotective fragment resulting from APP processing by α-secretase [373]. TTR up-regulation was also reported in situations of exposure of AD transgenic mice to an "enriched environment," also resulting in pronounced reductions in cerebral Aβ levels and amyloid deposits, compared to animals raised under "standard housing" conditions [375]. Later on, AD transgenic models with genetic reduction of TTR and/or overexpression of human TTR [372] further showed the ability of TTR to modulate Aβ aggregation and toxicity. While the overexpression of human TTR ameliorated AD features in APP transgenic mice [372], the ablation of the mouse TTR gene resulted in accelerated amyloid deposition and increased Aβ brain levels [372, 376, 377]. In vitro studies further demonstrated that a direct interaction between TTR and Aβ abrogated the noxious properties of Aβ oligomers [378].

Animal models, in particular mice models, also provided evidence for a gender-associated modulation of brain Aβ levels [377] as elevated brain levels of Aβ42 were observed in AD female mice with only one copy of TTR when compared to female with the two copies of the TTR gene, while no significant differences were observed in males. Additionally, this work also indicated that reduced levels of brain testosterone and 17β-estradiol in female mice with TTR genetic reduction might underlie their increased AD-like neuropathology [377]. Interestingly, estradiol was found to be decreased in female AD patients when compared to healthy age and gender-matched controls [114], which in conjunction with TTR regulation by sex hormones, as already described, can account for TTR lowering in AD and the prevalence of this disease in women. In fact, plasma TTR levels were found decreased in AD women, as compared to healthy age- and gender-matched controls, whereas plasma TTR levels in AD men were not significantly different from their respective controls [114], further confirming the gender modulation by TTR.

6.1.1. TTR and Aβ interaction

TTR and Aβ binding was initially demonstrated by adding radiolabelled Aβ1-28 synthetic peptide to human CSF and subsequent analysis by SDS-PAGE [365]. Later on, the TTR/Aβ complex was also demonstrated in plasma [379], although the details of the interaction as well as the effects in Aβ fibrillogenesis and toxicity were not known.

In 2008, Costa and colleagues characterized the TTR/Aβ interaction by competition-binding assays using synthetic Aβ42, which revealed that the WT TTR binds to different Aβ peptide species: soluble (with a Kd of 28 ± 5 nM), oligomers, and fibrils [378]. Other studies showed that TTR drastically decreased the rate of aggregation without affecting the fraction of Aβ in the aggregate pool and an estimated apparent KS of 2300 M^{-1} was calculated [380]. These data support a hypothesis, wherein TTR preferentially binds to aggregated rather than monomeric Aβ and arrests further growth of the aggregates. Recent work indicates that the intensity of TTR binding to Aβ peptide is highest for partially aggregated materials and decreased for freshly prepared or heavily aggregated Aβ, suggesting that TTR binds selectively to soluble toxic Aβ aggregates [381]. Although Schwarzman and colleagues had shown in 1994 that TTR is capable of inhibiting Aβ1-28 aggregation [365], Costa and co-workers showed by transmission electron microscopy (TEM) analysis that TTR is capable of interfering with Aβ fibrillization, both at inhibiting its aggregation and at disrupting pre-formed Aβ fibrils [378]. Thus, new and innovative studies are necessary to clarify the details of this interaction.

Another point of controversy refers to the TTR species involved in Aβ binding. Some studies support that the TTR monomer rather than the tetramer binds more strongly to Aβ [382], and it is even suggested that while the TTR monomer arrests Aβ aggregate growth, the tetramer modestly enhances the peptide aggregation [382]. Another study performed using diverse natural TTR mutants showed that different TTR variants bind differentially to Aβ in the following manner: T119M>WT>V30M³Y78F>L55P TTR [378], indicating the lower the amyloidogenic potential of TTR, the stronger the affinity toward the peptide. Since the amyloidogenic potential correlates inversely with TTR tetrameric stability, authors concluded that the TTR tetramer is the species binding to Aβ peptide. Previous work had already shown that amyloidogenic TTR mutants such as L55P and E42G, the only ones able to form TTR amyloid fibrils at pH 6.8 amongst the forty-seven variants tested, were unable to bind Aβ [383].

Given the above considerations, it is therefore conceivable that mutations of the TTR gene could alter the TI'R/Aβ sequestration properties. However, the screening study in AD patients found no correlation between TTR variants and AD [384], and therefore other factors, namely conformational changes resulting from aging, should be affecting TTR levels and its binding properties towards Aβ.

Computer-assisted modelling was developed to determine the possible key residues participating in the interaction and the data suggested that residues 38–42, Asparagine 62 (E62) and E66 of each TTR monomer had a central role in the interaction [365]. Later studies have confirmed that only the residues 38–42 of TTR were important for the interaction [366]. More recently, Du and Murphy, identified the A strand, in the inner β-sheet of TTR, as well as the EF helix, as regions of TTR that are involved with Aβ [382] association. New data from the same group now indicates the involvement of the G strand of TTR with the particular involvement of L82A and L110A, suggesting that Aβ binding to TTR is mediated through these bulky hydrophobic leucines [385].

6.1.2. *Effects of TTR stabilization in AD*

The decrease in TTR levels in the context of AD is found early in disease development as indicated by the lower levels also found in plasma TTR in MCI patients [114]. TTR levels continue to decrease as disease progresses correlating negatively with disease severity, both in CSF [115] and plasma [114], and with senile plaque burden [386]. Similar results were found in AD transgenic mice as TTR was decreased as early as 3 months of age [377], well before amyloid deposition. Mice, however, seem to be able to compensate and female showed restored TTR levels at the age of 10 months [377].

The reason for TTR decrease is not known, but its tetrameric stability seems to play an important role. An unstable TTR can result in accelerated clearance, accounting for the lower levels observed. Further, such instability can also affect the Aβ sequestration properties of TTR. Supporting this stability hypothesis is the observation that plasma TTR from AD patients presents impaired ability to carry T_4. This also supports that it is the TTR tetramer that binds Aβ, since T_4 binding to TTR implies that the tetramer is assembled. Very interestingly, TTR genetic stabilization, that is, the presence of the T119M allele, was associated to decreased cerebrovascular disease and increased life expectancy [387]. In the context of AD, and arguing in favor of the stability hypothesis is the observation that the TTR/Aβ interaction can be improved in vitro in the presence of small chemical molecules known to bind to the T_4-binding channel and to stabilize its tetrameric fold [388]. Importantly, in vivo studies using one of such stabilizer—iododiflunisal, known to be a very potent TTR stabilizer [389] and shown to improve TTR/Aβ interaction [388]—administrated to AD transgenic mice resulted in amelioration of AD features such as cognitive function and Aβ brain deposition [390]. In addition, plasma levels of Aβ42 were decreased upon iododiflunisal administration. These results opened the possibility for the use of TTR stabilizers in AD therapeutic drug development.

6.1.3. *Mechanisms of TTR protection in AD*

Aβ sequestration by TTR and other extracellular proteins was the first hypothesis proposed to explain why CSF is able to inhibit Aβ amyloid formation, implying that, when sequestered, Aβ cannot aggregate to form amyloid [362, 365]. However, the precise mechanism leading to final Aβ removal is not yet elucidated.

Following the identification of the TTR proteolytic activity, it was also described that Aβ peptide is cleaved by TTR, in vitro, with consequent generation of non-amyloidogenic fragments or fragments with amyloidogenic potential inferior to the full-length peptide [347]. Since clearance of Aβ from the brain can occur via proteolytic degradation of the peptide by several enzymes, such as neprilysin (NEP), insulin-degrading enzyme (IDE), Endothelin-converting enzyme (ECE), angiotensin-converting enzyme (ACE), uPA/tPA-plasmin system, cathepsin D, and matrix metalloendopeptidase 9 [391, 392], lower levels of TTR or inhibition of its proteolytic activity would result in less Aβ peptide eliminated by the cells, and therefore in its accumulation and amyloid formation. Interestingly, several sites of Aβ cleavage by TTR are common to several of the proteases mentioned [347]. Further, NEP is known to cleave not only monomeric but also oligomeric forms of Aβ localized intra and extracellularly, as determined in vitro and in vivo [393, 394]; similarly, TTR was shown to degrade both monomers and aggregates of Aβ in vitro. Nevertheless, Aβ degradation by TTR was not yet shown in vivo. It is also not known if binding/sequestration of Aβ and its degradation by TTR are part of the same mechanism or are independent processes.

In addition to the peptidolytic removal of Aβ, clearance of the peptide from the brain also occurs via active transport at the BBB and BCSFB, as already discussed. The receptors for Aβ at the BBB bind Aβ directly, or bind to one of its carrier proteins, and transport it across the endothelial cell. The first hint pointing to the involvement of TTR in Aβ transport and clearance came from the analysis of brain and plasma levels of the peptide in mice with different TTR genetic backgrounds. Results showed that AD transgenic mice with just one copy of TTR had lower brain and plasma Aβ levels, as compared to animals with two TTR gene copies, raising the hypothesis that TTR might be involved both in Aβ brain efflux and in its peripheral removal at the liver. Very recently, it has been showed that TTR promotes Aβ internalization and efflux in hCMEC/D3 cells, a BBB cellular model widely used. Importantly, TTR stimulated brain-to-blood Aβ permeability in hCMEC/D3 which in turn can be explained because TTR itself can only cross the BBB only in the brain-to-blood direction [290, 332]. Thus, TTR can transport Aβ from, but not into the brain, acting as a neuroprotective molecule.

The presence of TTR in brain areas other than its site of synthesis and secretion—CP and CSF, respectively—has been already shown. In situations of injury, such as ischemia, TTR was detected at the local of infarct and shown to derive from CSF TTR [360]. However, other studies demonstrated TTR synthesis by cortical [395] or hippocampal neurons both in vitro [396], and in vivo [397] showing that TTR expression in the brain can be regulated [396]. For instance, Kerridge and colleagues showed that TTR expressed in SH-SY5Y neuroblastoma cell line is up-regulated by the AICD fragment of amyloid precursor protein (APP), specifically derived from the APP695 isoform [396]. Induced accumulation of functional AICD resulted in TTR up-regulation with concomitant Aβ decreased levels. Wang and colleagues reported that TTR expression in SH-SY5Y cells, primary hippocampal neurons, and the hippocampus of APP23 mice is significantly enhanced by HSF1 [397]. In any case, TTR is available in the brain and might participate in brain Aβ efflux by promoting BBB permeability to the peptide. It is also possible that TTR contributes to Aβ clearance from the brain through the BCSFB.

TTR was also able to increase Aβ internalization by hepatocytes prompting TTR as an Aβ transporter both in the brain and at periphery. Previous work showed that TTR is internalized by hepatocytes using a RAP-sensitive receptor, which together with the knowledge that as follows: (1) LRP1 is the main Aβ receptor both at the BBB and at the liver, (2) LRP1 is preferentially expressed at the basolateral membrane of the endothelial cells of the BBB, and (3) TTR can only cross the BBB in the brain-to-blood direction, indicates this receptor is involved in TTR-assisted Aβ transport. So far, it has been shown that mice with TTR genetic ablation present decrease levels of brain and liver LRP1 and that TTR added to hCMEC/D3 cells results in increased LRP1 expression. These findings open new perspectives for TTR/LRP-related therapeutic interventions in AD. However, a direct interaction between LRP1 and TTR is yet to be demonstrated. TTR has also been suggested to act in a chaperone-like manner by binding toxic or pretoxic Aβ aggregates in both the intracellular and extracellular environment [372].

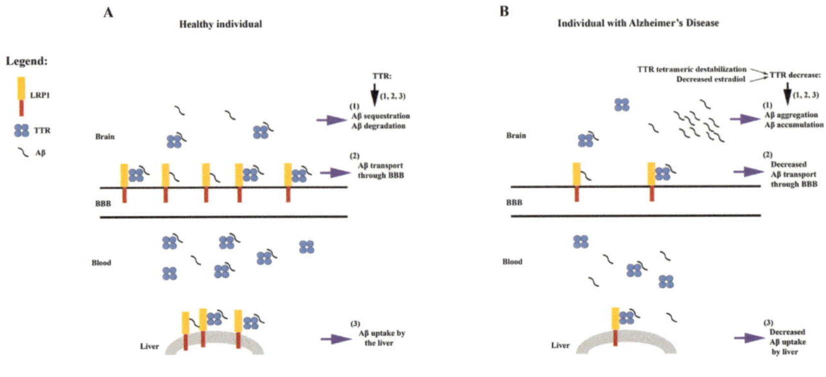

Figure 3. Schematic representation of the proposed mechanisms underlying TTR Protection in AD. (A) In a healthy individual, TTR binds Aβ peptide in the brain at the CSF promoting its degradation and elimination through the epithelial cells of the CP. At the BBB, Aβ effluxes through LRP1 to the blood, a process in which TTR also participates. At the periphery, TTR and other Aβ bindable substances create a peripheral sink avoiding the return of Aβ to the brain, and transport the peptide to the liver, where it will be internalized by liver LRP1 for final degradation. (B) In AD patients, TTR decreased tetrameric stability for yet unknown reasons, and decreased expression due to decreased sex hormones, result in lower protein levels in the brain and plasma. In turn, this contributes to failure in Aβ sequestration, efflux at the BBB, and peripheral transport to the liver. Impaired Aβ transport at the BBB and internalization/degradation by the liver is aggravated by LRP1 decreased expression, modulated by TTR.

Therefore, more studies are necessary to unravel the mechanism(s) underlying TTR protection in AD, and to clarify how the hypothesis presented so far fit together (**Figure 3**).

Acknowledgements

This work was funded by national funds through FCT—Fundação para a Ciência e a Tecnologia/MEC—Ministério da Educação e Ciência and when applicable co-funded by FEDER funds within the partnership agreement PT2020 related with the research unit number 4293, and by FEDER funds through the Operational Competitiveness Programme—COMPETE and by National Funds through FCT—Fundação para a Ciência e a Tecnologia under the projects FCOMP-01-0124-FEDER-037277 (PEst-C/SAU/LA0002/2013).

Author details

Isabel Cardoso[1,2*], Luis Miguel Santos[1,2] and Mobina Alemi[1,2,3]

*Address all correspondence to: icardoso@ibmc.up.pt

1 IBMC-Instituto de Biologia Molecular e Celular, Porto, Portugal

2 i3S-Instituto de Investigação e Inovação em Saúde, Universidade do Porto, Porto, Portugal

3 Faculdade de Medicina, Universidade do Porto, Porto, Portugal

References

[1] Westermark GT, Fändrich M, Westermark P. AA amyloidosis: pathogenesis and targeted therapy. Annu Rev Pathol [Internet]. 2015;10:321–44 [cited 2015 Dec 10]. http://www.ncbi.nlm.nih.gov/pubmed/25387054

[2] Virchow R. Zur Cellulose—Frage. Arch für Pathol Anat und Physiol und für Klin Med [Internet]. 1854;6(3):416–26 [cited 2016 Jan 5]. http://link.springer.com/10.1007/BF02116546

[3] Sipe JD, Benson MD, Buxbaum JN, Ikeda S, Merlini G, Saraiva MJM, et al. Nomenclature 2014: amyloid fibril proteins and clinical classification of the amyloidosis. Amyloid [Internet]. 2014;21(4):221–4 [cited 2015 May 28]. http://www.ncbi.nlm.nih.gov/pubmed/25263598

[4] Westermark P. Quantitative studies on amyloid in the islets of Langerhans. Ups J Med Sci [Internet]. 1972;77(2):91–4 [cited 2015 Oct 28]. http://www.ncbi.nlm.nih.gov/pubmed/4116019

[5] Prusiner SB. Novel proteinaceous infectious particles cause scrapie. Science [Internet]. 1982;216(4542):136–44 [cited 2015 Aug 2]. http://www.ncbi.nlm.nih.gov/pubmed/6801762

[6] Andrade C. A peculiar form of peripheral neuropathy; familiar atypical generalized amyloidosis with special involvement of the peripheral nerves. Brain [Internet]. 1952;75(3):408–27 [cited 2016 Jan 13]. http://www.ncbi.nlm.nih.gov/pubmed/12978172

[7] Glenner GG, Wong CW. Alzheimer's disease: initial report of the purification and characterization of a novel cerebrovascular amyloid protein. Biochem Biophys Res Commun [Internet]. 1984;120(3):885–90 [cited 2015 Jan 26]. http://www.ncbi.nlm.nih.gov/pubmed/6375662

[8] Stelzmann R a., Schnitzlein HN, Murtagh FR. An English translation of Alzheimer's 1907 paper, "uber eine eigenartige erkankung der hirnrinde." Clin Anat. 1995;8(6):429–31.

[9] Pimplikar SW. Reassessing the amyloid cascade hypothesis of Alzheimer's disease. Int J Biochem Cell Biol [Internet]. 2009;41(6):1261–8. http://www.pubmedcentral.nih.gov/articlerender.fcgi?artid=2680505&tool=pmcentrez&rendertype=abstract

[10] Alzheimer A, Stelzmann RA, Schnitzlein HN, Murtagh FR. An English translation of Alzheimer's 1907 paper, "Uber eine eigenartige Erkankung der Hirnrinde". Clin Anat [Internet]. 1995;8(6):429–31 [cited 2015 Mar 10]. http://www.ncbi.nlm.nih.gov/pubmed/8713166

[11] Kumar A, Singh A. A review on Alzheimer's disease pathophysiology and its management: an update. Pharmacol Rep [Internet]. 2015;67(2):195–203 [cited 2015 Jan 9]. http://www.ncbi.nlm.nih.gov/pubmed/25712639

[12] Burns A, Byrne EJ, Maurer K. Alzheimer's disease. Lancet (London, England) [Internet] (Elsevier). 2002;360(9327):163–5 [cited 2016 Jan 6]. http://www.thelancet.com/article/S0140673602094205/fulltext

[13] van der Linde RM, Dening T, Matthews FE, Brayne C. Grouping of behavioural and psychological symptoms of dementia. Int J Geriatr Psychiatry [Internet]. 2014;29(6): 562–8 [cited 2015 Oct 20]. http://www.pubmedcentral.nih.gov/articlerender.fcgi?artid=4255309&tool=pmcentrez&rendertype=abstract

[14] Petrovic M, Hurt C, Collins D, Burns A, Camus V, Liperoti R, et al. Clustering of behavioural and psychological symptoms in dementia (BPSD): a European Alzheimer's disease consortium (EADC) study. Acta Clin Belg [Internet]. 2016;62(6):426–32 [cited 2016 Jan 6]. http://www.ncbi.nlm.nih.gov/pubmed/18351187

[15] 2015 Alzheimer's disease facts and figures. Alzheimers Dement [Internet]. 2015;11(3): 332–84 [cited 2015 Jun 2]. http://www.ncbi.nlm.nih.gov/pubmed/25984581

[16] Reitz C, Mayeux R. Alzheimer disease: epidemiology, diagnostic criteria, risk factors and biomarkers. Biochem Pharmacol [Internet] (NIH Public Access) 2014;88(4):640–51 [cited 2014 Jul 10]. http:/pmc/articles/PMC3992261/?report=abstract

[17] McKhann G, Drachman D, Folstein M, Katzman R, Price D, Stadlan EM. Clinical diagnosis of Alzheimer's disease: report of the NINCDS-ADRDA Work Group* under the auspices of Department of Health and Human Services Task Force on Alzheimer's Disease. Neurology [Internet]. 1984;34(7):939–939 [cited 2015 Jun 7]. http://www.neurology.org/content/34/7/939

[18] McKhann GM, Knopman DS, Chertkow H, Hyman BT, Jack CR, Kawas CH, et al. The diagnosis of dementia due to Alzheimer's disease: recommendations from the National Institute on Aging-Alzheimer's Association workgroups on diagnostic guidelines for Alzheimer's disease. Alzheimers Dement [Internet] (Elsevier). 2011;7(3):263–9 [cited 2014 Jul 9]. http://www.alzheimersanddementia.com/article/S1552526011001014/fulltext

[19] Hyman BT, Phelps CH, Beach TG, Bigio EH, Cairns NJ, Carrillo MC, et al. National Institute on Aging-Alzheimer's Association guidelines for the neuropathologic assessment of Alzheimer's disease. Alzheimers Dement [Internet]. 2012;8(1):1–13 [cited 2015 Aug 6]. http://www.sciencedirect.com/science/article/pii/S1552526011029803

[20] 2013 Alzheimer's disease facts and figures. Alzheimers Dement [Internet]. 2013;9(2): 208–45 [cited 2015 Sep 2]. http://www.sciencedirect.com/science/article/pii/S1552526013000769

[21] Gaugler JE, Kane RL, Johnston J a, Sarsour K. Sensitivity and specificity of diagnostic accuracy in Alzheimer´s disease: a synthesis of existing evidence. Am J Alzheimer´s Dis Other Dement. 2013;28(4):337–47.

[22] Bertram L, Lill CM, Tanzi RE. The genetics of Alzheimer disease: back to the future. Neuron [Internet]. 2010;68(2):270–81 [cited 2015 Jun 14]. http://www.sciencedirect.com/science/article/pii/S0896627310008378

[23] Goate A, Chartier-Harlin MC, Mullan M, Brown J, Crawford F, Fidani L, et al. Segregation of a missense mutation in the amyloid precursor protein gene with familial Alzheimer's disease. Nature [Internet]. 1991;349(6311):704–6 [cited 2014 Dec 28]. http://www.ncbi.nlm.nih.gov/pubmed/1671712

[24] Scheuner D, Eckman C, Jensen M, Song X, Citron M, Suzuki N, et al. Secreted amyloid beta-protein similar to that in the senile plaques of Alzheimer's disease is increased in vivo by the presenilin 1 and 2 and APP mutations linked to familial Alzheimer's disease. Nat Med [Internet]. 1996;2(8):864–70 [cited 2015 Aug 4]. http://www.ncbi.nlm.nih.gov/pubmed/8705854

[25] Grundke-Iqbal I, Iqbal K, Quinlan M, Tung YC, Zaidi MS, Wisniewski HM. Microtubule-associated protein tau. A component of Alzheimer paired helical filaments. J Biol Chem [Internet]. 1986;261(13):6084–9 [cited 2016 Jan 8]. http://www.ncbi.nlm.nih.gov/pubmed/3084478

[26] Spillantini MG, Goedert M. Tau protein pathology in neurodegenerative diseases. Trends Neurosci [Internet]. 1998;21(10):428–33 [cited 2016 Jan 8]. http://www.sciencedirect.com/science/article/pii/S016622369801337X

[27] Lee VM, Goedert M, Trojanowski JQ. Neurodegenerative tauopathies. Annu Rev Neurosci [Internet].2011;24:1121–59 (Annual Reviews 4139 El Camino Way, P.O. Box 10139, Palo Alto, CA 94303-0139, USA; 2001 Jan 28 [cited 2015 Nov 22]). http://www.annualreviews.org/doi/full/10.1146/annurev.neuro.24.1.1121?url_ver=Z39.88-2003&rfr_id=ori%3Arid%3Acrossref.org&rfr_dat=cr_pub%3Dpubmed&

[28] Iwatsubo T, Odaka A, Suzuki N, Mizusawa H, Nukina N, Ihara Y. Visualization of A beta 42(43) and A beta 40 in senile plaques with end-specific A beta monoclonals: evidence that an initially deposited species is A beta 42(43). Neuron [Internet]. 1994;13(1):45–53 [cited 2015 Nov 18]. http://www.ncbi.nlm.nih.gov/pubmed/8043280

[29] Selkoe DJ. Alzheimer's disease: genes, proteins, and therapy. Physiol Rev [Internet]. 2001;81(2):741–66 [cited 2015 Dec 12]. http://www.ncbi.nlm.nih.gov/pubmed/11274343

[30] Dickson DW. The pathogenesis of senile plaques. J Neuropathol Exp Neurol [Internet]. 1997;56(4):321–39 [cited 2015 Nov 29]. http://www.ncbi.nlm.nih.gov/pubmed/9100663

[31] Nalivaeva NN, Turner AJ. The amyloid precursor protein: a biochemical enigma in brain development, function and disease. FEBS Lett [Internet]. 2013;587(13):2046–54 [cited 2016 Jan 10]. http://www.sciencedirect.com/science/article/pii/S0014579313003529

[32] Yoshikai S, Sasaki H, Doh-ura K, Furuya H, Sakaki Y. Genomic organization of the human amyloid beta-protein precursor gene. Gene [Internet]. 1990;87(2):257–63 [cited 2015 Dec 31]. http://www.ncbi.nlm.nih.gov/pubmed/2110105

[33] Zhang Y, Thompson R, Zhang H, Xu H. APP processing in Alzheimer's disease. Mol Brain [Internet]. 2011;4:3 [cited 2015 Nov 18]. http://www.pubmedcentral.nih.gov/articlerender.fcgi?artid=3022812&tool=pmcentrez&rendertype=abstract

[34] Zhou Z, Chan CH, Ma Q, Xu X, Xiao Z, Tan E. The roles of amyloid precursor protein (APP) in neurogenesis: implications to pathogenesis and therapy of Alzheimer disease. Cell Adh Migr. 2016;5(4):280–92.

[35] Musa A, Lehrach H, Russo VA. Distinct expression patterns of two zebrafish homologues of the human APP gene during embryonic development. Dev Genes Evol [Internet]. 2001;211(11):563–7 [cited 2015 Nov 18]. http://www.ncbi.nlm.nih.gov/pubmed/11862463

[36] Xiao Q, Gil S-C, Yan P, Wang Y, Han S, Gonzales E, et al. Role of phosphatidylinositol clathrin assembly lymphoid-myeloid leukemia (PICALM) in intracellular amyloid precursor protein (APP) processing and amyloid plaque pathogenesis. J Biol Chem [Internet]. 2012;287(25):21279–89 [cited 2016 Jan 10]. http://www.pubmedcentral.nih.gov/articlerender.fcgi?artid=3375549&tool=pmcentrez&rendertype=abstract

[37] Cirrito JR, Kang J-E, Lee J, Stewart FR, Verges DK, Silverio LM, et al. Endocytosis is required for synaptic activity-dependent release of amyloid-beta in vivo. Neuron [Internet]. 2008;58(1):42–51 [cited 2015 Nov 1]. http://www.pubmedcentral.nih.gov/articlerender.fcgi?artid=2390913&tool=pmcentrez&rendertype=abstract

[38] Seubert P, Vigo-Pelfrey C, Esch F, Lee M, Dovey H, Davis D, et al. Isolation and quantification of soluble Alzheimer's beta-peptide from biological fluids. Nature [Internet]. 1992;359(6393):325–7 [cited 2015 Dec 4]. http://www.ncbi.nlm.nih.gov/pubmed/1406936

[39] Querfurth HW, LaFerla FM. Alzheimer's disease. N Engl J Med [Internet]. 2010;362(4):329–44 [cited 2014 Nov 18]. http://www.ncbi.nlm.nih.gov/pubmed/20107219

[40] Selkoe DJ. Alzheimer disease: mechanistic understanding predicts novel therapies. Ann Intern Med [Internet]. 2004;140(8):627–38 [cited 2016 Jan 10]. http://www.ncbi.nlm.nih.gov/pubmed/15096334

[41] Jarrett JT, Berger EP, Lansbury PT. The carboxy terminus of the beta amyloid protein is critical for the seeding of amyloid formation: implications for the pathogenesis of Alzheimer's disease. Biochemistry [Internet]. 1993;32(18):4693–7 [cited 2015 Oct 5]. http://www.ncbi.nlm.nih.gov/pubmed/8490014

[42] Rossner S. New players in old amyloid precursor protein-processing pathways. Int J Dev Neurosci [Internet]. 2004;22(7):467–74 [cited 2016 Jan 11]. http://www.sciencedirect.com/science/article/pii/S0736574804000899

[43] Yu G, Nishimura M, Arawaka S, Levitan D, Zhang L, Tandon A, et al. Nicastrin modulates presenilin-mediated notch/glp-1 signal transduction and betaAPP processing. Nature [Internet]. 2000;407(6800):48–54 [cited 2015 Dec 9]. http://www.ncbi.nlm.nih.gov/pubmed/10993067

[44] Esler WP, Kimberly WT, Ostaszewski BL, Ye W, Diehl TS, Selkoe DJ, et al. Activity-dependent isolation of the presenilin—secretase complex reveals nicastrin and a substrate. Proc Natl Acad Sci [Internet]. 2002;99(5):2720–5 [cited 2016 Jan 11]. http://www.pubmedcentral.nih.gov/articlerender.fcgi?artid=122414&tool=pmcentrez&rendertype=abstract

[45] Francis R, McGrath G, Zhang J, Ruddy DA, Sym M, Apfeld J, et al. aph-1 and pen-2 are required for Notch pathway signaling, gamma-secretase cleavage of betaAPP, and presenilin protein accumulation. Dev Cell [Internet]. 2002;3(1):85–97 [cited 2016 Jan 11]. http://www.ncbi.nlm.nih.gov/pubmed/12110170

[46] Helm K von der, Korant BD, Cheronis JCD. Proteases as targets for therapy, Issue 146 [Internet]. Springer Science & Business Media; 2000; p. 410 [cited 2016 Jan 11]. https://books.google.com/books?id=a5_eckV79UEC&pgis=1

[47] Esposito LA. Measuring APP carboxy-terminal fragments. Methods Mol Biol [Internet]. 2011;670:71–84 [cited 2016 Jan 11]. http://www.ncbi.nlm.nih.gov/pubmed/20967584

[48] Multhaup G, Huber O, Buée L, Galas M-C. Amyloid precursor protein (APP) metabolites APP intracellular fragment (AICD), Aβ42, and Tau in nuclear roles. J Biol Chem [Internet]. 2015;290(39):23515–22 [cited 2016 Jan 11]. http://www.jbc.org/content/290/39/23515.long

[49] Makarova A, Williams SE, Strickland DK. Proteases and lipoprotein receptors in Alzheimer's disease. Cell Biochem Biophys [Internet]. 2004;41(1):139–78 [cited 2016 Jan 11]. http://www.ncbi.nlm.nih.gov/pubmed/15371644

[50] Vingtdeux V, Hamdane M, Gompel M, Bégard S, Drobecq H, Ghestem A, et al. Phosphorylation of amyloid precursor carboxy-terminal fragments enhances their processing by a gamma-secretase-dependent mechanism. Neurobiol Dis [Internet]. 2005;20(2):625–37 [cited 2016 Jan 11]. http://www.ncbi.nlm.nih.gov/pubmed/15936948

[51] Haass C, Selkoe DJ. Soluble protein oligomers in neurodegeneration: lessons from the Alzheimer's amyloid beta-peptide. Nat Rev Mol Cell Biol [Internet]. Nature Publishing Group; 2007;8(2):101–12 [cited 2014 Jul 9]. doi:10.1038/nrm2101

[52] Thinakaran G. The role of presenilins in Alzheimer's disease. J Clin Invest [Internet]. 1999;104(10):1321–7 [cited 2016 Jan 11]. http://www.pubmedcentral.nih.gov/articlerender.fcgi?artid=409849&tool=pmcentrez&rendertype=abstract

[53] Shoji M, Golde TE, Ghiso J, Cheung TT, Estus S, Shaffer LM, et al. Production of the Alzheimer amyloid β protein by normal proteolytic processing. Science (80). 1992;258(5079):126–9.

[54] Bennett DA, Schneider JA, Arvanitakis Z, Kelly JF, Aggarwal NT, Shah RC, et al. Neuropathology of older persons without cognitive impairment from two community-based studies. Neurology. 2006;66(12):1837–44.

[55] Hardy JA, Higgins GA. Alzheimer's disease: the amyloid cascade hypothesis. Science. 1992;256(5054):184–5.

[56] Reitz C. Alzheimer's disease and the amyloid cascade hypothesis: a critical review. Int J Alzheimers Dis [Internet]. 2012;2012:369808. http://www.pubmedcentral.nih.gov/articlerender.fcgi?artid=3313573&tool=pmcentrez&rendertype=abstract

[57] Mudher A, Lovestone S. Alzheimer's disease - Do tauists and baptists finally shake hands? Trends Neurosci. 2002;25(1):22–6.

[58] Chételat G. Alzheimer disease: aβ-independent processes-rethinking preclinical AD. Nat Rev Neurol [Internet]. 2013;9(3):123–4. http://www.pubmedcentral.nih.gov/articlerender.fcgi?artid=3935395&tool=pmcentrez&rendertype=abstract

[59] Klein WL, Krafft G a., Finch CE. Targeting small A β oligomers: the solution to an Alzheimer's disease conundrum? Trends Neurosci. 2001;24(4):219–24.

[60] Gilbert BJ. The role of amyloid β in the pathogenesis of Alzheimer's disease. J Clin Pathol [Internet]. 2013;66(5):362–6 [cited 2016 Jan 16]. http://www.ncbi.nlm.nih.gov/pubmed/23526599

[61] Jin M, Shepardson N, Yang T, Chen G, Walsh D, Selkoe DJ. Soluble amyloid beta-protein dimers isolated from Alzheimer cortex directly induce Tau hyperphosphorylation and neuritic degeneration. Proc Natl Acad Sci USA [Internet]. 2011;108(14):5819–24. http://www.pubmedcentral.nih.gov/articlerender.fcgi?artid=3078381&tool=pmcentrez&rendertype=abstract

[62] Jan A, Adolfsson O, Allaman I, Buccarello AL, Magistretti PJ, Pfeifer A, et al. Aβ42 neurotoxicity is mediated by ongoing nucleated polymerization process rather than by discrete Aβ42 species. J Biol Chem. 2011;286(10):8585–96.

[63] Puzzo D, Arancio O. Amyloid-β peptide: Dr. Jekyll or Mr. Hyde? J Alzheimers Dis [Internet]. 2013;33 Suppl 1:S111–20 [cited 2016 Jan 30]. http://www.pubmedcentral.nih.gov/articlerender.fcgi?artid=3696497&tool=pmcentrez&rendertype=abstract

[64] Robinson SR, Bishop GM. Aβ as a bioflocculant: implications for the amyloid hypothesis of Alzheimer's disease. Neurobiol Aging [Internet] (Elsevier). 2002;23(6):1051–72 [cited 2016 Jan 30]. http://www.neurobiologyofaging.org/article/S0197458001003426/fulltext

[65] Lee H, Zhu X, Castellani RJ, Nunomura A, Perry G, Smith MA. Amyloid-beta in Alzheimer disease: the null versus the alternate hypotheses. J Pharmacol Exp Ther [Internet]. 2007;321(3):823–9. http://www.ncbi.nlm.nih.gov/pubmed/17229880

[66] Maccioni RB, Farías G, Morales I, Navarrete L. The revitalized tau hypothesis on Alzheimer's disease. Arch Med Res [Internet]. 2010;41(3):226–31. http://www.sciencedirect.com/science/article/pii/S0188440910000500

[67] Nagy Z, Esiri MM, Jobst KA, Morris JH, King EM, McDonald B, et al. Relative roles of plaques and tangles in the dementia of Alzheimer's disease: correlations using three sets of neuropathological criteria. Dementia. 1995;6(1):21–31.

[68] Goedert M, Jakes R. Mutations causing neurodegenerative tauopathies. Biochim Biophys Acta Mol Basis Dis. 2005;1739(2):240–50.

[69] Hashiguchi M, Hashiguchi T. Kinase-Kinase interaction and modulation of Tau phosphorylation. Int Rev Cell Mol Biol. 2013;300:121–60.

[70] Hooper C, Killick R, Lovestone S. The GSK3 hypothesis of Alzheimer's disease. J Neurochem. 2008;104(6):1433–9.

[71] Hernández F, Borrell J, Guaza C, Avila J, Lucas JJ. Spatial learning deficit in transgenic mice that conditionally over-express GSK-3β in the brain but do not form tau filaments. J Neurochem. 2002;83:1529–33.

[72] DaRocha-Souto B, Coma M, Pérez-Nievas BG, Scotton TC, Siao M, Sánchez-Ferrer P, et al. Activation of glycogen synthase kinase-3 beta mediates β-amyloid induced neuritic damage in Alzheimer's disease. Neurobiol Dis [Internet]. 2012;45(1):425–37. doi: 10.1016/j.nbd.2011.09.002

[73] Hernández F, Gómez de Barreda E, Fuster-Matanzo A, Lucas JJ, Avila J. GSK3: a possible link between beta amyloid peptide and tau protein. Exp Neurol [Internet]. 2010;223(2):322–5. doi: 10.1016/j.expneurol.2009.09.011

[74] Hoshi M, Takashima a, Noguchi K, Murayama M, Sato M, Kondo S, et al. Regulation of mitochondrial pyruvate dehydrogenase activity by tau protein kinase I/glycogen synthase kinase 3beta in brain. Proc Natl Acad Sci USA. 1996;93(7):2719–23.

[75] Hetman M, Cavanaugh JE, Kimelman D, Xia Z. Role of glycogen synthase kinase-3beta in neuronal apoptosis induced by trophic withdrawal. J Neurosci. 2000;20(7):2567–74.

[76] Lucas JJ, Hernández F, Gómez-Ramos P, Morán MA, Hen R, Avila J. Decreased nuclear beta-catenin, tau hyperphosphorylation and neurodegeneration in GSK-3beta conditional transgenic mice. EMBO J [Internet]. 2001;20(1–2):27–39. http://www.pubmedcentral.nih.gov/articlerender.fcgi?artid=140191&tool=pmcentrez&rendertype=abstract

[77] Takashima A, Noguchi K, Michel G, Mercken M, Hoshi M, Ishiguro K, et al. Exposure of rat hippocampal neurons to amyloid◎?? peptide (25-35) induces the inactivation of phosphatidyl inositol-3 kinase and the activation of tau protein kinase I/glycogen synthase kinase-3?? Neurosci Lett. 1996;203:33–6.

[78] Lei P, Ayton S, Bush AI, Adlard P a. GSK-3 in Neurodegenerative Diseases. Int J Alzheimers Dis. 2011;2011:189246.

[79] Padurariu M, Ciobica A, Lefter R, Serban IL, Stefanescu C, Chirita R. The oxidative stress hypothesis in Alzheimer's disease. Psychiatr Danub [Internet]. 2013;25(4):401–9. http://www.ncbi.nlm.nih.gov/pubmed/24247053

[80] Markesbery WR. Oxidative stress hypothesis in Alzheimer's disease. Free Radic Biol Med. 1997;23(1):134–47.

[81] Graham SF, Nasaruddin M Bin, Carey M, Holscher C, McGuinness B, Kehoe PG, et al. Age-associated changes of brain copper, iron, and zinc in Alzheimer's disease and dementia with Lewy bodies. J Alzheimers Dis [Internet]. 2014;42(4):1407–13. http://content.iospress.com/articles/journal-of-alzheimers-disease/jad140684

[82] Deibel MA, Ehmann WD, Markesbery WR. Copper, iron, and zinc imbalances in severely degenerated brain regions in Alzheimer's disease: possible relation to oxidative stress. J Neurol Sci. 1996;143(606):137–42.

[83] Schrag M, Mueller C, Oyoyo U, Smith M a., Kirsch WM. Iron, zinc and copper in the Alzheimer's disease brain: a quantitative meta-analysis. Some insight on the influence of citation bias on scientific opinion. Prog Neurobiol [Internet]. 2011;94(3):296–306. doi: 10.1016/j.pneurobio.2011.05.001

[84] Tiiman A, Palumaa P, Tõugu V. The missing link in the amyloid cascade of Alzheimer's disease-Metal ions. Neurochem Int [Internet]. 2013;62(4):367–78. doi:10.1016/j.neuint.2013.01.023

[85] Mold M, Ouro-Gnao L, Wieckowski BM, Exley C. Copper prevents amyloid-β(1-42) from forming amyloid fibrils under near-physiological conditions in vitro. Sci Rep. 2013;3(Ii):1256.

[86] Mayes J, Tinker-Mill C, Kolosov O, Zhang H, Tabner BJ, Allsop D. Amyloid fibrils in alzheimer disease are not inert when bound to copper ions but can degrade hydrogen peroxide and generate reactive oxygen species. J Biol Chem. 2014;289(17):12052–62.

[87] Swerdlow RH, Khan SM. A "mitochondrial cascade hypothesis" for sporadic Alzheimer's disease. Med Hypotheses. 2004;63(1):8–20.

[88] Grimm A, Friedland K, Eckert A. Mitochondrial dysfunction: the missing link between aging and sporadic Alzheimer's disease. Biogerontology [Internet]. 2015 [cited 2015 Oct 16]. http://www.ncbi.nlm.nih.gov/pubmed/26468143

[89] Russell H. Swerdlow SMK. The Alzheimer's Disease mitochondrial cascade hypothesis: an update. Exp Neurol. 2009;218(2):308–15.

[90] Perry E, Perry R, Blessed G, Tomlinson B. Necropsy evidence of central cholinergic deficits in senile dementia. Lancet [Internet]. 1977;309(8004):189 [cited 2016 Jan 15]. http://www.sciencedirect.com/science/article/pii/S0140673677917809

[91] Pinto T, Lanctôt KL, Herrmann N. Revisiting the cholinergic hypothesis of behavioral and psychological symptoms in dementia of the Alzheimer's type. Ageing Res Rev [Internet]. 2011;10(4):404–12. doi:10.1016/j.arr.2011.01.003

[92] Coyle JT, Price DL, DeLong MR. Alzheimer's disease: a disorder of cortical cholinergic innervation. Science. 1983;219(4589):1184–90.

[93] Pákáski M, Kálmán J. Interactions between the amyloid and cholinergic mechanisms in Alzheimer's disease. Neurochem Int. 2008;53(3):103–11.

[94] Gilmor ML, Erickson JD, Varoqui H, Hersh LB, Bennett DA, Cochran EJ, et al. Preservation of nucleus basalis neurons containing choline acetyltransferase and the vesicular acetylcholine transporter in the elderly with mild cognitive impairment and early Alzheimer's disease. J Comp Neurol [Internet]. 1999;411(4):693–704. http://www.ncbi.nlm.nih.gov/pubmed/10421878

[95] DeKosky ST, Ikonomovic MD, Styren SD, Beckett L, Wisniewski S, Bennett DA, et al. Upregulation of choline acetyltransferase activity in hippocampus and frontal cortex of elderly subjects with mild cognitive impairment. Ann Neurol [Internet]. 2002;51(2): 145–55. http://www.ncbi.nlm.nih.gov/pubmed/11835370

[96] Di Santo SG, Prinelli F, Adorni F, Caltagirone C, Musicco M. A meta-analysis of the efficacy of donepezil, rivastigmine, galantamine, and memantine in relation to severity of Alzheimer's disease. J Alzheimer's Dis. 2013;35(2):349–61.

[97] Craig L a., Hong NS, McDonald RJ. Revisiting the cholinergic hypothesis in the development of Alzheimer's disease. Neurosci Biobehav Rev [Internet]. 2011;35(6): 1397–409. doi:10.1016/j.neubiorev.2011.03.001

[98] Khachaturian ZS. Calcium, membranes, aging, and Alzheimer's disease. Introduction and overview. Ann N Y Acad Sci [Internet]. 1989;568:1–4 [cited 2016 Jan 16]. http://www.ncbi.nlm.nih.gov/pubmed/2629579

[99] Berridge MJ. Calcium signalling and Alzheimer's disease. Neurochem Res. 2011;36(7): 1149–56.

[100] LaFerla FM. Calcium dyshomeostasis and intracellular signalling in Alzheimer's disease. Nat Rev Neurosci. 2002;3(11):862–72.

[101] Pierrot N, Ghisdal P, Caumont A-S, Octave J-N. Intraneuronal amyloid-beta1-42 production triggered by sustained increase of cytosolic calcium concentration induces neuronal death. J Neurochem. 2004;88(5):1140–50.

[102] Mattson MP, Cheng B, Davis D, Bryant K, Lieberburg I, Rydel RE. beta-Amyloid peptides destabilize calcium homeostasis and render human cortical neurons vulnerable to excitotoxicity. J Neurosci. 1992;12(2):376–89.

[103] Pierrot N, Santos SF, Feyt C, Morel M, Brion JP, Octave JN. Calcium-mediated transient phosphorylation of tau and amyloid precursor protein followed by intraneuronal amyloid-β accumulation. J Biol Chem. 2006;281(52):39907–14.

[104] Glabe CG. Common mechanisms of amyloid oligomer pathogenesis in degenerative disease. Neurobiol Aging. 2006;27(4):570–5.

[105] Strimbu K, Tavel JA. What are biomarkers? Curr Opin HIV AIDS [Internet]. 2010;5(6): 463–6. http://www.pubmedcentral.nih.gov/articlerender.fcgi?artid=3078627&tool=pmcentrez&rendertype=abstract

[106] Rosén C, Hansson O, Blennow K, Zetterberg H. Fluid biomarkers in Alzheimer's disease—current concepts. Mol Neurodegener [Internet]. 2013;8(1):20. http://www.molecularneurodegeneration.com/content/8/1/20

[107] Hansson O, Zetterberg H, Buchhave P, Londos E, Blennow K, Minthon L. Association between CSF biomarkers and incipient Alzheimer's disease in patients with mild cognitive impairment: a follow-up study. Lancet Neurol. 2006;5(3):228–34.

[108] Andreasson U, Lautner R, Schott JM, Mattsson N, Hansson O, Herukka S-K, et al. CSF biomarkers for Alzheimer's pathology and the effect size of APOE ◎4. Mol Psychiatry [Internet]. 2014;19(2):148–9 [cited 2016 Jan 17]. http://www.pubmedcentral.nih.gov/articlerender.fcgi?artid=3903112&tool=pmcentrez&rendertype=abstract

[109] Ringman JM, Younkin SG, Pratico D, Seltzer W, Cole GM, Geschwind DH, et al. Biochemical markers in persons with preclinical familial Alzheimer disease. Neurology. 2008;71(2):85–92.

[110] Graff-Radford NR, Crook JE, Lucas J, Boeve BF, Knopman DS, Ivnik RJ, et al. Association of low plasma Abeta42/Abeta40 ratios with increased imminent risk for mild cognitive impairment and Alzheimer disease. Arch Neurol [Internet]. 2007;64(3):354–62. http://archneur.jamanetwork.com/article.aspx?articleid=793567

[111] Verheijen JH, Huisman LGM, van Lent N, Neumann U, Paganetti P, Hack CE, et al. Detection of a soluble form of BACE-1 in human cerebrospinal fluid by a sensitive activity assay. Clin Chem [Internet]. 2006;52(6):1168–74. http://www.ncbi.nlm.nih.gov/pubmed/16614000

[112] Perneczky R, Tsolakidou a., Arnold a., Diehl-Schmid J, Grimmer T, Förstl H, et al. CSF soluble amyloid precursor proteins in the diagnosis of incipient Alzheimer disease. Neurology. 2011;77(1):35–8.

[113] Lopez-Font I, Cuchillo-Ibañez I, Sogorb-Esteve A, García-Ayllón M-S, Sáez-Valero J. Transmembrane amyloid-related proteins in CSF as potential biomarkers for Alzheimer's disease. Front Neurol [Internet]. 2015;6(June):125. http://www.pubmedcentral.nih.gov/articlerender.fcgi?artid=4451586&tool=pmcentrez&rendertype=abstract

[114] Ribeiro CA, Santana I, Oliveira C, Baldeiras I, Moreira J, Saraiva MJ, et al. Transthyretin decrease in plasma of MCI and AD patients: investigation of mechanisms for disease

modulation. Curr Alzheimer Res [Internet]. 2012;9(8):881–9. http://www.ncbi.nlm.nih.gov/pubmed/22698061

[115] Gloeckner SF, Meyne F, Wagner F, Heinemann U, Krasnianski A, Meissner B, et al. Quantitative analysis of transthyretin, tau and amyloid-beta in patients with dementia. J Alzheimers Dis [Internet]. 2008;14(1):17–25 [cited 2016 Jan 5]. http://www.ncbi.nlm.nih.gov/pubmed/18525124

[116] Fagan AM, Perrin RJ. Upcoming candidate cerebrospinal fluid biomarkers of Alzheimer's disease. Biomark Med [Internet]. 2012;6(4):455–76. http://www.ncbi.nlm.nih.gov/pubmed/22917147

[117] Petersen RC, Jack Jr. CR. Imaging and biomarkers in early Alzheimer's disease and mild cognitive impairment. Clin Pharmacol Ther [Internet]. 2009;86(4):438–41. http://www.nature.com/clpt/journal/v86/n4/pdf/clpt2009166a.pdf

[118] Klunk WE, Engler H, Nordberg A, Wang Y, Blomqvist G, Holt DP, et al. Imaging brain amyloid in Alzheimer's disease with Pittsburgh compound-B. Ann Neurol. 2004;55(3):306–19.

[119] Trzepacz PT, Yu P, Sun J, Schuh K, Case M, Witte MM, et al. Comparison of neuroimaging modalities for the prediction of conversion from mild cognitive impairment to alzheimer's dementia. Neurobiol Aging. 2014;35(1):143–51.

[120] Castellani RJ, Rolston RK, Smith MA. Alzheimer disease. Dis Mon [Internet]. 2010;56(9):484–546 [cited 2015 Dec 11]. http://www.pubmedcentral.nih.gov/articlerender.fcgi?artid=2941917&tool=pmcentrez&rendertype=abstract

[121] Brys M, Glodzik L, Mosconi L, Switalski R, De Santi S, Pirraglia E, et al. Magnetic resonance imaging improves cerebrospinal fluid biomarkers in the early detection of Alzheimer's disease. J Alzheimer's Dis. 2009;16(2):351–62.

[122] Herrup K. Reimagining Alzheimer's disease—an age-based hypothesis. J Neurosci [Internet]. 2010;30(50):16755–62. http://www.pubmedcentral.nih.gov/articlerender.fcgi?artid=3004746&tool=pmcentrez&rendertype=abstract

[123] Viña J, Lloret A. Why women have more Alzheimer's disease than men: gender and mitochondrial toxicity of amyloid-beta peptide. J Alzheimers Dis [Internet]. 2010;20 Suppl 2(S2):S527–33. http://content.iospress.com/articles/journal-of-alzheimers-disease/jad100501?resultNumber=0&totalResults=105&start=0&q=Why+women+have+more+Alzheimer%27s+disease+than+men%3A+gender+and+mitochondrial+toxicity+of+amyloid-beta+peptid&resultsPageSize=10&rows=1

[124] Li R, Singh M. Sex differences in cognitive impairment and Alzheimer's disease. Front Neuroendocrinol [Internet]. 2014;35(3):385–403. doi:10.1016/j.yfrne.2014.01.002

[125] Arvanitakis Z, Wilson RS, Bienias JL, Evans D a, Bennett D a. Diabetes mellitus and risk of Alzheimer disease and decline in cognitive function. Arch Neurol. 2004;61(5):661–6.

[126] Vuorinen M, Solomon A, Rovio S, Nieminen L, Kåreholt I, Tuomilehto J, et al. Changes in vascular risk factors from midlife to late life and white matter lesions: a 20-year follow-up study. Dement Geriatr Cogn Disord. 2011;31(2):119–25.

[127] Imtiaz B, Tolppanen A-M, Kivipelto M, Soininen H. Future directions in Alzheimer's disease from risk factors to prevention. Biochem Pharmacol [Internet]. 2014;88(4):661–70. http://www.ncbi.nlm.nih.gov/pubmed/24418410

[128] Shepardson NE, Shankar GM, Selkoe DJ. Cholesterol level and statin use in Alzheimer disease: II. Review of human trials and recommendations. Arch Neurol [Internet]. 2011;68(11):1385–92. http://eutils.ncbi.nlm.nih.gov/entrez/eutils/elink.fcgi?dbfrom=pubmed&id=22084122&retmode=ref&cmd=prlinks\npapers3://publication/doi/10.1001/archneurol.2011.242

[129] Lindsay J, Laurin D, Verreault R, Hébert R, Helliwell B, Hill GB, et al. Risk factors for Alzheimer's disease: a prospective analysis from the Canadian Study of Health and Aging. Am J Epidemiol. 2002;156(5):445–53.

[130] Corder EH, Saunders a M, Strittmatter WJ, Schmechel DE, Gaskell PC, Small GW, et al. Gene dose of apolipoprotein E type 4 allele and the risk of Alzheimer's disease in late onset families. Science. 1993;261(5123):921–3.

[131] Tanzi RE, Bertram L. Twenty years of the Alzheimer's disease amyloid hypothesis: a genetic perspective. Cell. 2005;120(4):545–55.

[132] Rinne JO, Brooks DJ, Rossor MN, Fox NC, Bullock R, Klunk WE, et al. 11C-PiB PET assessment of change in fibrillar amyloid-beta load in patients with Alzheimer's disease treated with bapineuzumab: a phase 2, double-blind, placebo-controlled, ascending-dose study. Lancet Neurol [Internet]. 2010;9(4):363–72 [cited 2015 Aug 12]. http://www.ncbi.nlm.nih.gov/pubmed/20189881

[133] Gandy S, DeKosky ST. Toward the treatment and prevention of Alzheimer's disease: rational strategies and recent progress. Annu Rev Med [Internet]. 2013;64:367–83. http://www.pubmedcentral.nih.gov/articlerender.fcgi?artid=3625402&tool=pmcentrez&rendertype=abstract

[134] Watt AD, Crespi GAN, Down RA, Ascher DB, Gunn A, Perez KA, et al. Do current therapeutic anti-Aβ antibodies for Alzheimer's disease engage the target? Acta Neuropathol. 2014;127(6):803–10.

[135] Gong B, Pan Y, Zhao W, Knable L, Vempati P, Begum S, et al. IVIG immunotherapy protects against synaptic dysfunction in Alzheimer's disease through complement anaphylatoxin C5a-mediated AMPA-CREB-C/EBP signaling pathway. Mol Immunol. 2013;56(4):619–29.

[136] Laxton AW, Tang-Wai DF, McAndrews MP, Zumsteg D, Wennberg R, Keren R, et al. A phase I trial of deep brain stimulation of memory circuits in Alzheimer's disease.

Ann Neurol [Internet]. 2010;68(4):521–34 [cited 2016 Jan 18]. http://www.ncbi.nlm.nih.gov/pubmed/20687206

[137] Laxton AW, Lozano AM. Deep brain stimulation for the treatment of alzheimer disease and dementias. World Neurosurg [Internet]. 2013;80(3–4):S28.e1–S28.e8. doi: 10.1016/j.wneu.2012.06.028

[138] Zlokovic BV. The blood-brain barrier in health and chronic neurodegenerative disorders. Neuron [Internet]. 2008;57(2):178–201 [cited 2015 Jul 15]. http://www.ncbi.nlm.nih.gov/pubmed/18215617

[139] Ehrlich P. Das sauerstufbudurfnis des organismus. Eine Farbenanalytische Stud. 1885

[140] Goldmann E. Vitalfarbung am zentralnervensystem. Abh Preuss Akd Wiss Phys Math. 1913;1(1):1–13.

[141] Lewandowsky M. Zur lehre von der cerebrospinalflussigkeit. Z Klin Med. 1900;40:480–94.

[142] Hawkins BT, Davis TP. The blood-brain barrier/neurovascular unit in health and disease. Pharmacol Rev [Internet]. 2005;57(2):173–85. http://www.ncbi.nlm.nih.gov/pubmed/15914466

[143] Brightman MW, Reese TS. Junctions between intimately apposed cell membranes in the vertebrate brain. J Cell Biol. 1969;40(3):648–77.

[144] Reese TS, Karnovsky MJ. Fine structural localization of a blood-brain barrier to exogenous peroxidase. J Cell Biol [Internet]. 1967;34(1):207–17. http://www.pubmedcentral.nih.gov/articlerender.fcgi?artid=2107213&tool=pmcentrez&rendertype=abstract

[145] Bates KA, Verdile G, Li Q-X, Ames D, Hudson P, Masters CL, et al. Clearance mechanisms of Alzheimer's amyloid-beta peptide: implications for therapeutic design and diagnostic tests. Mol Psychiatry [Internet]. Nature Publishing Group; 2009;14(5):469–86 [cited 2015 Dec 28]. doi: 10.1038/mp.2008.96

[146] Pardridge WM. Molecular biology of the blood-brain barrier. Mol Biotechnol [Internet]. 2005;30(1):57–70. http://www.ncbi.nlm.nih.gov/pubmed/15805577

[147] Oldendorf WH, Cornford ME, Brown WJ. The large apparent work capability of the blood-brain barrier: a study of the mitochondrial content of capillary endothelial cells in brain and other tissues of the rat. Ann Neurol [Internet]. 1977;1(5):409–17 [cited 2015 Dec 1]. http://www.ncbi.nlm.nih.gov/pubmed/617259

[148] Fenstermacher J, Gross P, Sposito N, Acuff V, Pettersen S, Gruber K. Structural and functional variations in capillary systems within the brain. Ann N Y Acad Sci. 1988;529:21–30.

[149] Sedlakova R, Shivers RR, Del Maestro RF. Ultrastructure of the blood-brain barrier in the rabbit. J Submicrosc Cytol Pathol. 1999;31:149–61.

[150] Kniesel U, Wolburg H. Tight junctions of the blood-brain barrier. Cell Mol Neurobiol. 2000;20(1):57–76.

[151] Ohtsuki S, Terasaki T. Contribution of carrier-mediated transport systems to the blood-brain barrier as a supporting and protecting interface for the brain; importance for CNS drug discovery and development. Pharm Res. 2007;24(9):1745–58.

[152] Tagami M, Nara Y, Kubota A, Fujino H, Yamori Y. Ultrastructural changes in cerebral pericytes and astrocytes of stroke-prone spontaneously hypertensive rats. Stroke. 1990;21:1064–71.

[153] Farkas E, Luiten PGM. Cerebral microvascular pathology in aging and Alzheimer's disease. Vol. 64, Progress in Neurobiology. 2001. 575-611 p.

[154] Ramsauer M, Krause D, Dermietzel R. Angiogenesis of the blood-brain barrier in vitro and the function of cerebral pericytes. FASEB J. 2002;16(10):1274–6.

[155] Gonul E, Duz B, Kahraman S, Kayali H, Kubar A, Timurkaynak E. Early pericyte response to brain hypoxia in cats: an ultrastructural study. Microvasc Res [Internet]. 2002;64(1):116–9. http://www.ncbi.nlm.nih.gov/pubmed/12074637

[156] Dore-Duffy P, Owen C, Balabanov R, Murphy S, Beaumont T, Rafols JA. Pericyte migration from the vascular wall in response to traumatic brain injury. Microvasc Res [Internet]. 2000;60(1):55–69. http://www.ncbi.nlm.nih.gov/pubmed/10873515

[157] Hori S, Ohtsuki S, Hosoya K, Nakashima E, Terasaki T. A pericyte-derived angiopoietin-1 multimeric complex induces occludin gene expression in brain capillary endothelial cells through Tie-2 activation in vitro. J Neurochem [Internet]. 2004;89(2):503–13. http://www.ncbi.nlm.nih.gov/pubmed/15056293

[158] Davson H, Oldendorf WH. Symposium on membrane transport. Transport in the central nervous system. Proc R Soc Med [Internet]. 1967;60(4):326–9 [cited 2016 Jan 12]. http://www.pubmedcentral.nih.gov/articlerender.fcgi?artid=1901728&tool=pmcentrez&rendertype=abstract

[159] Tao-Cheng JH, Nagy Z, Brightman MW. Tight junctions of brain endothelium in vitro are enhanced by astroglia. J Neurosci [Internet]. 1987;7(10):3293–9 [cited 2016 Jan 12]. http://www.ncbi.nlm.nih.gov/pubmed/3668629

[160] Maxwell K, Berliner JA, Cancilla PA. Induction of gamma-glutamyl transpeptidase in cultured cerebral endothelial cells by a product released by astrocytes. Brain Res [Internet]. 1987;410(2):309–14 [cited 2016 Jan 12]. http://www.ncbi.nlm.nih.gov/pubmed/2885071

[161] Ballabh P, Braun A, Nedergaard M. The blood-brain barrier: an overview: structure, regulation, and clinical implications. Neurobiol Dis [Internet]. 2004;16(1):1–13 [cited 2014 Jul 11]. http://www.ncbi.nlm.nih.gov/pubmed/15207256

[162] Braet K, Paemeleire K, D'Herde K, Sanderson MJ, Leybaert L. Astrocyte-endothelial cell calcium signals conveyed by two signalling pathways. Eur J Neurosci. 2001;13(1): 79–91.

[163] Zonta M, Angulo MC, Gobbo S, Rosengarten B, Hossmann K-A, Pozzan T, et al. Neuron-to-astrocyte signaling is central to the dynamic control of brain microcirculation. Nat Neurosci [Internet]. 2003;6(1):43–50 [cited 2016 Jan 12]. http://www.ncbi.nlm.nih.gov/pubmed/12469126

[164] Anderson CM, Nedergaard M. Astrocyte-mediated control of cerebral microcirculation. Trends Neurosci [Internet]. 2003;26(7):340–4 [cited 2016 Jan 12] (author reply 344–5). http://www.ncbi.nlm.nih.gov/pubmed/12850427

[165] Alliot F, Godin I, Pessac B. Microglia derive from progenitors, originating from the yolk sac, and which proliferate in the brain. Brain Res Dev Brain Res [Internet]. 1999;117(2): 145–52 [cited 2015 Dec 20]. http://www.ncbi.nlm.nih.gov/pubmed/10567732

[166] Hickey WF, Kimura H. Perivascular microglial cells of the CNS are bone marrow-derived and present antigen in vivo. Science [Internet]. 1988;239(4837):290–2 [cited 2015 Dec 20]. http://www.ncbi.nlm.nih.gov/pubmed/3276004

[167] Fantin A, Vieira JM, Gestri G, Denti L, Schwarz Q, Prykhozhij S, et al. Tissue macrophages act as cellular chaperones for vascular anastomosis downstream of VEGF-mediated endothelial tip cell induction. Blood [Internet]. 2010;116(5):829–40 [cited 2015 Dec 8]. http://www.pubmedcentral.nih.gov/articlerender.fcgi?artid=2938310&tool=pmcentrez&rendertype=abstract

[168] Nayak D, Roth TL, McGavern DB. Microglia development and function. Annu Rev Immunol [Internet]. 2014;32:367–402 [cited 2015 Nov 24]. http://www.ncbi.nlm.nih.gov/pubmed/24471431

[169] Espinosa-Heidmann DG, Suner IJ, Hernandez EP, Monroy D, Csaky KG, Cousins SW. Macrophage depletion diminishes lesion size and severity in experimental choroidal neovascularization. Invest Ophthalmol Vis Sci [Internet]. 2003;44(8):3586–92 [cited 2016 Jan 13]. http://www.ncbi.nlm.nih.gov/pubmed/12882811

[170] Sumi N, Nishioku T, Takata F, Matsumoto J, Watanabe T, Shuto H, et al. Lipopolysaccharide-activated microglia induce dysfunction of the blood-brain barrier in rat microvascular endothelial cells co-cultured with microglia. Cell Mol Neurobiol [Internet]. 2010;30(2):247–53 [cited 2016 Jan 13]. http://www.ncbi.nlm.nih.gov/pubmed/19728078

[171] Nishioku T, Matsumoto J, Dohgu S, Sumi N, Miyao K, Takata F, et al. Tumor necrosis factor-alpha mediates the blood-brain barrier dysfunction induced by activated microglia in mouse brain microvascular endothelial cells. J Pharmacol Sci [Internet]. 2010;112(2):251–4 [cited 2016 Jan 13]. http://www.ncbi.nlm.nih.gov/pubmed/20118615

[172] Obermeier B, Daneman R, Ransohoff RM. Development, maintenance and disruption of the blood-brain barrier. Nat Med [Internet]. 2013;19(12):1584–96 [cited 2014 Jul 10].

http://www.pubmedcentral.nih.gov/articlerender.fcgi?artid=4080800&tool=pmcentrez&rendertype=abstract

[173] Bolton SJ, Anthony DC, Perry VH. Loss of the tight junction proteins occludin and zonula occludens-1 from cerebral vascular endothelium during neutrophil-induced blood-brain barrier breakdown in vivo. Neuroscience [Internet]. 1998;86(4):1245–57 [cited 2016 Jan 13]. http://www.ncbi.nlm.nih.gov/pubmed/9697130

[174] da Fonseca ACC, Matias D, Garcia C, Amaral R, Geraldo LH, Freitas C, et al. The impact of microglial activation on blood-brain barrier in brain diseases. Front Cell Neurosci [Internet]. 2014;8:362 [cited 2016 Jan 13]. http://www.pubmedcentral.nih.gov/articlerender.fcgi?artid=4217497&tool=pmcentrez&rendertype=abstract

[175] Bazzoni G, Dejana E. Endothelial cell-to-cell junctions: molecular organization and role in vascular homeostasis. Physiol Rev [Internet]. 2004;84(3):869–901 [cited 2015 Aug 6]. http://www.ncbi.nlm.nih.gov/pubmed/15269339

[176] Furuse M, Hirase T, Itoh M, Nagafuchi A, Yonemura S, Tsukita S. Occludin: a novel integral membrane protein localizing at tight junctions. J Cell Biol [Internet]. 1993;123(6 Pt 2):1777–88 [cited 2015 Mar 19]. http://www.pubmedcentral.nih.gov/articlerender.fcgi?artid=2290891&tool=pmcentrez&rendertype=abstract

[177] Lippoldt A, Kniesel U, Liebner S, Kalbacher H, Kirsch T, Wolburg H, et al. Structural alterations of tight junctions are associated with loss of polarity in stroke-prone spontaneously hypertensive rat blood-brain barrier endothelial cells. Brain Res [Internet]. 2000;885(2):251–61 [cited 2016 Jan 13]. http://www.ncbi.nlm.nih.gov/pubmed/11102579

[178] Hawkins BT, Abbruscato TJ, Egleton RD, Brown RC, Huber JD, Campos CR, et al. Nicotine increases in vivo blood-brain barrier permeability and alters cerebral microvascular tight junction protein distribution. Brain Res [Internet]. 2004;1027(1–2):48–58 [cited 2015 Dec 22]. http://www.ncbi.nlm.nih.gov/pubmed/15494156

[179] Hirase T, Staddon JM, Saitou M, Ando-Akatsuka Y, Itoh M, Furuse M, et al. Occludin as a possible determinant of tight junction permeability in endothelial cells. J Cell Sci [Internet]. 1997;110(Pt 1):1603–13 [cited 2016 Jan 13]. http://www.ncbi.nlm.nih.gov/pubmed/9247194

[180] Bamforth SD, Kniesel U, Wolburg H, Engelhardt B, Risau W. A dominant mutant of occludin disrupts tight junction structure and function. J Cell Sci [Internet]. 1999;112(Pt 1):1879–88. http://www.ncbi.nlm.nih.gov/pubmed/10341207

[181] Saitou M, Furuse M, Sasaki H, Schulzke JD, Fromm M, Takano H, et al. Complex phenotype of mice lacking occludin, a component of tight junction strands. Mol Biol Cell. 2000;11(12):4131–42.

[182] Schulzke JD, Gitter a. H, Mankertz J, Spiegel S, Seidler U, Amasheh S, et al. Epithelial transport and barrier function in occludin-deficient mice. Biochim Biophys Acta Biomembr. 2005;1669(1):34–42.

[183] Murata M, Kojima T, Yamamoto T, Go M, Takano KI, Osanai M, et al. Down-regulation of survival signaling through MAPK and Akt in occludin-deficient mouse hepatocytes in vitro. Exp Cell Res. 2005;310:140–51.

[184] Morgan L, Shah B, Rivers LE, Barden L, Groom AJ, Chung R, et al. Inflammation and dephosphorylation of the tight junction protein occludin in an experimental model of multiple sclerosis. Neuroscience [Internet]. 2007;147(3):664–73. http://www.sciencedirect.com/science/article/pii/S030645220700468X

[185] Rosenberg GA, Yang Y. Vasogenic edema due to tight junction disruption by matrix metalloproteinases in cerebral ischemia. Neurosurg Focus [Internet]. 2007;22(5):E4 [cited 2016 Jan 14]. http://www.ncbi.nlm.nih.gov/pubmed/17613235

[186] Piontek J, Winkler L, Wolburg H, Müller SL, Zuleger N, Piehl C, et al. Formation of tight junction: determinants of homophilic interaction between classic claudins. FASEB J. 2008;22(1):146–58.

[187] Rolf Dermietzel, David C. Spray MN, editor. Blood-brain barriers: from ontogeny to artificial interfaces, vol 1. Wiley Online Library. Wiley-VCH Verlag GmbH & Co. KGaA; 2007. 741 p.

[188] Nitta T, Hata M, Gotoh S, Seo Y, Sasaki H, Hashimoto N, et al. Size-selective loosening of the blood-brain barrier in claudin-5-deficient mice. J Cell Biol [Internet]. 2003;161(3): 653–60. http://jcb.rupress.org/content/161/3/653.long

[189] Kubota K, Furuse M, Sasaki H, Sonoda N, Fujita K, Nagafuchi A, et al. Ca(2+)-independent cell-adhesion activity of claudins, a family of integral membrane proteins localized at tight junctions. Curr Biol [Internet]. 1999;9(18):1035–8 [cited 2016 Jan 14]. http://www.ncbi.nlm.nih.gov/pubmed/10508613

[190] Jia W, Martin TA, Zhang G, Jiang WG. Junctional adhesion molecules in cerebral endothelial tight junction and brain metastasis. Anticancer Res [Internet]. 2013;33(6): 2353–9 [cited 2016 Jan 14]. http://www.ncbi.nlm.nih.gov/pubmed/23749882

[191] Martìn-Padura I, Lostaglio S, Schneemann M, Williams L, Romano M, Fruscella P, et al. Junctional adhesion molecule, a novel member of the immunoglobulin superfamily that distributes at intercellular junctions and modulates monocyte transmigration. J Cell Biol [Internet]. 1998;142(1):117–27 [cited 2016 Jan 14]. http://www.pubmedcentral.nih.gov/articlerender.fcgi?artid=2133024&tool=pmcentrez&rendertype=abstract

[192] Dejana E, Lampugnani MG, Martinez-Estrada O, Bazzoni G. The molecular organization of endothelial junctions and their functional role in vascular morphogenesis and permeability. Int J Dev Biol [Internet]. 2000;44(6):743–8 [cited 2016 Jan 14]. http://www.ncbi.nlm.nih.gov/pubmed/11061439

[193] Yeung D, Manias JL, Stewart DJ, Nag S. Decreased junctional adhesion molecule-A expression during blood-brain barrier breakdown. Acta Neuropathol [Internet]. 2008;115(6):635–42 [cited 2016 Jan 14]. http://www.ncbi.nlm.nih.gov/pubmed/18357461

[194] Vincent PA, Xiao K, Buckley KM, Kowalczyk AP. VE-cadherin: adhesion at arm's length. Am J Physiol Cell Physiol [Internet]. 2004;286(5):C987–97 [cited 2016 Jan 14]. http://www.ncbi.nlm.nih.gov/pubmed/15075197

[195] Lampugnani MG, Dejana E. Adherens junctions in endothelial cells regulate vessel maintenance and angiogenesis. Thromb Res [Internet]. 2007;120 Suppl :S1–6 [cited 2016 Jan 14]. http://www.ncbi.nlm.nih.gov/pubmed/18023702

[196] Abbruscato TJ, Davis TP. Protein expression of brain endothelial cell E-cadherin after hypoxia/aglycemia: influence of astrocyte contact. Brain Res [Internet]. 1999;842(2): 277–86 [cited 2016 Jan 14]. http://www.ncbi.nlm.nih.gov/pubmed/10526124

[197] Romero IA, Radewicz K, Jubin E, Michel CC, Greenwood J, Couraud P-O, et al. Changes in cytoskeletal and tight junctional proteins correlate with decreased permeability induced by dexamethasone in cultured rat brain endothelial cells. Neurosci Lett [Internet]. 2003;344(2):112–6 [cited 2015 Dec 8]. http://www.ncbi.nlm.nih.gov/pubmed/12782340

[198] Privratsky JR, Newman PJ. PECAM-1: regulator of endothelial junctional integrity. Cell Tissue Res [Internet]. 2014;355(3):607–19 [cited 2016 Jan 14]. http://www.pubmedcentral.nih.gov/articlerender.fcgi?artid=3975704&tool=pmcentrez&rendertype=abstract

[199] Graesser D, Solowiej A, Bruckner M, Osterweil E, Juedes A, Davis S, et al. Altered vascular permeability and early onset of experimental autoimmune encephalomyelitis in PECAM-1-deficient mice. J Clin Invest [Internet]. 2002;109(3):383–92 [cited 2016 Jan 14]. http://www.pubmedcentral.nih.gov/articlerender.fcgi?artid=150854&tool=pmcentrez&rendertype=abstract

[200] Tietz S, Engelhardt B. Brain barriers: crosstalk between complex tight junctions and adherens junctions. J Cell Biol [Internet]. 2015;209(4):493–506 [cited 2016 Jan 14]. http://www.pubmedcentral.nih.gov/articlerender.fcgi?artid=4442813&tool=pmcentrez&rendertype=abstract

[201] Fanning AS, Jameson BJ, Jesaitis LA, Anderson JM. The tight junction protein ZO-1 establishes a link between the transmembrane protein occludin and the actin cytoskeleton. J Biol Chem [Internet]. 1998;273(45):29745–53 [cited 2016 Jan 15]. http://www.ncbi.nlm.nih.gov/pubmed/9792688

[202] Van Itallie CM, Anderson JM. Architecture of tight junctions and principles of molecular composition. Semin Cell Dev Biol [Internet]. 2014;36:157–65 [cited 2016 Jan 6]. ttp://www.pubmedcentral.nih.gov/articlerender.fcgi?artid=4254347&tool=pmcentrez&rendertype=abstract

[203] Kirk J, Plumb J, Mirakhur M, McQuaid S. Tight junctional abnormality in multiple sclerosis white matter affects all calibres of vessel and is associated with blood-brain

barrier leakage and active demyelination. J Pathol [Internet]. 2003;201(2):319–27 [cited 2016 Jan 15]. http://www.ncbi.nlm.nih.gov/pubmed/14517850

[204] Stevenson BR, Siliciano JD, Mooseker MS, Goodenough DA. Identification of ZO-1: a high molecular weight polypeptide associated with the tight junction (zonula occludens) in a variety of epithelia. J Cell Biol [Internet]. 1986;103(3):755–66 [cited 2016 Jan 15]. http://www.pubmedcentral.nih.gov/articlerender.fcgi?artid=2114282&tool=pmcentrez&rendertype=abstract

[205] Howarth AG, Hughes MR, Stevenson BR. Detection of the tight junction-associated protein ZO-1 in astrocytes and other nonepithelial cell types. Am J Physiol [Internet]. 1992;262(2 Pt 1):C461–9 [cited 2016 Jan 15]. http://www.ncbi.nlm.nih.gov/pubmed/1539634

[206] Itoh M, Morita K, Tsukita S. Characterization of ZO-2 as a MAGUK family member associated with tight as well as adherens junctions with a binding affinity to occludin and alpha catenin. J Biol Chem [Internet]. 1999;274(9):5981–6 [cited 2016 Jan 15]. http://www.ncbi.nlm.nih.gov/pubmed/10026224

[207] Toyofuku T, Yabuki M, Otsu K, Kuzuya T, Hori M, Tada M. Direct association of the gap junction protein connexin-43 with ZO-1 in cardiac myocytes. J Biol Chem [Internet]. 1998;273(21):12725–31 [cited 2016 Jan 15]. http://www.ncbi.nlm.nih.gov/pubmed/9582296

[208] Abbruscato TJ, Lopez SP, Mark KS, Hawkins BT, Davis TP. Nicotine and cotinine modulate cerebral microvascular permeability and protein expression of ZO-1 through nicotinic acetylcholine receptors expressed on brain endothelial cells. J Pharm Sci [Internet]. 2002;91(12):2525–38 [cited 2016 Jan 15]. http://www.ncbi.nlm.nih.gov/pubmed/12434396

[209] Gumbiner B, Lowenkopf T, Apatira D. Identification of a 160-kDa polypeptide that binds to the tight junction protein ZO-1. Proc Natl Acad Sci USA [Internet]. 1991;88(8):3460–4 [cited 2016 Jan 15]. http://www.pubmedcentral.nih.gov/articlerender.fcgi?artid=51467&tool=pmcentrez&rendertype=abstract

[210] Umeda K, Matsui T, Nakayama M, Furuse K, Sasaki H, Furuse M, et al. Establishment and characterization of cultured epithelial cells lacking expression of ZO-1. J Biol Chem [Internet]. 2004;279(43):44785–94 [cited 2016 Jan 15]. http://www.ncbi.nlm.nih.gov/pubmed/15292177

[211] Dejana E, Tournier-Lasserve E, Weinstein BM. The control of vascular integrity by endothelial cell junctions: molecular basis and pathological implications. Dev Cell [Internet]. 2009;16(2):209–21 [cited 2015 Sep 8]. http://www.ncbi.nlm.nih.gov/pubmed/19217423

[212] Nico B, Frigeri A, Nicchia GP, Corsi P, Ribatti D, Quondamatteo F, et al. Severe alterations of endothelial and glial cells in the blood-brain barrier of dystrophic mdx

mice. Glia [Internet]. 2003;42(3):235–51 [cited 2016 Jan 16]. http://www.ncbi.nlm.nih.gov/pubmed/12673830

[213] Shiu C, Barbier E, Di Cello F, Choi HJ, Stins M. HIV-1 gp120 as well as alcohol affect blood-brain barrier permeability and stress fiber formation: involvement of reactive oxygen species. Alcohol Clin Exp Res [Internet]. 2007;31(1):130–7 [cited 2016 Jan 16]. http://www.ncbi.nlm.nih.gov/pubmed/17207111

[214] Davson H. Review lecture. The blood-brain barrier. J Physiol [Internet]. 1976;255(1):1–28 [cited 2016 Jan 17]. http://www.pubmedcentral.nih.gov/articlerender.fcgi?artid=1309232&tool=pmcentrez&rendertype=abstract

[215] Wong AD, Ye M, Levy AF, Rothstein JD, Bergles DE, Searson PC. The blood-brain barrier: an engineering perspective. Front Neuroeng [Internet]. 2013;6:7 [cited 2016 Jan 16]. http://journal.frontiersin.org/article/10.3389/fneng.2013.00007/abstract

[216] Abbott NJ, Patabendige AAK, Dolman DEM, Yusof SR, Begley DJ. Structure and function of the blood-brain barrier. Neurobiol Dis [Internet]. 2010;37(1):13–25 [cited 2014 Jul 15]. http://www.ncbi.nlm.nih.gov/pubmed/19664713

[217] Taylor CJ, Nicola PA, Wang S, Barrand MA, Hladky SB. Transporters involved in regulation of intracellular pH in primary cultured rat brain endothelial cells. J Physiol [Internet]. 2006;576(Pt 3):769–85 [cited 2016 Jan 17]. http://www.pubmedcentral.nih.gov/articlerender.fcgi?artid=1890423&tool=pmcentrez&rendertype=abstract

[218] Giacomini KM, Huang S-M, Tweedie DJ, Benet LZ, Brouwer KLR, Chu X, et al. Membrane transporters in drug development. Nat Rev Drug Discov [Internet]. 2010;9(3):215–36 [cited 2014 Jul 11]. http://www.pubmedcentral.nih.gov/articlerender.fcgi?artid=3326076&tool=pmcentrez&rendertype=abstract

[219] Ueno M. Mechanisms of the penetration of blood-borne substances into the brain. Curr Neuropharmacol [Internet]. 2009;7(2):142–9 [cited 2016 Jan 16]. http://www.pubmedcentral.nih.gov/articlerender.fcgi?artid=2730006&tool=pmcentrez&rendertype=abstract

[220] Enerson BE, Drewes LR. The rat blood-brain barrier transcriptome. J Cereb Blood Flow Metab. 2006;26(7):959–73.

[221] Abbott NJ, Rönnbäck L, Hansson E. Astrocyte-endothelial interactions at the blood-brain barrier. Nat Rev Neurosci [Internet]. 2006;7(1):41–53 [cited 2014 Jul 9]. http://www.ncbi.nlm.nih.gov/pubmed/16371949

[222] Dauchy S, Dutheil F, Weaver RJ, Chassoux F, Daumas-Duport C, Couraud P-O, et al. ABC transporters, cytochromes P450 and their main transcription factors: expression at the human blood-brain barrier. J Neurochem [Internet]. 2008;107(6):1518–28 [cited 2016 Jan 17]. http://www.ncbi.nlm.nih.gov/pubmed/19094056

[223] Begley DJ. ABC transporters and the blood-brain barrier. Curr Pharm Des [Internet]. 2004;10(12):1295–312 [cited 2016 Jan 17]. http://www.ncbi.nlm.nih.gov/pubmed/15134482

[224] Dallas S, Miller DS, Bendayan R. Multidrug resistance-associated proteins: expression and function in the central nervous system. Pharmacol Rev [Internet]. 2006;58(2):140–61 [cited 2016 Jan 17]. ttp://www.ncbi.nlm.nih.gov/pubmed/16714484

[225] Bendayan R, Ronaldson PT, Gingras D, Bendayan M. In situ localization of P-glycoprotein (ABCB1) in human and rat brain. J Histochem Cytochem [Internet]. 2006;54(10):1159–67 [cited 2016 Jan 12]. http://www.pubmedcentral.nih.gov/articlerender.fcgi?artid=3957801&tool=pmcentrez&rendertype=abstract

[226] Banks WA. The CNS as a target for peptides and peptide-based drugs. Expert Opin Drug Deliv [Internet]. 2006;3(6):707–12 [cited 2016 Jan 17]. http://www.ncbi.nlm.nih.gov/pubmed/17076593

[227] Lajoie P, Nabi IR. Regulation of raft-dependent endocytosis. J Cell Mol Med [Internet]. 2016;11(4):644–53 [cited 2016 Jan 17]. http://www.pubmedcentral.nih.gov/articlerender.fcgi?artid=3823247&tool=pmcentrez&rendertype=abstract

[228] Parton RG, Richards AA. Lipid rafts and caveolae as portals for endocytosis: new insights and common mechanisms. Traffic [Internet]. 2003;4(11):724–38 [cited 2016 Jan 17]. http://www.ncbi.nlm.nih.gov/pubmed/14617356

[229] Wolburg H. Blood-Brain Barriers. In: Dermietzel R, Spray DC, Nedergaard M, editors. Weinheim, Germany: Wiley-VCH Verlag GmbH & Co. KGaA; 2006 [cited 2016 Jan 17]. doi: 10.1002/9783527611225

[230] Song L, Ge S, Pachter JS. Caveolin-1 regulates expression of junction-associated proteins in brain microvascular endothelial cells. Blood [Internet]. 2007;109(4):1515–23 [cited 2016 Jan 17]. http://www.pubmedcentral.nih.gov/articlerender.fcgi?artid=1794065&tool=pmcentrez&rendertype=abstract

[231] Nahirney PC, Reeson P, Brown CE. Ultrastructural analysis of blood-brain barrier breakdown in the peri-infarct zone in young adult and aged mice. J Cereb Blood Flow Metab [Internet]. 2015 [cited 2016 Jan 1]. http://www.ncbi.nlm.nih.gov/pubmed/26661190

[232] Ueno M, Chiba Y, Matsumoto K, Nakagawa T, Miyanaka H. Clearance of beta-amyloid in the brain. Curr Med Chem [Internet]. 2014;21(35):4085–90 [cited 2016 Jan 17]. http://www.ncbi.nlm.nih.gov/pubmed/25312211

[233] Citron M, Oltersdorf T, Haass C, McConlogue L, Hung AY, Seubert P, et al. Mutation of the beta-amyloid precursor protein in familial Alzheimer's disease increases beta-protein production. Nature [Internet]. 1992;360(6405):672–4 [cited 2015 Dec 29]. http://www.ncbi.nlm.nih.gov/pubmed/1465129

[234] Tanzi RE, Moir RD, Wagner SL. Clearance of Alzheimer's Abeta peptide: the many roads to perdition. Neuron [Internet]. 2004;43(5):605–8 [cited 2016 Jan 17]. http://www.ncbi.nlm.nih.gov/pubmed/15339642

[235] Zlokovic B V, Yamada S, Holtzman D, Ghiso J, Frangione B. Clearance of amyloid beta-peptide from brain: transport or metabolism? Nat Med [Internet]. 2000;6(7):718–9 [cited 2016 Jan 17]. http://www.ncbi.nlm.nih.gov/pubmed/10888892

[236] Hardy J. Amyloid double trouble. Nat Genet [Internet]. 2006;38(1):11–2 [cited 2016 Jan 17]. http://www.ncbi.nlm.nih.gov/pubmed/16380721

[237] Ballatore C, Lee VM-Y, Trojanowski JQ. Tau-mediated neurodegeneration in Alzheimer's disease and related disorders. Nat Rev Neurosci [Internet]. 2007;8(9):663–72 [cited 2014 Jul 21]. doi: 10.1038/nrn2194

[238] Selkoe DJ. Clearing the brain's amyloid cobwebs. Neuron [Internet]. 2001;32(2):177–80 [cited 2016 Jan 17]. http://www.ncbi.nlm.nih.gov/pubmed/11683988

[239] Shibata M, Yamada S, Kumar SR, Calero M, Bading J, Frangione B, et al. Clearance of Alzheimer's amyloid-ss(1-40) peptide from brain by LDL receptor-related protein-1 at the blood-brain barrier. J Clin Invest [Internet]. 2000;106(12):1489–99 [cited 2015 Dec 14]. http://www.pubmedcentral.nih.gov/articlerender.fcgi?artid=387254&tool=pmcentrez&rendertype=abstract

[240] Deane R, Wu Z, Sagare A, Davis J, Du Yan S, Hamm K, et al. LRP/amyloid beta-peptide interaction mediates differential brain efflux of Abeta isoforms. Neuron [Internet]. 2004;43(3):333–44 [cited 2015 Nov 26]. http://www.ncbi.nlm.nih.gov/pubmed/15294142

[241] Deane R, Du Yan S, Submamaryan RK, LaRue B, Jovanovic S, Hogg E, et al. RAGE mediates amyloid-beta peptide transport across the blood-brain barrier and accumulation in brain. Nat Med [Internet]. 2003;9(7):907–13 [cited 2015 Sep 21]. http://www.ncbi.nlm.nih.gov/pubmed/12808450

[242] Pascale CL, Miller MC, Chiu C, Boylan M, Caralopoulos IN, Gonzalez L, et al. Amyloid-beta transporter expression at the blood-CSF barrier is age-dependent. Fluids Barriers CNS [Internet]. 2011;8:21 [cited 2015 Dec 5]. http://www.pubmedcentral.nih.gov/articlerender.fcgi?artid=3162580&tool=pmcentrez&rendertype=abstract

[243] Deane R, Bell RD, Sagare A, Zlokovic B V. Clearance of amyloid-beta peptide across the blood-brain barrier: implication for therapies in Alzheimer's disease. CNS Neurol Disord Drug Targets [Internet]. 2009;8(1):16–30 [cited 2015 Oct 5]. http://www.pubmedcentral.nih.gov/articlerender.fcgi?artid=2872930&tool=pmcentrez&rendertype=abstract

[244] Bell RD, Sagare AP, Friedman AE, Bedi GS, Holtzman DM, Deane R, et al. Transport pathways for clearance of human Alzheimer's amyloid β-peptide and apolipoproteins E and J in the mouse central nervous system. J Cereb Blood Flow Metab [Internet].

2007;27(5):909–18 [cited 2015 Oct 22]. http://www.pubmedcentral.nih.gov/articlerender.fcgi?artid=2853021&tool=pmcentrez&rendertype=abstract

[245] Deane R, Sagare A, Hamm K, Parisi M, Lane S, Finn MB, et al. apoE isoform–specific disruption of amyloid β peptide clearance from mouse brain. J Clin Invest [Internet]. 2008;118(12):4002–13 [cited 2015 Oct 17]. http://www.pubmedcentral.nih.gov/articlerender.fcgi?artid=2582453&tool=pmcentrez&rendertype=abstract

[246] Herz J, Strickland DK. LRP: a multifunctional scavenger and signaling receptor. J Clin Invest [Internet]. 2001;108(6):779–84 [cited 2015 Nov 12]. http://www.pubmedcentral.nih.gov/articlerender.fcgi?artid=200939&tool=pmcentrez&rendertype=abstract

[247] Nazer B, Hong S, Selkoe DJ. LRP promotes endocytosis and degradation, but not transcytosis, of the amyloid-beta peptide in a blood-brain barrier in vitro model. Neurobiol Dis [Internet]. 2008;30(1):94–102 [cited 2016 Jan 17]. http://www.pubmedcentral.nih.gov/articlerender.fcgi?artid=2376120&tool=pmcentrez&rendertype=abstract

[248] Pflanzner T, Janko MC, André-Dohmen B, Reuss S, Weggen S, Roebroek AJM, et al. LRP1 mediates bidirectional transcytosis of amyloid-β across the blood-brain barrier. Neurobiol Aging [Internet]. 2011;32(12):2323.e1–11 [cited 2016 Jan 17]. http://www.ncbi.nlm.nih.gov/pubmed/20630619

[249] von Arnim CAF, Kinoshita A, Peltan ID, Tangredi MM, Herl L, Lee BM, et al. The low density lipoprotein receptor-related protein (LRP) is a novel beta-secretase (BACE1) substrate. J Biol Chem [Internet]. 2005;280(18):17777–85 [cited 2015 Dec 15]. http://www.ncbi.nlm.nih.gov/pubmed/15749709

[250] Koistinaho M, Lin S, Wu X, Esterman M, Koger D, Hanson J, et al. Apolipoprotein E promotes astrocyte colocalization and degradation of deposited amyloid-beta peptides. Nat Med [Internet]. 2004;10(7):719–26 [cited 2016 Jan 18]. http://www.ncbi.nlm.nih.gov/pubmed/15195085

[251] Yan S Du, Chen X, Fu J, Chen M, Zhu H, Roher A, et al. RAGE and amyloid-β peptide neurotoxicity in Alzheimer's disease. Nature [Internet]. 1996;382(6593):685–91 [cited 2016 Jan 14]. http://www.ncbi.nlm.nih.gov/pubmed/8751438

[252] Zlokovic B V, Ghiso J, Mackic JB, McComb JG, Weiss MH, Frangione B. Blood-brain barrier transport of circulating Alzheimer's amyloid beta. Biochem Biophys Res Commun [Internet]. 1993;197(3):1034–40 [cited 2016 Jan 18]. http://www.ncbi.nlm.nih.gov/pubmed/8280117

[253] Correale J, Villa A. The blood-brain-barrier in multiple sclerosis: functional roles and therapeutic targeting. Autoimmunity [Internet]. 2007;40(2):148–60 [cited 2016 Jan 13]. http://www.ncbi.nlm.nih.gov/pubmed/17453713

[254] Kaur C, Ling EA. Blood brain barrier in hypoxic-ischemic conditions. Curr Neurovasc Res [Internet]. 2008;5(1):71–81 [cited 2016 Jan 18]. http://www.ncbi.nlm.nih.gov/pubmed/18289024

[255] Desai BS, Monahan AJ, Carvey PM, Hendey B. Blood-brain barrier pathology in Alzheimer's and Parkinson's disease: implications for drug therapy. Cell Transplant [Internet]. 2007;16(3):285–99 [cited 2016 Jan 18]. http://www.ncbi.nlm.nih.gov/pubmed/17503739

[256] Förster C. Tight junctions and the modulation of barrier function in disease. Histochem Cell Biol [Internet]. 2008;130(1):55–70 [cited 2015 Nov 30]. http://www.pubmedcentral.nih.gov/articlerender.fcgi?artid=2413111&tool=pmcentrez&rendertype=abstract

[257] Wardlaw JM, Sandercock PAG, Dennis MS, Starr J. Is breakdown of the blood-brain barrier responsible for lacunar stroke, leukoaraiosis, and dementia? Stroke [Internet]. 2003;34(3):806–12 [cited 2015 Dec 5]. http://www.ncbi.nlm.nih.gov/pubmed/12624314

[258] Zlokovic B V. Clearing amyloid through the blood-brain barrier. J Neurochem [Internet]. 2004;89(4):807–11 [cited 2016 Jan 14]. http://www.ncbi.nlm.nih.gov/pubmed/15140180

[259] Owen JB, Sultana R, Aluise CD, Erickson MA, Price TO, Bu G, et al. Oxidative modification to LDL receptor-related protein 1 in hippocampus from subjects with Alzheimer disease: implications for Aβ accumulation in AD brain. Free Radic Biol Med [Internet]. 2010;49(11):1798–803 [cited 2016 Jan 18]. http://www.pubmedcentral.nih.gov/articlerender.fcgi?artid=2970765&tool=pmcentrez&rendertype=abstract

[260] Cirrito JR, Deane R, Fagan AM, Spinner ML, Parsadanian M, Finn MB, et al. P-glycoprotein deficiency at the blood-brain barrier increases amyloid-beta deposition in an Alzheimer disease mouse model. J Clin Invest [Internet]. 2005;115(11):3285–90 [cited 2016 Jan 18]. http://www.pubmedcentral.nih.gov/articlerender.fcgi?artid=1257538&tool=pmcentrez&rendertype=abstract

[261] Landau SM, Harvey D, Madison CM, Koeppe RA, Reiman EM, Foster NL, et al. Associations between cognitive, functional, and FDG-PET measures of decline in AD and MCI. Neurobiol Aging [Internet]. 2011;32(7):1207–18 [cited 2016 Jan 18]. http://www.pubmedcentral.nih.gov/articlerender.fcgi?artid=2891865&tool=pmcentrez&rendertype=abstract

[262] Harik SI. Changes in the glucose transporter of brain capillaries. Can J Physiol Pharmacol [Internet]. 1992;70 Suppl:S113–7 [cited 2016 Jan 18]. http://www.ncbi.nlm.nih.gov/pubmed/1295661

[263] Mooradian AD, Chung HC, Shah GN. GLUT-1 expression in the cerebra of patients with Alzheimer's disease. Neurobiol Aging [Internet]. 2016;18(5):469–74 [cited 2016 Jan 18]. http://www.ncbi.nlm.nih.gov/pubmed/9390772

[264] Sagare AP, Bell RD, Zlokovic BV. Neurovascular dysfunction and faulty amyloid β-peptide clearance in Alzheimer disease. Cold Spring Harb Perspect Med. 2012 Oct

1;2(10). pii: a011452. doi: 10.1101/cshperspect.a011452. Review. PubMed PMID: 23028132; PubMed Central PMCID: PMC3475405.

[265] Claudio L. Ultrastructural features of the blood-brain barrier in biopsy tissue from Alzheimer's disease patients. Acta Neuropathol [Internet]. 1996;91(1):6–14 [cited 2016 Feb 5]. http://www.ncbi.nlm.nih.gov/pubmed/8773140

[266] Bailey TL, Rivara CB, Rocher AB, Hof PR. The nature and effects of cortical microvascular pathology in aging and Alzheimer's disease. Neurol Res [Internet]. 2004;26(5): 573–8 [cited 2016 Jan 8]. http://www.ncbi.nlm.nih.gov/pubmed/15265277

[267] Romanitan MO, Popescu BO, Winblad B, Bajenaru OA, Bogdanovic N. Occludin is overexpressed in Alzheimer's disease and vascular dementia. J Cell Mol Med [Internet]. 2016;11(3):569–79 [cited 2016 Jan 18]. http://www.pubmedcentral.nih.gov/articlerender.fcgi?artid=3922362&tool=pmcentrez&rendertype=abstract

[268] Wu Z, Guo H, Chow N, Sallstrom J, Bell RD, Deane R, et al. Role of the MEOX2 homeobox gene in neurovascular dysfunction in Alzheimer disease. Nat Med [Internet]. 2005;11(9):959–65 [cited 2016 Jan 18]. doi: 10.1038/nm1287

[269] Rogers J, Luber-Narod J, Styren SD, Civin WH. Expression of immune system-associated antigens by cells of the human central nervous system: relationship to the pathology of Alzheimer's disease. Neurobiol Aging. Jan 1988; ;9(4):339–49.

[270] Mehta PD, Pirttilä T, Mehta SP, Sersen EA, Aisen PS, Wisniewski HM. Plasma and cerebrospinal fluid levels of amyloid beta proteins 1-40 and 1-42 in Alzheimer disease. Arch Neurol [Internet]. 2000;57(1):100–5 [cited 2016 Jan 18]. http://www.ncbi.nlm.nih.gov/pubmed/10634455

[271] Pesaresi M, Lovati C, Bertora P, Mailland E, Galimberti D, Scarpini E, et al. Plasma levels of beta-amyloid (1-42) in Alzheimer's disease and mild cognitive impairment. Neurobiol Aging [Internet]. 2006;27(6):904–5 [cited 2016 Jan 18]. http://www.ncbi.nlm.nih.gov/pubmed/16638622

[272] Hansson O, Zetterberg H, Vanmechelen E, Vanderstichele H, Andreasson U, Londos E, et al. Evaluation of plasma Abeta(40) and Abeta(42) as predictors of conversion to Alzheimer's disease in patients with mild cognitive impairment. Neurobiol Aging [Internet]. 2010;31(3):357–67 [cited 2016 Jan 18]. http://www.ncbi.nlm.nih.gov/pubmed/18486992

[273] Roher AE, Esh CL, Kokjohn TA, Castaño EM, Van Vickle GD, Kalback WM, et al. Amyloid beta peptides in human plasma and tissues and their significance for Alzheimer's disease. Alzheimers Dement [Internet]. 2009;5(1):18–29 [cited 2016 Jan 18]. http://www.pubmedcentral.nih.gov/articlerender.fcgi?artid=2663406&tool=pmcentrez&rendertype=abstract

[274] Li QX, Whyte S, Tanner JE, Evin G, Beyreuther K, Masters CL. Secretion of Alzheimer's disease Abeta amyloid peptide by activated human platelets. Lab Invest [Internet]. 1998;78(4):461–9 [cited 2016 Jan 18]. http://www.ncbi.nlm.nih.gov/pubmed/9564890

[275] Kuo YM, Kokjohn TA, Watson MD, Woods AS, Cotter RJ, Sue LI, et al. Elevated abeta42 in skeletal muscle of Alzheimer disease patients suggests peripheral alterations of AbetaPP metabolism. Am J Pathol [Internet]. 2000;156(3):797–805 [cited 2016 Jan 18]. http://www.pubmedcentral.nih.gov/articlerender.fcgi?artid=1876838&tool=pmcentrez&rendertype=abstract

[276] Kuo YM, Kokjohn TA, Kalback W, Luehrs D, Galasko DR, Chevallier N, et al. Amyloid-beta peptides interact with plasma proteins and erythrocytes: implications for their quantitation in plasma. Biochem Biophys Res Commun [Internet]. 2000;268(3):750–6 [cited 2016 Jan 18]. http://www.ncbi.nlm.nih.gov/pubmed/10679277

[277] Biere AL, Ostaszewski B, Stimson ER, Hyman BT, Maggio JE, Selkoe DJ. Amyloid beta-peptide is transported on lipoproteins and albumin in human plasma. J Biol Chem [Internet]. 1996;271(51):32916–22 [cited 2016 Jan 18]. http://www.ncbi.nlm.nih.gov/pubmed/8955133

[278] Strittmatter WJ, Weisgraber KH, Huang DY, Dong LM, Salvesen GS, Pericak-Vance M, et al. Binding of human apolipoprotein E to synthetic amyloid beta peptide: isoform-specific effects and implications for late-onset Alzheimer disease. Proc Natl Acad Sci U S A [Internet]. 1993;90(17):8098–102 [cited 2016 Jan 18]. http://www.pubmedcentral.nih.gov/articlerender.fcgi?artid=47295&tool=pmcentrez&rendertype=abstract

[279] Sagare A, Deane R, Bell RD, Johnson B, Hamm K, Pendu R, et al. Clearance of amyloid-beta by circulating lipoprotein receptors. Nat Med [Internet]. 2007;13(9):1029–31 [cited 2015 Oct 1]. http://www.pubmedcentral.nih.gov/articlerender.fcgi?artid=2936449&tool=pmcentrez&rendertype=abstract

[280] Pan W, Solomon B, Maness LM, Kastin AJ. Antibodies to beta-amyloid decrease the blood-to-brain transfer of beta-amyloid peptide. Exp Biol Med (Maywood) [Internet]. 2002;227(8):609–15 [cited 2016 Jan 18]. http://www.ncbi.nlm.nih.gov/pubmed/12192102

[281] Erickson MA, Banks WA. Blood-brain barrier dysfunction as a cause and consequence of Alzheimer's disease. J Cereb Blood Flow Metab [Internet]. 2013;33(10):1500–13 [cited 2016 Jan 16]. http://www.pubmedcentral.nih.gov/articlerender.fcgi?artid=3790938&tool=pmcentrez&rendertype=abstract

[282] Geroldi D, Falcone C, Emanuele E. Soluble receptor for advanced glycation end products: from disease marker to potential therapeutic target. Curr Med Chem [Internet]. 2006;13(17):1971–8 [cited 2016 Jan 18]. http://www.ncbi.nlm.nih.gov/pubmed/16842191

[283] Marchi N, Fazio V, Cucullo L, Kight K, Masaryk T, Barnett G, et al. Serum transthyretin monomer as a possible marker of blood-to-CSF barrier disruption. J Neurosci [Internet]. 2003;23(5):1949–55 [cited 2016 Jan 18]. http://www.ncbi.nlm.nih.gov/pubmed/12629200

[284] Kapural M, Krizanac-Bengez L, Barnett G, Perl J, Masaryk T, Apollo D, et al. Serum S-100beta as a possible marker of blood-brain barrier disruption. Brain Res [Internet]. 2002;940(1–2):102–4 [cited 2016 Jan 19]. http://www.ncbi.nlm.nih.gov/pubmed/12020881

[285] Tamaki C, Ohtsuki S, Iwatsubo T, Hashimoto T, Yamada K, Yabuki C, et al. Major involvement of low-density lipoprotein receptor-related protein 1 in the clearance of plasma free amyloid beta-peptide by the liver. Pharm Res [Internet]. 2006;23(7):1407–16 [cited 2015 Dec 15]. http://www.ncbi.nlm.nih.gov/pubmed/16779710

[286] Sagare AP, Deane R, Zlokovic B V. Low-density lipoprotein receptor-related protein 1: a physiological Aβ homeostatic mechanism with multiple therapeutic opportunities. Pharmacol Ther [Internet]. 2012;136(1):94–105. doi: 10.1016/j.pharmthera.2012.07.008

[287] Kandimalla KK, Curran GL, Holasek SS, Gilles EJ, Wengenack TM, Poduslo JF. Pharmacokinetic analysis of the blood-brain barrier transport of 125I-amyloid beta protein 40 in wild-type and Alzheimer's disease transgenic mice (APP,PS1) and its implications for amyloid plaque formation. J Pharmacol Exp Ther. 2005;313(3):1370–8.

[288] Ghiso J, Shayo M, Calero M, Ng D, Tomidokoro Y, Gandy S, et al. Systemic catabolism of Alzheimer's Abeta40 and Abeta42. J Biol Chem [Internet]. 2004;279(44):45897–908 [cited 2016 Jan 19]. http://www.ncbi.nlm.nih.gov/pubmed/15322125

[289] Tamaki C, Ohtsuki S, Terasaki T. Insulin facilitates the hepatic clearance of plasma amyloid beta-peptide (1 40) by intracellular translocation of low-density lipoprotein receptor-related protein 1 (LRP-1) to the plasma membrane in hepatocytes. Mol Pharmacol [Internet]. 2007;72(4):850–5 [cited 2016 Jan 19]. http://www.ncbi.nlm.nih.gov/pubmed/17609417

[290] Alemi M, Gaiteiro C, Ribeiro CA, Santos LM, Gomes JR, Oliveira SM, et al. Transthyretin participates in beta-amyloid transport from the brain to the liver- involvement of the low-density lipoprotein receptor-related protein 1? Sci Rep [Internet]. 2016;6:20164 [cited 2016 Feb 4]. http://www.ncbi.nlm.nih.gov/pubmed/26837706

[291] Duckworth WC, Bennett RG, Hamel FG. Insulin degradation: progress and potential. Endocr Rev [Internet]. 1998;19(5):608–24 [cited 2016 Jan 19]. http://www.ncbi.nlm.nih.gov/pubmed/9793760

[292] Wang D-S, Dickson DW, Malter JS. beta-Amyloid degradation and Alzheimer's disease. J Biomed Biotechnol [Internet]. 2006;2006(3):58406 [cited 2016 Jan 19]. http://www.pubmedcentral.nih.gov/articlerender.fcgi?artid=1559921&tool=pmcentrez&rendertype=abstract

[293] Ghersi-Egea JF, Gorevic PD, Ghiso J, Frangione B, Patlak CS, Fenstermacher JD. Fate of cerebrospinal fluid-borne amyloid beta-peptide: rapid clearance into blood and appreciable accumulation by cerebral arteries. J Neurochem [Internet]. 1996;67(2):880–3 [cited 2016 Jan 19]. http://www.ncbi.nlm.nih.gov/pubmed/8764620

[294] Soprano DR, Herbert J, Soprano KJ, Schon EA, Goodman DS. Demonstration of transthyretin mRNA in the brain and other extrahepatic tissues in the rat. J Biol Chem [Internet]. 1985;260(21):11793–8 [cited 2015 Dec 30]. http://www.ncbi.nlm.nih.gov/pubmed/4044580

[295] Woeber KA, Ingbar SH. The contribution of thyroxine-binding prealbumin to the binding of thyroxine in human serum, as assessed by immunoadsorption. J Clin Invest. 1968;47(7):1710–21.

[296] Goodman D. Retinoids and retinol-binding proteins. Harvey Lect. 1987;Series 81:111–32.

[297] Kabat EA, Moore DH, Landow H. An electrophoretic study of the protein components in cerebrospinal fluid and their relationship to the serum proteins. J Clin Invest [Internet]. 1942;21(5):571–7 [cited 2015 Dec 30]. http://www.pubmedcentral.nih.gov/articlerender.fcgi?artid=435175&tool=pmcentrez&rendertype=abstract

[298] Seibert FB NJ. Electrophoretic study of the blood response in tuberculosis. J Biol Chem. 1942;143:29–38.

[299] Wallace MR, Naylor SL, Kluve-Beckerman B, Long GL, McDonald L, Shows TB, et al. Localization of the human prealbumin gene to chromosome 18. Biochem Biophys Res Commun [Internet]. 1985;129(3):753–8. http://www.ncbi.nlm.nih.gov/pubmed/2990465

[300] Sasaki H, Yoshioka N, Takagi Y, Sakaki Y. Structure of the chromosomal gene for human serum prealbumin. Gene [Internet]. 1985;37(1–3):191–7 [cited 2015 Dec 30]. http://www.ncbi.nlm.nih.gov/pubmed/4054629

[301] Tsuzuki T, Mita S, Maeda S, Araki S, Shimada K. Structure of the human prealbumin gene. J Biol Chem. 1985;260(22):12224–7.

[302] Whitehead AS, Skinner M, Bruns GA, Costello W, Edge MD, Cohen AS, et al. Cloning of human prealbumin complementary DNA. Localization of the gene to chromosome 18 and detection of a variant prealbumin allele in a family with familial amyloid polyneuropathy. Mol Biol Med [Internet]. 1984;2(6):411–23 [cited 2015 Dec 30]. http://www.ncbi.nlm.nih.gov/pubmed/6100724

[303] Mita S, Maeda S, Shimada K, Araki S. Cloning and sequence analysis of cDNA for human prealbumin. Biochem Biophys Res Commun [Internet]. 1984;124(2):558–64. http://www.sciencedirect.com/science/article/pii/0006291X84915900

[304] Sundelin J, Melhus H, Das S, Eriksson U, Lind P, Trägårdh L, et al. The primary structure of rabbit and rat prealbumin and a comparison with the tertiary structure of human prealbumin [Internet]. J Biol Chem. 1985;260:6481–7. http://www.ncbi.nlm.nih.gov/entrez/query.fcgi?db=pubmed&cmd=Retrieve&dopt=AbstractPlus&list_uids=3922975\nhttp://www.jbc.org/cgi/reprint/260/10/6481

[305] Dickson PW, Howlett GJ, Schreiber G. Rat transthyretin (prealbumin). Molecular cloning, nucleotide sequence, and gene expression in liver and brain. J Biol Chem [Internet]. 1985;260(13):8214–9. http://www.ncbi.nlm.nih.gov/pubmed/3839240

[306] Costa RH, Lai E, Darnell JE. Transcriptional control of the mouse prealbumin (transthyretin) gene: both promoter sequences and a distinct enhancer are cell specific. Mol Cell Biol. 1986;6(12):4697–708.

[307] Andreoli M, Robbins J. Serum proteins and thyroxineprotein interaction in early human fetuses. J Clin Invest [Internet]. 1962;41:1070–7 [cited 2015 Dec 30]. http://www.pubmedcentral.nih.gov/articlerender.fcgi?artid=291012&tool=pmcentrez&rendertype=abstract

[308] Stabilini R, Vergani C, Agostoni A, Agostoni RP. Influence of age and sex on prealbumin levels. Clin Chim Acta [Internet]. 1968;20(2):358–9 [cited 2015 Dec 30]. http://www.ncbi.nlm.nih.gov/pubmed/4968450

[309] Vahlquist A, Rask L, Peterson PA, Berg T. The concentrations of retinol-binding protein, prealbumin, and transferrin in the sera of newly delivered mothers and children of various ages. Scand J Clin Lab Invest [Internet]. 1975;35(6):569–75 [cited 2015 Dec 30]. http://www.ncbi.nlm.nih.gov/pubmed/1239075

[310] Weisner B, Roethig HJ. The concentration of prealbumin in cerebrospinal fluid (CSF), indicator of CSF circulation disorders. Eur Neurol [Internet]. 1983;22(2):96–105 [cited 2016 Jan 12]. http://www.ncbi.nlm.nih.gov/pubmed/6840150

[311] Gonçalves I, Alves CH, Quintela T, Baltazar G, Socorro S, Saraiva MJ, et al. Transthyretin is up-regulated by sex hormones in mice liver. Mol Cell Biochem [Internet]. 2008;317(1–2):137–42 [cited 2016 Feb 2]. http://www.ncbi.nlm.nih.gov/pubmed/18568387

[312] Quintela T, Gonçalves I, Martinho A, Alves CH, Saraiva MJ, Rocha P, et al. Progesterone enhances transthyretin expression in the rat choroid plexus in vitro and in vivo via progesterone receptor. J Mol Neurosci. 2011;44(3):152–8.

[313] Martinho A, Gonçalves I, Costa M, Santos CR. Stress and glucocorticoids increase transthyretin expression in rat choroid plexus via mineralocorticoid and glucocorticoid receptors. J Mol Neurosci. 2012;48(1):1–13.

[314] Kanda Y, Goodman DS, Canfield RE, Morgan FJ. The amino acid sequence of human plasma prealbumin. J Biol Chem [Internet]. 1974;249(21):6796–805 [cited 2016 Jan 12]. http://www.ncbi.nlm.nih.gov/pubmed/4607556

[315] Blake CC, Geisow MJ, Oatley SJ, Rérat B, Rérat C. Structure of prealbumin: secondary, tertiary and quaternary interactions determined by Fourier refinement at 1.8 A. J Mol Biol [Internet]. 1978;121(3):339–56 [cited 2015 Dec 31]. http://www.ncbi.nlm.nih.gov/pubmed/671542

[316] Loun B, Hage DS. Characterization of thyroxine-albumin binding using high-performance affinity chromatography. I. Interactions at the warfarin and indole sites of

albumin. J Chromatogr [Internet]. 1992;579(2):225–35 [cited 2016 Jan 12]. http://www.ncbi.nlm.nih.gov/pubmed/1429970

[317] Ferguson RN, Edelhoch H, Saroff HA, Robbins J, Cahnmann HJ. Negative cooperativity in the binding of thyroxine to human serum prealbumin. Preparation of tritium-labeled 8-anilino-1-naphthalenesulfonic acid. Biochemistry. 1975;14(2):282–9.

[318] Richardson SJ, Wijayagunaratne RC, D'Souza DG, Darras VM, Van Herck SLJ. Transport of thyroid hormones via the choroid plexus into the brain: The roles of transthyretin and thyroid hormone transmembrane transporters. Vol. 9, Frontiers in Neuroscience. 2015.

[319] Manral P, Reixach N. Amyloidogenic and non-amyloidogenic transthyretin variants interact differently with human cardiomyocytes: insights into early events of non-fibrillar tissue damage. Biosci Rep. 2015 Jan 14;35(1). pii: e00172. doi: 10.1042/BSR20140155. PubMed PMID: 25395306; PubMed Central PMCID: PMC4293901.

[320] Palha JA, Hays MT, Morreale de Escobar G, Episkopou V, Gottesman ME, Saraiva MJ. Transthyretin is not essential for thyroxine to reach the brain and other tissues in transthyretin-null mice. Am J Physiol [Internet]. 1997;272(3 Pt 1):E485–93 [cited 2016 Jan 13]. http://www.ncbi.nlm.nih.gov/pubmed/9124556

[321] Palha JA, Episkopou V, Maeda S, Shimada K, Gottesman ME, Saraiva MJ. Thyroid hormone metabolism in a transthyretin-null mouse strain. J Biol Chem [Internet]. 1994;269(52):33135–9 [cited 2016 Jan 13]. http://www.ncbi.nlm.nih.gov/pubmed/7806543

[322] Palha JA, Fernandes R, de Escobar GM, Episkopou V, Gottesman M, Saraiva MJ. Transthyretin regulates thyroid hormone levels in the choroid plexus, but not in the brain parenchyma: study in a transthyretin-null mouse model. Endocrinology [Internet]. 2000;141(9):3267–72 [cited 2016 Jan 13]. http://www.ncbi.nlm.nih.gov/pubmed/10965897

[323] Rask L, Anundi H, Peterson PA. The primary structure of the human retinol-binding protein. FEBS Lett [Internet]. 1979;104(1):55–8 [cited 2016 Jan 13]. http://www.ncbi.nlm.nih.gov/pubmed/573217

[324] Newcomer ME, Jones TA, Aqvist J, Sundelin J, Eriksson U, Rask L, et al. The three-dimensional structure of retinol-binding protein. EMBO J [Internet]. 1984;3(7):1451–4 [cited 2016 Jan 13]. http://www.pubmedcentral.nih.gov/articlerender.fcgi?artid=557543&tool=pmcentrez&rendertype=abstract

[325] Blaner WS. Retinol-binding protein: the serum transport protein for vitamin A. Endocr Rev [Internet]. 1989;10(3):308–16 [cited 2015 Dec 12]. http://www.ncbi.nlm.nih.gov/pubmed/2550213

[326] Kopelman M, Cogan U, Mokady S, Shinitzky M. The interaction between retinol-binding proteins and prealbumins studied by fluorescence polarization. Biochim

Biophys Acta [Internet]. 1976;439(2):449–60 [cited 2016 Jan 13]. http://www.ncbi.nlm.nih.gov/pubmed/986177

[327] van Jaarsveld PP, Edelhoch H, Goodman DS, Robbins J. The interaction of human plasma retinol-binding protein and prealbumin. J Biol Chem [Internet]. 1973;248(13): 4698–705 [cited 2016 Jan 13]. http://www.ncbi.nlm.nih.gov/pubmed/4718739

[328] Vahlquist A, Peterson PA, Wibell L. Metabolism of the viatmin A transporting protein complex. I. Turnover studies in normal persons and in patients with chronic renal failure. Eur J Clin Invest [Internet]. 1973;3(4):352–62 [cited 2016 Jan 13]. http://www.ncbi.nlm.nih.gov/pubmed/4760057

[329] Socolow EL, Woeber KA, Purdy RH, Holloway MT, Ingbar SH. Preparation of I-131-labeled human serum prealbumin and its metabolism in normal and sick patients. J Clin Invest [Internet]. 1965;44(10):1600–9 [cited 2016 Jan 13]. http://www.pubmedcentral.nih.gov/articlerender.fcgi?artid=292644&tool=pmcentrez&rendertype=abstract

[330] Vahlquist A, Peterson PA. Comparative studies on the vitamin A transporting protein complex in human and cynomolgus plasma. Biochemistry [Internet]. 1972;11(24):4526–32 [cited 2016 Jan 13]. http://www.ncbi.nlm.nih.gov/pubmed/4631638

[331] Peterson PA, Nilsson SF, Ostberg L, Rask L, Vahlquist A. Aspects of the metabolism of retinol-binding protein and retinol. Vitam Horm [Internet]. 1974;32:181–214 [cited 2016 Jan 13]. http://www.ncbi.nlm.nih.gov/pubmed/4617399

[332] Makover A, Moriwaki H, Ramakrishnan R, Saraiva MJ, Blaner WS, Goodman DS. Plasma transthyretin. Tissue sites of degradation and turnover in the rat. J Biol Chem. 1988;263:8598–603.

[333] Receptor-mediated uptake and internalization of transthyretin. PubMed—NCBI [Internet]. 2016 [cited 2016 Jan 14]. http://www.ncbi.nlm.nih.gov/pubmed/2153133

[334] Vieira A V, Sanders EJ, Schneider WJ. Transport of serum transthyretin into chicken oocytes. A receptor-mediated mechanism. J Biol Chem [Internet]. 1995;270(7):2952–6 [cited 2016 Jan 14]. http://www.ncbi.nlm.nih.gov/pubmed/7852374

[335] Sousa MM, Norden AG, Jacobsen C, Willnow TE, Christensen EI, Thakker R V, et al. Evidence for the role of megalin in renal uptake of transthyretin. J Biol Chem [Internet]. 2000;275(49):38176–81 [cited 2016 Jan 14]. http://www.ncbi.nlm.nih.gov/pubmed/10982792

[336] Sousa MM, Saraiva MJ. Internalization of transthyretin. Evidence of a novel yet unidentified receptor-associated protein (RAP)-sensitive receptor. J Biol Chem [Internet]. 2001;276(17):14420–5. http://www.ncbi.nlm.nih.gov/pubmed/11278770

[337] Divino CM, Schussler GC. Transthyretin receptors on human astrocytoma cells. J Clin Endocrinol Metab [Internet]. 1990;71(5):1265–8 [cited 2016 Jan 14]. http://www.ncbi.nlm.nih.gov/pubmed/2172276

[338] Bourgault S, Choi S, Buxbaum JN, Kelly JW, Price JL, Reixach N. Mechanisms of transthyretin cardiomyocyte toxicity inhibition by resveratrol analogs. Biochem Biophys Res Commun [Internet]. 2011;410(4):707–13 [cited 2016 Jan 14]. http://www.pubmedcentral.nih.gov/articlerender.fcgi?artid=3145458&tool=pmcentrez&rendertype=abstract

[339] Manral P, Reixach N. Amyloidogenic and non-amyloidogenic transthyretin variants interact differently with human cardiomyocytes: insights into early events of non-fibrillar tissue damage. Biosci Rep [Internet]. 2015;35(1) [cited 2016 Jan 14]. http://www.pubmedcentral.nih.gov/articlerender.fcgi?artid=4293901&tool=pmcentrez&rendertype=abstract

[340] Fleming CE, Mar FM, Franquinho F, Saraiva MJ, Sousa MM. Transthyretin internalization by sensory neurons is megalin mediated and necessary for its neuritogenic activity. J Neurosci [Internet]. 2009;29(10):3220–32 [cited 2016 Jan 14]. http://www.ncbi.nlm.nih.gov/pubmed/19279259

[341] Vieira M, Gomes JR, Saraiva MJ. Transthyretin Induces Insulin-like Growth Factor I Nuclear Translocation Regulating Its Levels in the Hippocampus. Mol Neurobiol [Internet]. 2015;51(3):1468–79. http://link.springer.com/10.1007/s12035-014-8824-4

[342] Liz MA, Faro CJ, Saraiva MJ, Sousa MM. Transthyretin, a new cryptic protease. J Biol Chem [Internet]. 2004;279(20):21431–8 [cited 2016 Jan 13]. http://www.ncbi.nlm.nih.gov/pubmed/15033978

[343] Liz MA, Gomes CM, Saraiva MJ, Sousa MM. ApoA-I cleaved by transthyretin has reduced ability to promote cholesterol efflux and increased amyloidogenicity. J Lipid Res [Internet]. 2007;48(11):2385–95 [cited 2016 Jan 13]. http://www.ncbi.nlm.nih.gov/pubmed/17693625

[344] Liz MA, Fleming CE, Nunes AF, Almeida MR, Mar FM, Choe Y, et al. Substrate specificity of transthyretin: identification of natural substrates in the nervous system. Biochem J [Internet]. 2009;419(2):467–74 [cited 2016 Jan 13]. http://www.pubmedcentral.nih.gov/articlerender.fcgi?artid=4153561&tool=pmcentrez&rendertype=abstract

[345] Liz MA, Leite SC, Juliano L, Saraiva MJ, Damas AM, Bur D, et al. Transthyretin is a metallopeptidase with an inducible active site. Biochem J [Internet]. 2012;443(3):769–78 [cited 2016 Jan 13]. http://www.ncbi.nlm.nih.gov/pubmed/22332999

[346] Gouvea IE, Kondo MY, Assis DM, Alves FM, Liz MA, Juliano MA, et al. Studies on the peptidase activity of transthyretin (TTR). Biochimie [Internet]. 2013;95(2):215–23 [cited 2016 Jan 13]. http://www.ncbi.nlm.nih.gov/pubmed/23000319

[347] Costa R, Ferreira-da-Silva F, Saraiva MJ, Cardoso I. Transthyretin protects against A-beta peptide toxicity by proteolytic cleavage of the peptide: a mechanism sensitive to the Kunitz protease inhibitor. PLoS One [Internet]. 2008;3(8):e2899 [cited 2015 Dec 9]. http://www.pubmedcentral.nih.gov/articlerender.fcgi?artid=2483353&tool=pmcentrez&rendertype=abstract

[348] Reilly MM, King RH. Familial amyloid polyneuropathy. Brain Pathol [Internet]. 1993;3(2):165–76 [cited 2016 Jan 14]. http://www.ncbi.nlm.nih.gov/pubmed/8293178

[349] Costa PP, Figueira AS, Bravo FR. Amyloid fibril protein related to prealbumin in familial amyloidotic polyneuropathy. Proc Natl Acad Sci USA [Internet]. 1978;75(9): 4499–503 [cited 2016 Jan 14]. http://www.pubmedcentral.nih.gov/articlerender.fcgi?artid=336143&tool=pmcentrez&rendertype=abstract

[350] Biochemical marker in familial amyloidotic polyneuropathy, Portuguese type. Family studies on the transthyretin (prealbumin)-methionine-30 variant. PubMed—NCBI [Internet]. 2016 [cited 2016 Jan 14]. http://www.ncbi.nlm.nih.gov/pubmed/?term=saraiva+mj+1985

[351] Maeda S, Mita S, Araki S, Shimada K. Structure and expression of the mutant prealbumin gene associated with familial amyloidotic polyneuropathy. Mol Biol Med [Internet]. 1986;3(4):329–38 [cited 2016 Jan 14]. http://www.ncbi.nlm.nih.gov/pubmed/3022108

[352] Sousa MM, Cardoso I, Fernandes R, Guimarães A, Saraiva MJ. Deposition of transthyretin in early stages of familial amyloidotic polyneuropathy: evidence for toxicity of nonfibrillar aggregates. Am J Pathol [Internet]. 2001;159(6):1993–2000 [cited 2016 Feb 2]. http://www.pubmedcentral.nih.gov/articlerender.fcgi?artid=1850610&tool=pmcentrez&rendertype=abstract

[353] Berk JL, Suhr OB, Obici L, Sekijima Y, Zeldenrust SR, Yamashita T, et al. Repurposing diflunisal for familial amyloid polyneuropathy: a randomized clinical trial. JAMA. 2013;310(24):2658–67.

[354] Sekijima Y, Tojo K, Morita H, Koyama J, Ikeda S. Safety and efficacy of long-term diflunisal administration in hereditary transthyretin (ATTR) amyloidosis. Amyloid. 2015;22(2):79–83.

[355] Sousa JC, Grandela C, Fernández-Ruiz J, de Miguel R, de Sousa L, Magalhães AI, et al. Transthyretin is involved in depression-like behaviour and exploratory activity. J Neurochem [Internet]. 2004;88(5):1052–8 [cited 2016 Jan 14]. http://www.ncbi.nlm.nih.gov/pubmed/15009661

[356] Heilig M. The NPY system in stress, anxiety and depression. Neuropeptides [Internet]. 2004;38(4):213–24 [cited 2016 Jan 14]. http://www.ncbi.nlm.nih.gov/pubmed/15337373

[357] Nunes AF, Saraiva MJ, Sousa MM. Transthyretin knockouts are a new mouse model for increased neuropeptide Y. FASEB J [Internet]. 2006;20(1):166–8 [cited 2016 Jan 14]. http://www.ncbi.nlm.nih.gov/pubmed/16263939

[358] Sousa JC, Marques F, Dias-Ferreira E, Cerqueira JJ, Sousa N, Palha JA. Transthyretin influences spatial reference memory. Neurobiol Learn Mem [Internet]. 2007;88(3):381–5. http://www.ncbi.nlm.nih.gov/pubmed/17698379

[359] Fleming CE, Saraiva MJ, Sousa MM. Transthyretin enhances nerve regeneration. J Neurochem. 2007;103(2):831–9.

[360] Santos SD, Lambertsen KL, Clausen BH, Akinc A, Alvarez R, Finsen B, et al. CSF transthyretin neuroprotection in a mouse model of brain ischemia. J Neurochem [Internet]. 2010;115(6):1434–44. http://www.ncbi.nlm.nih.gov/pubmed/21044072

[361] Kooijman R. Regulation of apoptosis by insulin-like growth factor (IGF)-I. Cytokine Growth Factor Rev [Internet]. 2006;17(4):305–23 [cited 2016 Jan 14]. http://www.ncbi.nlm.nih.gov/pubmed/16621671

[362] Wisniewski T, Castano E, Ghiso J, Frangione B. Cerebrospinal fluid inhibits Alzheimer®?-amyloid fibril formation in vitro. Ann Neurol [Internet]. 1993;34(4):631–3 [cited 2016 Jan 4]. http://www.ncbi.nlm.nih.gov/pubmed/8215255

[363] Ghiso J, Matsubara E, Koudinov A, Choi-Miura NH, Tomita M, Wisniewski T, et al. The cerebrospinal-fluid soluble form of Alzheimer's amyloid beta is complexed to SP-40,40 (apolipoprotein J), an inhibitor of the complement membrane-attack complex. Biochem J [Internet]. 1993;293(Pt 1):27–30 [cited 2016 Jan 4]. http://www.pubmedcentral.nih.gov/articlerender.fcgi?artid=1134315&tool=pmcentrez&rendertype=abstract

[364] Goldgaber D, Schwarzman AI, Bhasin R, Gregori L, Schmechel D, Saunders AM, et al. Sequestration of amyloid beta-peptide. Ann N Y Acad Sci [Internet]. 1993;695:139–43 [cited 2016 Jan 4]. http://www.ncbi.nlm.nih.gov/pubmed/8239272

[365] Schwarzman AL, Gregori L, Vitek MP, Lyubski S, Strittmatter WJ, Enghilde JJ, et al. Transthyretin sequesters amyloid beta protein and prevents amyloid formation. Proc Natl Acad Sci USA [Internet]. 1994;91(18):8368–72 [cited 2015 Dec 6]. http://www.pubmedcentral.nih.gov/articlerender.fcgi?artid=44607&tool=pmcentrez&rendertype=abstract

[366] Schwarzman AL, Goldgaber D. Interaction of transthyretin with amyloid beta-protein: binding and inhibition of amyloid formation. Ciba Found Symp [Internet]. 1996;199:146–60 [cited 2015 Nov 30]; discussion 160–4. http://www.ncbi.nlm.nih.gov/pubmed/8915609

[367] Serot JM, Christmann D, Dubost T, Couturier M. Cerebrospinal fluid transthyretin: aging and late onset Alzheimer's disease. J Neurol Neurosurg Psychiatry. 1997;63(4): 506–8.

[368] Han S-H, Jung ES, Sohn J-H, Hong HJS, Hong HJS, Kim JW, et al. Human serum transthyretin levels correlate inversely with Alzheimer's disease. J Alzheimers Dis [Internet]. 2011;25(1):77–84. http://www.ncbi.nlm.nih.gov/pubmed/21335655

[369] González-Marrero I, Giménez-Llort L, Johanson CE, Carmona-Calero EM, Castañeyra-Ruiz L, Brito-Armas JM, et al. Choroid plexus dysfunction impairs beta-amyloid clearance in a triple transgenic mouse model of Alzheimer's disease. Front Cell

Neurosci [Internet]. 2015;9:17. http://www.pubmedcentral.nih.gov/articlerender.fcgi?artid=4319477&tool=pmcentrez&rendertype=abstract

[370] Mazur-Kolecka B, Frackowiak J, Wiśniewski HM. Apolipoproteins E3 and E4 induce, and transthyretin prevents accumulation of the Alzheimer's beta-amyloid peptide in cultured vascular smooth muscle cells. Brain Res [Internet]. 1995;698(1–2):217–22 [cited 2016 Jan 4]. http://www.ncbi.nlm.nih.gov/pubmed/8581485

[371] Shirahama T, Skinner M, Westermark P, Rubinow A, Cohen AS, Brun A, et al. Senile cerebral amyloid. Prealbumin as a common constituent in the neuritic plaque, in the neurofibrillary tangle, and in the microangiopathic lesion. Am J Pathol. 1982;107(1):41–50.

[372] Buxbaum JN, Ye Z, Reixach N, Friske L, Levy C, Das P, et al. Transthyretin protects Alzheimer's mice from the behavioral and biochemical effects of Abeta toxicity. Proc Natl Acad Sci USA [Internet]. 2008;105(7):2681–6 [cited 2015 Dec 7]. http://www.pubmedcentral.nih.gov/articlerender.fcgi?artid=2268196&tool=pmcentrez&rendertype=abstract

[373] Stein TD, Anders NJ, DeCarli C, Chan SL, Mattson MP, Johnson JA. Neutralization of transthyretin reverses the neuroprotective effects of secreted amyloid precursor protein (APP) in APPSW mice resulting in tau phosphorylation and loss of hippocampal neurons: support for the amyloid hypothesis. J Neurosci [Internet]. 2004;24(35):7707–17 [cited 2016 Jan 4]. http://www.ncbi.nlm.nih.gov/pubmed/15342738

[374] Stein TD, Johnson JA. Lack of neurodegeneration in transgenic mice overexpressing mutant amyloid precursor protein is associated with increased levels of transthyretin and the activation of cell survival pathways. J Neurosci [Internet]. 2002;22(17):7380–8 [cited 2016 Jan 4]. http://www.ncbi.nlm.nih.gov/pubmed/12196559

[375] Lazarov O, Robinson J, Tang Y-P, Hairston IS, Korade-Mirnics Z, Lee VM-Y, et al. Environmental enrichment reduces Aβ levels and amyloid deposition in transgenic mice. Cell [Internet]. 2005;120(5):701–13 [cited 2015 Oct 7]. http://www.ncbi.nlm.nih.gov/pubmed/15766532

[376] Choi SH, Leight SN, Lee VM-Y, Li T, Wong PC, Johnson J a, et al. Accelerated Abeta deposition in APPswe/PS1deltaE9 mice with hemizygous deletions of TTR (transthyretin). J Neurosci. 2007;27(26):7006–10.

[377] Oliveira SM, Ribeiro CA, Cardoso I, Saraiva MJ. Gender-dependent transthyretin modulation of brain amyloid-β Levels: evidence from a mouse model of alzheimer's disease. J Alzheimer's Dis. 2011;27(2):429–39.

[378] Costa R, Gonçalves A, Saraiva MJ, Cardoso I. Transthyretin binding to A-Beta peptide —impact on a-beta fibrillogenesis and toxicity. FEBS Lett. 2008;582(6):936–42.

[379] Carro E, Trejo JL, Gomez-Isla T, LeRoith D, Torres-Aleman I. Serum insulin-like growth factor I regulates brain amyloid-beta levels. Nat Med [Internet]. 2002;8(12):1390–7 [cited 2015 Dec 29]. http://www.ncbi.nlm.nih.gov/pubmed/12415260

[380] Liu L, Murphy RM. Kinetics of inhibition of beta-amyloid aggregation by transthyretin. Biochemistry [Internet]. 2006;45(51):15702–9 [cited 2016 Jan 4]. http://www.ncbi.nlm.nih.gov/pubmed/17176092

[381] Yang DT, Joshi G, Cho PY, Johnson JA, Murphy RM. Transthyretin as both a sensor and a scavenger of β-amyloid oligomers. Biochemistry [Internet]. 2013;52(17):2849–61 [cited 2016 Jan 5]. http://www.pubmedcentral.nih.gov/articlerender.fcgi?artid=3658121&tool=pmcentrez&rendertype=abstract

[382] Du J, Murphy RM. Characterization of the interaction of β-amyloid with transthyretin monomers and tetramers. Biochemistry [Internet]. 2010;49(38):8276–89 [cited 2016 Jan 5]. http://www.pubmedcentral.nih.gov/articlerender.fcgi?artid=2943652&tool=pmcentrez&rendertype=abstract

[383] Schwarzman AL, Tsiper M, Wente H, Wang A, Vitek MP, Vasiliev V, et al. Amyloidogenic and anti-amyloidogenic properties of recombinant transthyretin variants. Amyloid [Internet]. 2004;11(1):1–9 [cited 2015 Dec 23]. http://www.ncbi.nlm.nih.gov/pubmed/15185492

[384] Palha JA, Moreira P, Wisniewski T, Frangione B, Saraiva MJ. Transthyretin gene in Alzheimer's disease patients. Neurosci Lett [Internet]. 1996;204(3):212–4 [cited 2016 Jan 5]. http://www.ncbi.nlm.nih.gov/pubmed/8938268

[385] Du J, Cho PY, Yang DT, Murphy RM. Identification of beta-amyloid-binding sites on transthyretin. Protein Eng Des Sel [Internet]. 2012;25(7):337–45 [cited 2016 Feb 1]. http://www.pubmedcentral.nih.gov/articlerender.fcgi?artid=3530273&tool=pmcentrez&rendertype=abstract

[386] Merched A, Serot JM, Visvikis S, Aguillon D, Faure G, Siest G. Apolipoprotein E, transthyretin and actin in the CSF of Alzheimer's patients: relation with the senile plaques and cytoskeleton biochemistry. FEBS Lett [Internet]. 1998;425(2):225–8 [cited 2016 Jan 5]. http://www.ncbi.nlm.nih.gov/pubmed/9559653

[387] Hornstrup LS, Frikke-Schmidt R, Nordestgaard BG, Tybjærg-Hansen A. Genetic stabilization of transthyretin, cerebrovascular disease, and life expectancy. Arterioscler Thromb Vasc Biol [Internet]. 2013;33(6):1441–7 [cited 2015 Oct 27]. http://www.ncbi.nlm.nih.gov/pubmed/23580146

[388] Ribeiro CA, Saraiva MJ, Cardoso I. Stability of the transthyretin molecule as a key factor in the interaction with a-beta peptide—relevance in Alzheimer's Disease. PLoS One [Internet]. 2012;7(9):e45368. http://www.pubmedcentral.nih.gov/articlerender.fcgi?artid=3444465&tool=pmcentrez&rendertype=abstract

[389] Cardoso I, Almeida MR, Ferreira N, Arsequell G, Valencia G, Saraiva MJ. Comparative in vitro and ex vivo activities of selected inhibitors of transthyretin aggregation: relevance in drug design. Biochem J. 2007;408(1):131–8.

[390] Ribeiro C a., Oliveira SM, Guido LF, Magalhães A, Valencia G, Arsequell G, et al. Transthyretin stabilization by iododiflunisal promotes amyloid-β peptide clearance, decreases its deposition, and ameliorates cognitive deficits in an Alzheimer's disease mouse model. J Alzheimer's Dis. 2014;39:357–70.

[391] Eckman EA, Reed DK, Eckman CB. Degradation of the Alzheimer's amyloid beta peptide by endothelin-converting enzyme. J Biol Chem [Internet]. 2001;276(27):24540–8 [cited 2015 Dec 27]. http://www.ncbi.nlm.nih.gov/pubmed/11337485

[392] Proteolytic mechanisms in amyloid-beta metabolism: therapeutic implications for Alzheimer's disease. PubMed—NCBI [Internet]. 2016 [cited 2016 Jan 6]. http://www.ncbi.nlm.nih.gov/pubmed/16153892

[393] Malito E, Hulse RE, Tang W-J. Amyloid beta-degrading cryptidases: insulin degrading enzyme, presequence peptidase, and neprilysin. Cell Mol Life Sci [Internet]. 2008;65(16):2574–85 [cited 2016 Jan 14]. http://www.pubmedcentral.nih.gov/articlerender.fcgi?artid=2756532&tool=pmcentrez&rendertype=abstract

[394] Wang Y-J, Zhou H-D, Zhou X-F. Clearance of amyloid-beta in Alzheimer's disease: progress, problems and perspectives. Drug Discov Today [Internet]. 2006;11(19–20): 931–8 [cited 2016 Jan 14]. http://www.ncbi.nlm.nih.gov/pubmed/16997144

[395] Li X, Masliah E, Reixach N, Buxbaum JN. Neuronal production of transthyretin in human and murine Alzheimer's disease: is it protective? J Neurosci [Internet]. 2011;31(35):12483–90 [cited 2015 Nov 16]. http://www.pubmedcentral.nih.gov/articlerender.fcgi?artid=3172869&tool=pmcentrez&rendertype=abstract

[396] Kerridge C, Belyaev ND, Nalivaeva NN, Turner AJ. The Aβ-clearance protein transthyretin, like neprilysin, is epigenetically regulated by the amyloid precursor protein intracellular domain. J Neurochem. 2014;130(3):419–31.

[397] Wang X, Cattaneo F, Ryno L, Hulleman J, Reixach N, Buxbaum JN. The systemic amyloid precursor transthyretin (TTR) behaves as a neuronal stress protein regulated by HSF1 in SH-SY5Y human neuroblastoma cells and APP23 Alzheimer's disease model mice. J Neurosci [Internet]. 2014;34(21):7253–65. http://www.jneurosci.org/content/34/21/7253.short

Chapter 2

Supramolecular Organization of Amyloid Fibrils

Dmitry Kurouski

Additional information is available at the end of the chapter

http://dx.doi.org/10.5772/62672

Abstract

The current chapter illustrates how both electron and scanning probe microscopy can be utilized to unravel the supramolecular organization of amyloid fibrils, β-sheet-rich protein aggregates, which are strongly associated with various neurodegenerative diseases. It also discusses why morphologically different fibrils can be grown from the same protein under slightly different experimental conditions, which is a phenomenon known as fibril polymorphism. Next, it establishes the high potential of vibrational circular dichroism (VCD) for unraveling the supramolecular organization of amyloid fibrils. Finally, it discusses several hypotheses of amyloid fibril formation that were developed based on numerous microscopic and spectroscopic studies.

Keywords: amyloid fibrils, supramolecular chirality, microscopy, VCD, polymorphism or fibril polymorphism

1. Introduction

Under normal physiological conditions, the native structure of partially unfolded proteins is restored by numerous self-sustaining pathways of cell homeostasis. However, under some pathological conditions, such as neurodegenerative diseases, partially unfolded proteins may adopt β-sheet structure [1, 2]. This primarily happens because the β-sheet structure is energetically more favorable when compared to the native structure of the protein. When two β-sheet moieties associate together plane-to-plane, they form a very stable structure, known as a cross-β-sheet. The cross-β-sheet is capable of templating the aggregation of misfolded or partially unfolded proteins. As a result, fibril filament, the simplest supramolecular architecture, is formed. It stretches microns in length in the direction perpendicular the peptide strands in the β-sheets [3–5]. Following electrostatic energy minimization, filaments tend to twist along their longitudinal axis. And as a result, local charges on the fibril surface increase their mutual distance.

Contrastingly, twisted filaments have much higher elastic energy than a flat structure. And consequently, the filaments tend to adopt becoming as relaxed and flat geometrically as possible to reach the elastic energy minimum. The net between these two competing energies, electrostatic and elastic, determines the degree of the filament twist [6, 7].

Twisted filaments also braid and coil with other filaments [8–10], forming higher hierarchical supramolecular structures named proto-fibrils and fibrils [11, 12]. Alternatively, twisted filaments may associate side-by-side, forming cross-β-sheet tape-like fibrils [10, 11]. Different filaments' propagation pathways result in a large diversity of fibril morphologies. This phenomenon is known as fibril polymorphism [3, 13]. *Post-mortem* microscopic examination of fibrils that were detected in the organs and tissue of patients, who were diagnosed with different neurodegenerative diseases, also revealed their morphological heterogeneity [14, 15]. Moreover, *in vitro* studies have demonstrated that morphologically or structurally different fibril polymorphs had different toxicity [16]. And as a result, a clear understanding of fibril supramolecular organization will help to unravel the origin of fibril toxicity.

Methodologically, unraveling the supramolecular organization of amyloid fibrils is a challenging task. This is primarily because fibrils are insoluble and cannot be crystalized, which unfortunately limits X-ray and NMR, classical tools of structural biology, for their studies [17, 18]. Historically, microscopy was the first, and most commonly utilized technique which is capable of unraveling supramolecular organization of amyloid fibrils. There are several microscopes that are effective in resolving amyloid aggregates which include: electron (EM), transmission (TEM), and scanning electron (SEM) microscopes, and lastly probe microscopes. In addition to microscopy, vibrational circular dichroism (VCD) can directly probe supramolecular organization of amyloid fibrils [11, 19]. It was recently discovered that VCD can detect the twist of the fibril filaments, which not always may be visualized using SEM or atomic force microscopy (AFM) [8]. The observed VCD intensities of fully developed fibrils and their filaments are one to two orders of magnitude larger than VCD intensities observed from solutions of individual proteins. This indicates that enhanced VCD arises from the long-range supramolecular chirality of fibrils, making VCD a unique *solution-phase*, stereospecific probe of protein fibril structure and chiral morphology. A growing body of literature indicates that VCD has already become a powerful and broadly used tool for the supramolecular characterization of amyloid aggregates [11, 20, 21].

2. Unraveling supramolecular chirality of amyloid fibrils using microscopy

Conventional light microscopy is not capable of visualizing individual amyloid aggregates due to their small sizes. According to Abbe diffraction limit, a resolution (d) directly depends on a wavelength of light (λ), where α is the half-angle of the maximum cone of light that can enter the microscope objective (1).

http://dx.doi.org/10.5772/62672

$$d = \frac{\lambda}{2\sin(\alpha)} \quad (1)$$

For a microscope objective, the aperture angle is described by the numerical aperture (NA), where NA = n•sinα (n is a media refractive index). Consequently, *d* of any confocal microscope can be expressed as (2).

$$d = \frac{0.61\lambda}{NA} \quad (2)$$

The expression 2 indicates that the resolution increase with the decrease in the wavelength and an increase in the NA of the objective. The best optical systems would be equipped with 100× oil immersed objective (NA=1.4) will give the resolution of ~200 nm. At the same time, amyloid fibrils, as we will discuss below, are only 10–20 nm in diameter. Nevertheless, it should be mentioned that the light microscopy is the most commonly utilized technique in the clinical practice for the confirmatory diagnostic of amyloid plaques. Upon staining with Congo-red, in the linearly polarized light, these amyloid deposits exhibit green birefringence.

Recently invented super-resolution microscopy, such as photoactivated localization microscopy (PALM) and direct stochastical optical reconstruction microscopy (d-STORM), allowed for overcoming the Abbe diffraction limit and reach 2–10 nm spatial resolution [22–24]. For example, d-STORM was capable of resolving individual amyloid β aggregates [25]. However, very limited information about their supramolecular organization could be obtained. Partially, because sample labeling with fluorophores is required, which obscures tiny details of fibril topology. Also, since there are only a few fluorophores are activated per every light exposure in super-resolution microscopy, long acquisition time is typically required for an image processing. Therefore, thermal drift of current super-resolution microscopes becomes the serious issue which limits their spatial resolution.

2.1. Unraveling the shape and localization of amyloid fibrils by TEM

The invention of the electron microscope, by Max Knoll and Ernst Ruska at the Berlin Technische Hochschule, in 1931, allowed for overcoming the limitation of a visible light in obtaining higher spatial resolution. Using TEM, the first morphological characterization of the individual amyloid fibrils was achieved [26, 30]. This microscopic technique is relatively facile when compared to other microscopic tools which will be discussed below. In most cases, only a drop of the analyzed sample is needed to be placed onto a carbon or formvar-coated Cu film support and dried under ambient conditions. Uranium or osmium salts are often applied to the dried sample to increase the contrast of biological samples. Alternatively, samples for TEM can be prepared by cutting plastic embedded biological samples. For example, TEM imaging of the thin-cut plastic embedded amyloid tissues revealed long unbranched rod-like aggregates that were named amyloid fibrils (**Figure 1A**) [26–29]. Aggregates with the same morphology were later reported by M. Kidd upon TEM imaging of the extract of amyloid-loaded liver tissue (**Figure 1B**) [30].

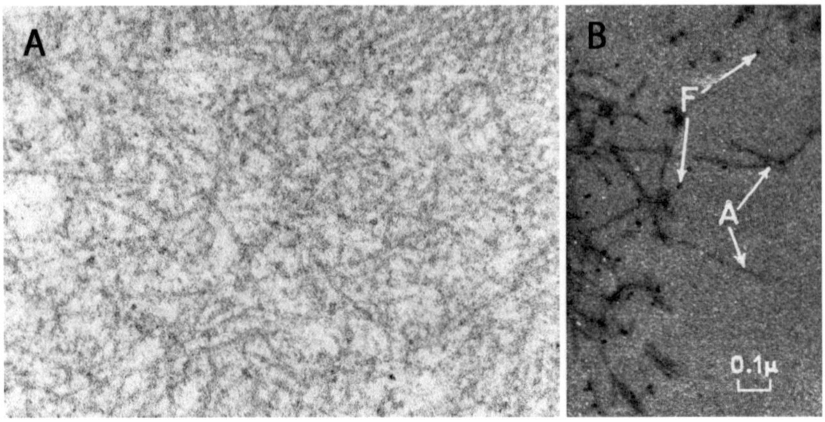

Figure 1. TEM images of amyloid fibrils in (A) thin-cut plastic embedded amyloid tissue (×50,000) and (B) extract of amyloid-loaded liver tissue. Locations of amyloid fibrils and their twisted filaments are marked by "A" and "F" respectively. Adapted from Tosoni et al. [26] and Kidd [30].

Aggregates of Tau proteins, histologically known as neurofibrillary tangles, are commonly co-present together with amyloid plaques in brains of patients, who have been diagnosed with Alzheimer's disease. Their detailed microscopic study conducted by Wischik et al. (**Figure 2**) [14, 15]. Using TEM, Wischik et al. studied the extracts from the human brains that contained neurofibrillary tangles. Authors observed fibrils with flat and twisted topologies. Using metal

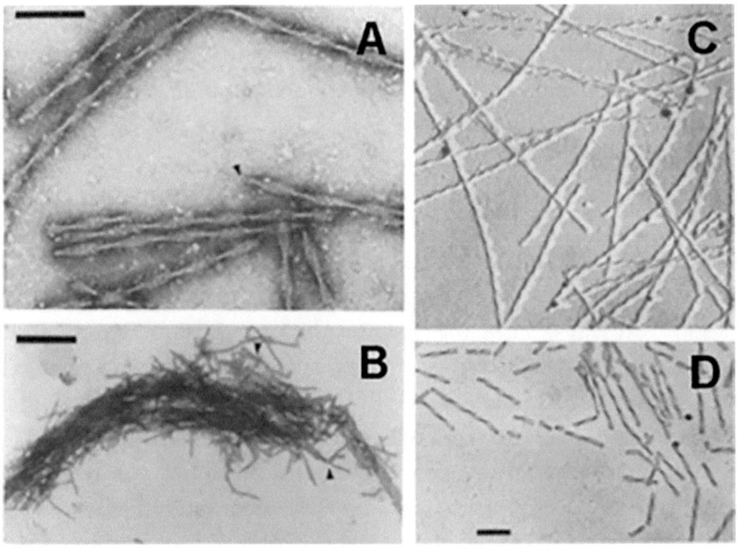

Figure 2. TEM images of uncoated (A, B) and metal coated (C, D) Tau fibrils extracted from the human brain. Scale bards are 100 nm (A, C, D) and 1000 nm (B) [14, 15].

shadowing, Wischik et al. determined the twist direction, which appeared to be left-handed. Additional, it was discovered that these left-twisted fibrils were composed of two intertwined left-handed proto-fibrils. The exposure of left-twisted fibrils to an alkali solution led to their untwining, which made Wischik et al. to conclude that the integrity of left-twisted fibrils was held by electrostatic interactions between their proto-fibrils.

These pioneering works were followed by numerous studies that report TEM microphotographs of various protein aggregates and amyloid fibrils [31, 32]. It has been demonstrated that TEM was capable of detecting twists in ribbon-like fibrils, curvature of fibrils, and the roughness of their surfaces. TEM images could also be used to obtain quantitative data, including dimensions of fibrils and their precursors, such as oligomers and filaments. In addition, TEM was able to reveal a number of filaments in the mature fibril, as well as the periodicity of the fibril twists. However, in most cases, TEM imaging was simply used to confirm a presence of fibril species rather than to provide their morphological characterization. This is in parts because such microscopic examination can be performed relatively quickly, allowing researchers to verify whether fibril formation has occurred or not.

In parallel, TEM was used to monitor changes in the structure of mature fibrils which were caused by various chemical and physical factors [33, 34]. For example, it has been demonstrated that integrity of insulin fibrils could be perturbed through alteration of fibril electrostatic interactions [33]. Shammas et al. exposed insulin fibrils which were grown at pH 2 to solutions with pH 4, 6, 8, 10, and 12. Using TEM, Shammas et al. found that at pH above 4 insulin fibrils drastically changed their morphology (**Figure 3**). Moreover, full disintegration of fibrils was observed if the solution pH was higher than pH 10. It has been concluded that these changes were caused by the strong electrostatic repulsion of the protein amino acid sequence in the fibril cross-β-sheet.

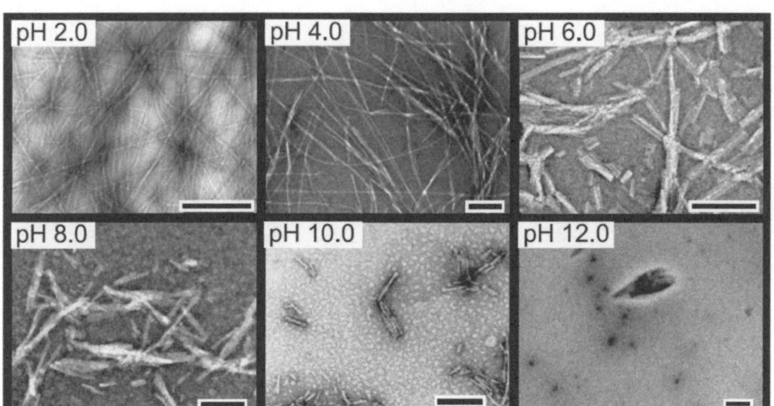

Figure 3. TEM images of insulin fibrils (pH 2.0) after prolong exposition in solvents with higher pHs. Scale bars are 200 nm [34].

Separately, using VCD, Kurouski et al. demonstrated that a small change in pH drastically changes morphology and supramolecular chirality of insulin fibrils [35]. This process was irreversible and occurred only when the pH was raised from 1.5 to 2.5. No effect of solution ionic strength was found. An addition of sodium chloride up to 1 M concentration to pH 1.5 fibrils did not change the kinetics of the polymorphs' inter-conversion.

2.2. Mass-per-length measurements of amyloid fibrils using scanning transmission electron microscopy

As the analog of TEM, scanning transmission electron microscopy (STEM) is often used to explore the morphological organization of amyloid aggregates. Similar to TEM, the background of STEM images has lower intensity than protein specimens. This is due to stronger electron scattering from protein aggregates comparing to a thin carbon film on which they are adsorbed on. As a result, STEM image intensities appear to be proportional to mass densities (per unit area). This can be used to determine mass-per-length (MPL) values of the analyzed specimens [17, 36, 37]. MPL can be determined directly by measuring the incident electron beam flux if the electron scattering cross-sections, as well as the detector geometry and sensitivity are known. Alternatively, MPL can be evaluated by a comparison of the intensities of the analyzed specimens with the intensities of objects with known mass densities. Tobacco mosaic virus (TMV) is the most commonly used reference for such a comparison-based MPL imaging. MPL values can be utilized to determine secondary structure of amyloid fibrils. For

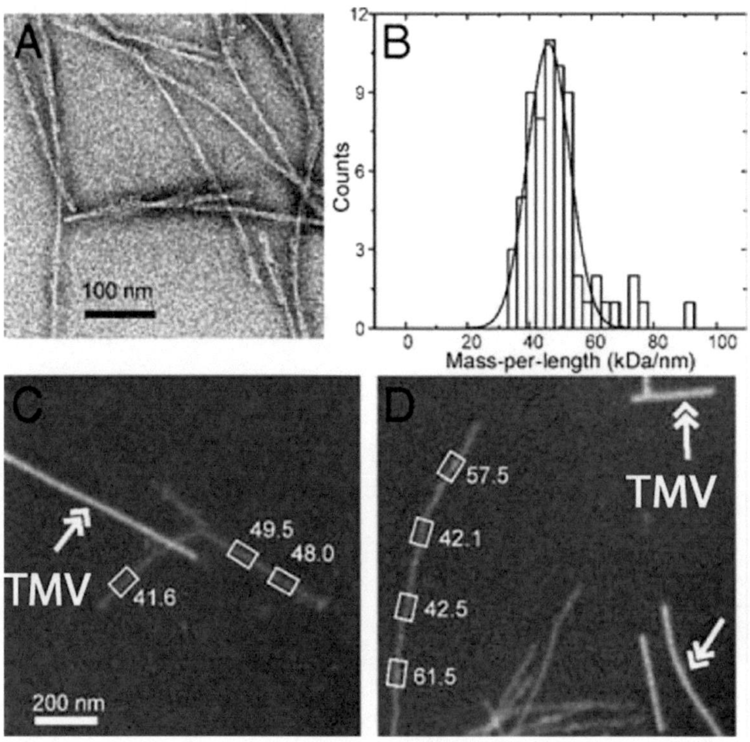

Figure 4. TEM microphotograph (A) of amyloid fibrils grown from Rnq1 prion and their MPL (B) histogram. STEM microphotographs (C and D) or the same fibrils and TMV rods (indicated by double-headed arrows). MPL values (kDa/nm) are shown for fibril segments enclosed in rectangles [39].

example, using MPL, it has been found that 40-residue amyloid β peptide (Aβ1–40) formed two distinct fibril polymorphs with 2- and 3-fold symmetry [36]. MPL measurements confirmed a β-helix-like structure of HET-s prion (HET-s218–289) protein fibrils, where each peptide molecule spanned two turns of the β-helix [38]. It has been also shown that MPL measurements could be used to investigate structural organization of fibrils formed by the yeast prion protein Rnq1 (**Figure 4**) [39]. Chen et al. found that the prion sequence was folded into in-register parallel β-sheet structure, with one Rnq1 molecule per 0.47-nm β-sheet repeat spacing.

2.3. Probing topology and supramolecular chirality of amyloids by SEM

In SEM, both detector and the electron source are located on the same side of the sample. Consequently, only scattered electrons (rather than electrons that go through the sample, as in the case of TEM) are used to obtain the image of the analyzed specimen. SEM also requires much lower energy of the electron beam (0.2–40 keV vs 100–120 keV, as used for TEM) to obtain the contrast image. Similar to TEM, protein samples, such as amyloid fibrils, are commonly stained with uranium or osmium salts prior to microscopic examination to gain a better contrast. While SEM is not capable of resolving amyloid fibrils in the fixed tissues, it provides excessive morphological information about the *in vitro* prepared or *ex vivo* extracted fibrils. One of the most valuable sides of SEM morphological examination is its capacity to determine the twist handedness of amyloid fibrils. For example, using SEM Rubin et al. evaluated supramolecular chirality of fibrils grown from short amino acid fragments of serum amyloid A (SAA) protein [40, 41]. SAA are a group of apolipoproteins associated with high-density

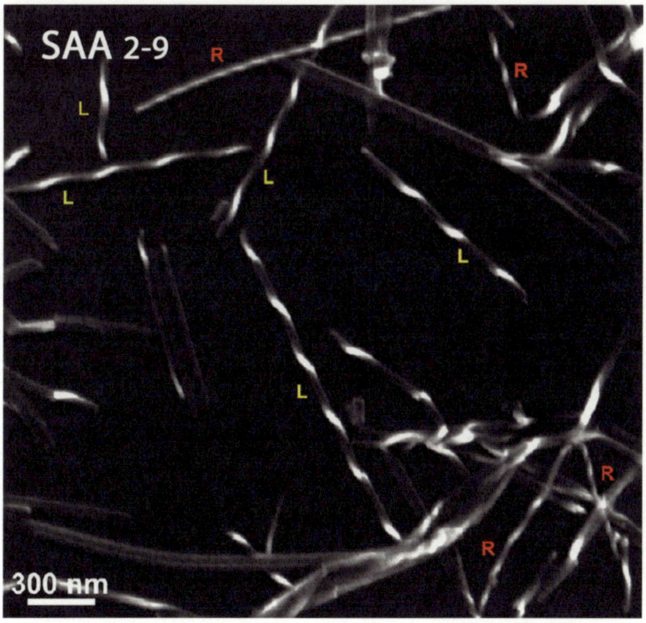

Figure 5. SEM image of simultaneously grown amyloid fibrils of serum amyloid A SAA_{2-6} peptide that exhibit left- and right-twisted fibrils [40].

lipoprotein (HDL) in blood plasma that are often expressed in response to inflammatory stimuli in liver.

Rubin et al. found that SAA fragment with the sequence SFFSFLG (SAA_{2-6}) simultaneously formed both left- and right-twisted fibrils (**Figure 5**). It was also found that fibrils with the same twist direction had different twist periodicity. Some of the right-twisted fibrils were highly twisted (**Figure 3**, fibril marked R at the top), while others had much more of a loose twist (**Figure 3**, fibrils marked R on the right and bottom). This indicated that several right-twisted fibril polymorphs have simultaneously grown. Rubin et al. also discovered that SAA_{2-12} with the sequence SFFSFLGEAFD exclusively formed right-twisted fibrils, while its analog with only two different amino acids, SAA_{1-11}RSFFSFLGEAF aggregated in 100% left-twisted fibrils [40]. This discovery suggested that amino acid sequence may control the supramolecular chirality of amyloid aggregates.

At the same time, Kurouski et al. demonstrated that fibril morphology and supramolecular chirality can be directly controlled by pH [8, 42]. Insulin and lysozyme aggregation at pH below 2 (25°C) led to a formation of tape-like flat fibrils [11]. At the same time, at pH above this point, both of these proteins formed left-twisted fibrils (**Figure 6**) [8]. A fragment of transthyretin (105–115) and HET-s prion (HET-s218–289) protein, on the opposite, formed left twisted fibrils at low pH (25°C), while their aggregation at pH above 2.5 resulted in flat tape-like fibrils [11]. HET-s is a prion protein of the fungus *Podospora anserine*, which C-terminus fragment is capable of forming amyloid fibrils at low pH. Authors suggested that protonation/deprotonation of aspartic and glutamic amino acid residues, as well as peptide C-termini, which was taking place around this pH, changed the charge on the surface of the filaments. As a result, filaments adopted either left-handed or right handed twist. Left twisted filaments tended to braid and coil forming left-handed fibrils. At the same time, right twisted filaments associated side-by-side forming tape-like fibrils [11].

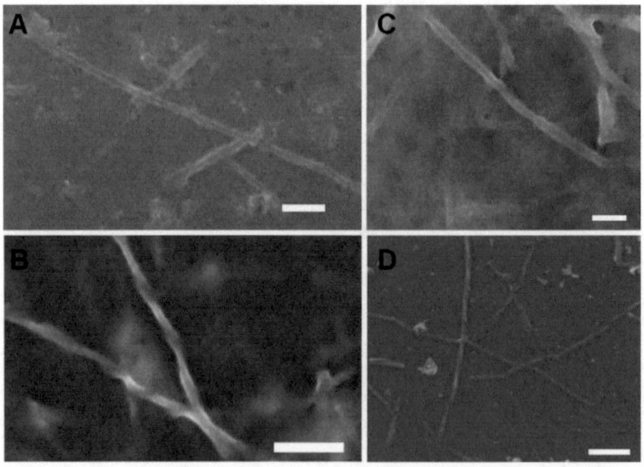

Figure 6. SEM images of insulin (A, B) and lysozyme (C and D) tape-like (top panel) and twisted (bottom panel) fibrils [8]. Twists on the fibril surface are marked by red arrows. Scale bars are 100 nm.

2.4. Application of cryo-SEM for determination of amyloid fibril topology

Typically, both TEM and SEM require sample dehydration. Protein specimens in general and amyloid fibrils in particular are very sensitive to dehydration, which may cause drastic changes in their morphology. To overcome this limitation, cryo-procedure of the sample preparation is often used. In cryo-SEM, protein specimens are imaged at temperature below ambient (typically between −100 and −175°C). This allows for the sample to be preserved and recorded in the fully hydrated and chemically unmodified state.

Cryo-SEM has been extensively used to investigate supramolecular organization of amyloid aggregates that strongly associated with Alzheimer's and Parkinson's diseases. For example, using cryo-EM, Meinhardt et al. found that Aβ(1–40) peptide could form amyloid fibrils with a range of different morphologies [43]. Authors showed that proto-fibrils could associate either side-by-side, forming tape-like fibrils, or coil (intertwine), forming twisted cables. It has been also shown that despite the width of the coiled fibrils varied from 10 to 21 nm, all of them exhibited the same left-handed twist with a turnover from 65 to 163 nm. It was concluded that such difference in the fibril thickness could be due to a different number of proto-filaments that were taking place in their formation [44].

Antzutkin et al. investigated an aggregation of Arctic mutant of Aβ(1–40). It has been shown that this peptide formed seven fibril polymorphs (three non-coiled and four coiled) if aggregated at pH 7.4, 22°C [45]. Moreover, Antzutkin et al. demonstrated that these fibril polymorphs with different morphologies had dramatically different growth rates. It has been found that Aβ(1–40) fibril morphologies could have significant variations in both width and twist tightness, depending on the ionic strength (and the nature of ions) in the aggregation solution [46]. Finally, Petkova et al. investigated the sample agitation impact on the morphology of Aβ(1–40) fibrils. Using microscopy and solid-state NMR (ss-NMR), significant structural differences between fibrils that were grown with and without agitation were found [47].

Supramolecular organization and polymorphism of Aβ(1–42) fibrils are much less investigated comparing to Aβ(1–40) fibrils. Using cryo-SEM, Lührs et al. investigated structural organization of Aβ(1–42) fibrils and found that they were composed of several filaments that had ~2.5 nm in height and around 4.5 nm in width [48]. These filaments braided and coiled together forming thick left-handed cables. Later, Zhang et al. confirmed that Aβ(1–42) formed exclusively left-handed fibrils [49]. It has been also suggested that Aβ(1–42) filaments intertwined around each other, forming a hollow core.

In 2008, Vilar et al. reported results of a very detailed investigation of supramolecular organization of α-synuclein fibrils [50]. Using cryo-SEM and ss-NMR, Vilar et al. found that α-synuclein aggregated formed straight filaments that were around 2 nm in width. These filaments tended to dimerize into thicker proto-fibrils via side-to-side association, forming straight tape-like fibrils. At the same time, they it has been noticed that these filaments could braid together forming left-handed proto-fibrils, with a diameter of ~6.5 nm, and fibrils with a diameter of 9.8 nm (**Figure 7**) [50]. In fact, both straight and twisted α-synuclein fibril polymorphs were detected upon the *post mortem* examination of brains of people who were diagnosed with Parkinson's disease [51, 52].

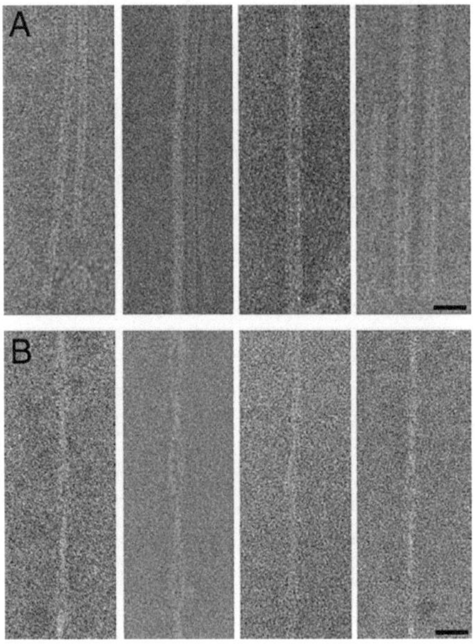

Figure 7. Cryo-SEM images of tape-like (top row) and twisted (bottom row) α-synuclein fibrils. Scale bars are 20 nm [50].

Recently, using cryo-SEM, Rubin et al. examined how the absolute chiral configuration of the amino acids in a peptide sequence impacts on the supramolecular organization of the peptide aggregates [41].

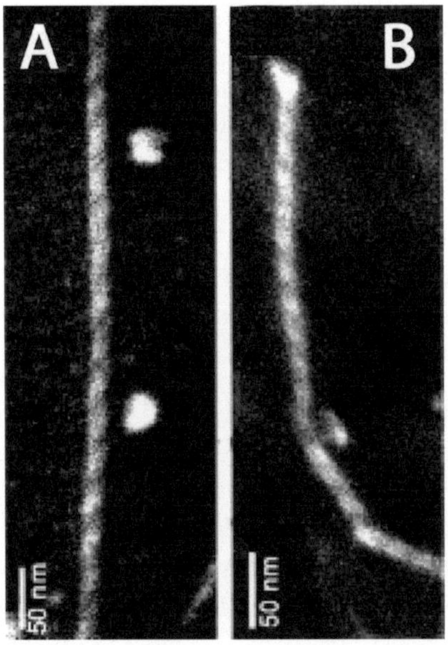

Figure 8. Cryo-SEM images of fibrils grown from all-L amino acid (A) and all-R (B) amino acid fragment of serum amyloid A (SAA_{1-12}) protein [41].

It has been found that all L amino acid peptide with the sequence RSFFSFLGEAFD (SAA_{1-12}) formed right-handed fibrils (**Figure 8**). At the same time, aggregation of the same amino acid sequence with all D amino acids led to a formation of exclusively left-twisted fibrils. Separately, Harper et al. demonstrated the same for $A\beta_{(1-40)}$ peptide. It has been found that all L amino acid $A\beta_{(1-40)}$ peptide formed left-handed fibrils twist. At the same time, aggregation of all D amino acid peptide $A\beta_{(1-40)}$ resulted in right-handed fibrils. These experimental pieces of evidence demonstrate that absolute chiral configuration of the peptide sequence may determine whether one or another chiral polymorph will be grown.

2.5. AFM is capable of unraveling mechanisms of fibril formation and structural organization of amyloids

In AFM, silicon or silicon nitride cantilever is used to image the sample. Changes in the frequency of tip oscillation, as it is moved across the surface (tapping mode AFM), are recorded by the laser that is reflected from the back side of the cantilever. As higher the object on the surface, as smaller becomes the amplitude of the tip oscillation. In another modification of AFM, known as contact-mode AFM (CM-AFM), the tip is not oscillating above the surface, but rather steadily kept at it. When CM-AFM tip is moved across the surface, it simply reflects its roughness, similar to a finger of a blind person who reads the Braille font. One can imagine that the CM-AFM cantilever can easily damage fine protein samples upon such microscopic examination. This much rarely happens in AC-AFM because the tip is being repulsed from the surface as soon as van der Waals forces appear between the two. Therefore, CM-AFM is much less frequently used for imaging biological samples, including amyloid fibrils.

One advantage of AFM over EM is its ability to image the specimen without any dehydration or fixation. This is extremely important for microscopic characterization of protein samples, such as amyloid fibrils. It should be noted that AFM provides an accurate height of the imaged specimen, while width often appear slightly larger than the real width of the imaged object. This error is known as the tip convolution effect. It arises from the tip that is used for the sample imaging: as larger the tip diameter and smaller the object on the surface, as larger the tip convolution error. Therefore, AFM and SEM are commonly used complimentary to each other for a determination of accurate height (AFM) and width (SEM) of the analyzed specimens [8, 11].

Using AFM, Mezenga group recently investigated aggregation of bovine serum albumin (BSA) [53]. Usov et al. found that BSA aggregated forming flexible filaments with left-handed twisted morphology. On later stages of fibril formation, they observed rigid fibrils that either had no twist or were right-twisted. Usov et al. proposed that tube-like structures could be formed if the left-twisted filaments would continue twisting along their longitudinal axis. Such super-twisting would finally result in a formation of a hollow tube. Usov et al. also proposed that observed right-handed twisted ribbons could be formed if left-handed filaments would continue to twist passing through the tube stage. This paradigm is very easy to visualize with a piece of rope. If a degree of left-handed twist will be increased, the left-twitted rope would suddenly start making right-handed twists. Therefore, Usov et al. concluded that observed right-twisted fibrils had the left-handed twist of their internal filaments [53].

Adamcik et al. recently demonstrated that the degree of the fibril twist could be changed by the solvent ionic strength. It has been shown that if β-lactoglobulin was aggregated in 100 mM NaCl, it formed tape-like fibrils. However, at 0 mM NaCl, grown fibrils tended to adopt a left-handed twist. It has been concluded that as lower the ionic strength, as higher the twist degree of the formed β-lactoglobulin fibrils [54].

Mezzenga group also explored how pH controlled supramolecular organization of amyloid fibril growth at water-air interface (AWI) [55, 56]. It was discovered that small change in pH caused significant differences in interfacial properties of β-lactoglobulin fibrils, such as their alignment, entanglement, multilayer formation, and fibril fracture. For example, at pH 2, β-lactoglobulin fibrils did not change their aggregation state after 5-hour exposition at AWI (**Figure 9**). However, at pH 3, these fibrils tended to associate into bundles rather than stay in nematic domains. It has been concluded that such drastic changes were caused by the change of the charge on the fibril surface [56].

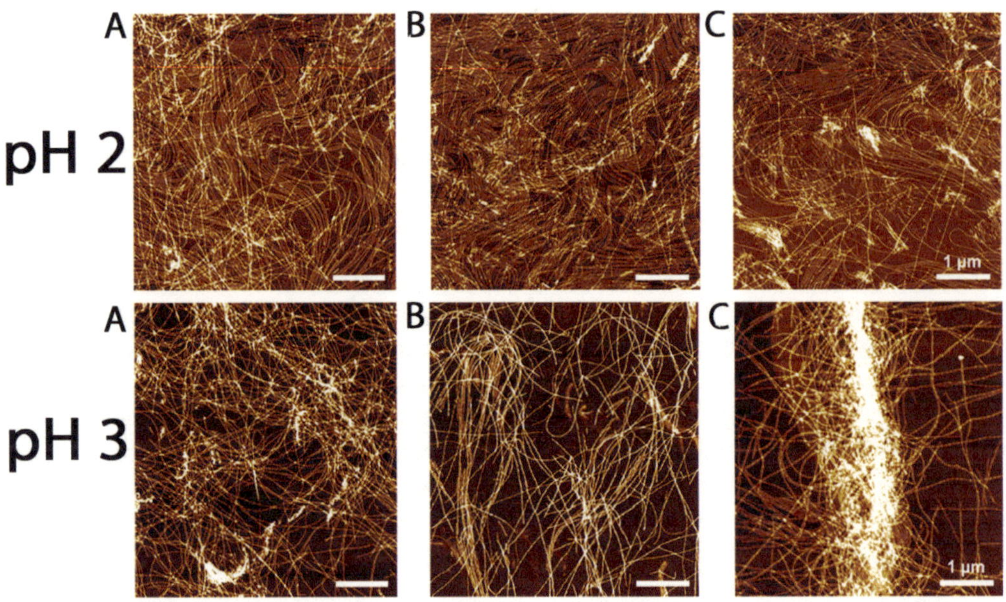

Figure 9. β-Lactoglobulin fibrils on water-air interface at pH 2 (top) and 3 (bottom) after (A) 1, (B) 2, and 5 hours (C). Modified from Jordens et al. [56].

Nearly a decade ago, it was demonstrated that vortexing of insulin solutions during protein aggregation at 60°C caused formation of similar bundled fibril superstructures [57, 58]. In addition to AFM, Dzwolak group explored chiroptical properties of these insulin bundles using induced circular dichroism (ICD) [59]. In ICD, an achiral chromophore is used to probe the structure of a chiral molecule that has very low intensity of circular dichroism signal. It has been found that these fibril superstructures are capable of binding thioflavin T (ThT), which results in a negative induced circular dichroism (−ICD). However, if the protein aggregation

http://dx.doi.org/10.5772/62672

was carried out at steady-state conditions, insulin fibrils did not form bundles and consequently no enhanced ICD signal was observed.

Mezzenga group also explored aggregation of α-synuclein at AWI and solid-liquid interfaces using AFM [60]. They found that at AWI, α-synuclein rapidly aggregated into amyloid fibrils that remained adsorbed to the AWI. Instead, when the protein aggregation was taken place at solid-liquid interface, α-synuclein aggregation is greatly reduced. This finding demonstrated that protein aggregation is a very complex process that can be altered by varying solution conditions and presence of interfaces that can either accelerate or decelerate fibril formation.

Separately, Qin et al. aggregated α-synuclein in similar conditions (10 mM phosphate buffer, pH 7.4) and found that mature fibrils have a left-handed twist [61]. They also elucidated the role of two terminal fragments of α-synuclein. It was found that the protein without the first 29 amino acids from the N terminus (syn30–140) formed fibrils similar to the intact α-synuclein. These fibrils had a right-twisted twist and were composed of two filaments and were around 107 nm in height (AFM), **Figure 10**.

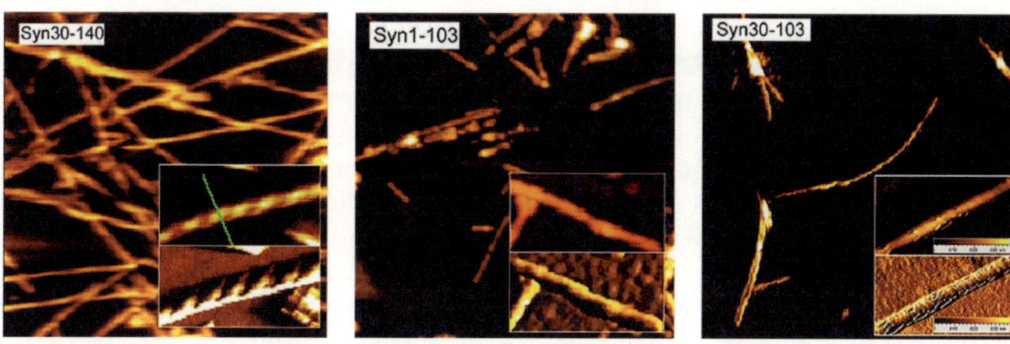

Figure 10. Morphology of the fibrils derived from three truncated α-synucleins. The inserted panels in each AFM image are a single fibril (upper) and its second derivative image (lower). Syn30–140 fibrils show long, straight morphology, and the double-filament twisted structure is observed in the enlarged fibril and its second derivative images (attributed to a pair of twisted protofibrils). Syn1–103 gives much thinner fibrils, but double-filament twisted structure is also observed (attributed to a protofibril consisting of two protofilaments). Syn30–103, however, shows very thin fibrils with a single filament and untwisted structure (attributed to a protofilament) [61].

Intriguingly, according to their AFM images, full-length α-synuclein fibrils were almost 140 nm in height. It has also been found that C-terminal truncated α-synuclein (syn1–103) was able to aggregate. However, this 103 amino acid peptide formed fibrils with smaller height (~57 nm). These fibrils, like syn30–140, also exhibited a right-handed twist. According to the Qin et al., syn1–103 fibrils looked rather like proto-fibrils than mature fibrils [61]. Based on this observation, authors made a conclusion that C-terminus of α-synuclein was highly important for the assembly of two proto-fibrils into a mature fibril. Finally, the central sequence fragment of α-synuclein that lacked both N- and C-termini, syn30–103, was found to be able to aggregate forming long un-branched fibrils. However, these fibrils were only 28.8 nm in height with no clear twist evident from the obtained AFM images.

Using AFM, Jansen et al. performed a detailed investigation of insulin aggregates that were grown at pH 1.6 [62]. It was determined that insulin proto-fibrils, which had around 1.2 nm in diameter, intertwined, forming left-handed fibrils with 3–7 nm in diameter. In addition, right-handed fibrils were simultaneously observed. Intriguingly, that it has been proposed that these right-handed fibrils were formed not as a result of proto-fibril coiling, but rather as a result of a lateral aggregation or small fibril blocks (10 × 60 nm). This aggregation mechanism will be further discussed in the last section of this chapter. This type (side-by-side) of aggregation was also proposed as the origin of binary, tape-like ribbons that were also observed upon insulin aggregation. Finally, authors observed that many insulin fibrils formed from small (~150 nm in length) subunits that are linearly extend one other. Based on this observation, Jansen et al. proposed that insulin fibrils can assemble via chainlike quenching of these subunits.

Human amylin is a 3.9 kDa protein secreted by islet β-cells of the pancreas. Together with insulin, it is involved in glucose metabolism. Amylin fibril aggregates are toxic and strongly associated with diabetes type II. Upon *invitro* aggregation at neutral pH (7.4), amylin forms thin proto-fibrils, which are around 5 nm in width and tend to aggregate further, forming two morphologically distinct polymorphs. In one case, proto-fibrils intertwine (coil), and form cable-like structures 8–10 nm in width with a distinct left-handed twist with a crossover of 25 nm. These cable-like structures could coil further, forming thick left-handed cables with larger widths. In addition, the height of these twisted fibrils has been determined. It has been shown that it varies from 3 (proto-fibrils) to 7 nm mature fibril cables [63]. Alternatively, three, four, or more proto-fibrils could aggregate side-by-side, forming flat, single-layer ribbons. Intriguing that the ribbons also twist at moderate regular intervals in a left-handed fashion [31]. Based on these observations, Goldsbury et al. proposed that amylin fibril polymorphism originated from different ways of proto-fibril associations, while all observed fibril polymorphs have the same structure [64]. There was no clear understanding about the nature of a force that determined the formation of either type of those polymorphs. Three years later, Goldsbury et al. investigated aggregation of the full-length amylin (37 amino acids) and two fragments of amylin: 8–37 and 20–29. It was found that 20–29 fragment formed exclusively flat-ribbons, which were around 40 nm in width. However, 8–37 fragment, similar to the full-length amylin, formed fibril polymorphs with variable morphologies. Most of them were left-handed cables with 25 or 50 nm cross-over and flat-like ribbons [32]. Thus, based on this observation, authors proposed that peptide sequence was directly responsible for the determination of the fibril morphology.

2.5.1. Changes in supramolecular chirality upon fibril disintegration

Recently, Kurouski et al. explored how supramolecular architecture of insulin fibrils could be changed by bacterial chaperonins. The interactions of heat shock proteins with amyloid fibrils have drawn significant attention in recently years. However, most of these studies focused on one group of heat shock proteins with small molecular mass, so called small heat shock proteins [65–67]. Many small heat shock proteins have been reported to disassemble fibrils or prevent the fibrillation process *in vitro* [68].

Kurouski et al. investigated the effect on the mutant chaperonin complex from *Pyrococcusfuriosus* (Pf) on insulin fibrils [69]. This chaperonin (Cpn) was composed of identical subunits and commonly found in most hyperthermophiles [70]. Cpn was mutated to reach its optimum activity below 50°C. Using AFM, Kurouski et al. found that after 5 min of incubation of insulin fibrils with Cpn, fibrils were found fragmented (**Figure 11**) [69].

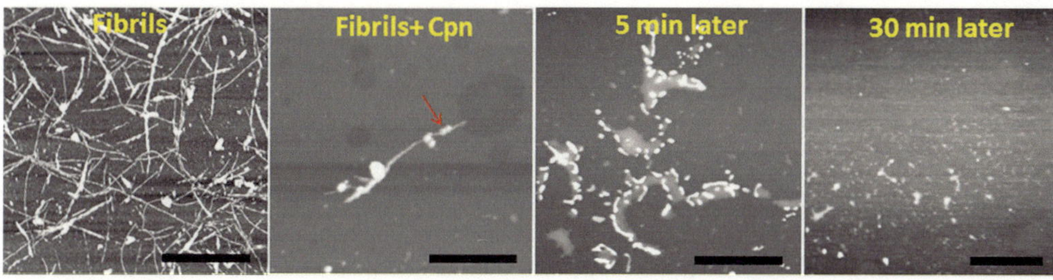

Figure 11. AFM kinetic examination of the insulin fibrils (Fibrils) mixed with Cpn and deposited right away (Fibrils + Cpn), five (5 min later) and half an hour (30 min later) later on mica surface. Immediately upon mixing, Cpn absorb on the fibril surfaces (shown with red arrow). As a result of these Cpn-Fibril interactions the last swell and break apart (5 min later). Even some fibril fragments that are evident on the early microscopic examination (5 min later) disappear after 30 min (30 min later). The scale bar is 1 μm [69].

The foreshortened fibrils looked like swollen clamps with significantly lower height (~6 nm) and width up to 200–400 nm. Interestingly, white image features on the edges of these clamps mimicked the outline of the original fibrils. Most likely they were fibrillar regions that were not melted by Cpn because the reaction was quickly terminated. These observations confirmed that Cpn was able to change the fibril architecture. Kurouski et al. concluded that Cpn melted the fibril core and formed an amorphous protein mass from regular β-sheet structure. Microscopic observations of this phenomenon also indicated a fibril swelling. Authors also found that longer exposure of insulin fibrils to Cpn resulted in their further fragmentation into smaller and smaller species with irregular shapes. These species coagulated during late stages, forming large amorphous aggregates. Most of the fibril-shaped species disappeared and predominantly amorphous objects form after 30 min of Cpn-fibril co-incubation were observed (**Figure 11**) [69].

In this section, supramolecular organization of amyloid fibrils that were formed by most of known amyloid-associated proteins was discussed. It was shown that an aggregation of these proteins may result in either flat, left- or right-twisted fibrils. Very often several different fibril polymorphs can be grown simultaneously. Numerous research findings indicate that fibril polymorphism can be controlled by pH. At the same time, there are several studies which showed that amino acid sequence can determine supramolecular organization of amyloid fibrils. This section also demonstrated that microscopy can be utilized to monitor changes in the fibril morphology during fibril formation. Moreover, microscopy can be used to monitor changes in the structure of mature fibrils, which can be initiated by chemical or physical factors, or triggered by biological molecules, such as chaperonins. Based on these finding one can envision that amyloid fibrils are dynamic rather than static thermodynamic systems and that small change in pH or salinity may change fibril morphology or aggregation state of fibrils at the interfaces.

3. Vibrational circular dichroism a unique tool for the determination of fibril supramolecular organization

VCD is a unique spectroscopic technique that is capable of probing supramolecular chirality of amyloid fibrils [19, 42, 71]. In VCD, left (L)- and right (R)-circularly polarized infra-red (IR) light pass through the sample. It is well known that solutions of two enantiomers have different absorption of left- vs right-circularly polarized light. This physical principle is used to determine the absolute configuration or small chiral molecules, as well as to unravel supramolecular organization of macromolecules. VCD probes deeper levels of fibril supramolecular chiral organization that may not be apparent to existing forms of microscopy [8]. It was also shown that enhanced VCD sensitivity arose directly from the long-range supramolecular chirality of fibril structures at all hierarchical levels [11]. Measey and Schweitzer-Stenner modeled VCD spectra of a fibril filament that had only two peptide units long, run perpendicular to the filament axis direction [72]. The model was based on exciton coupling among amide I transition dipoles arrayed as dual, stacked β-sheet ribbons. They introduced a 2° left-hand twist between the strands yielding a long-range gradual helical twist of the filament with a one full-turn distance of 180 strands. It was found that such a structure yields enhanced VCD with a negative VCD band near 1620 cm^{-1} and a positive VCD band to higher wavenumber frequencies. A corresponding 2° intrastrand helical twist in the opposite direction, corresponding to a right-hand helical filament, reversed the sign of the enhanced VCD couplet and corresponds to the reversed VCD. This theoretical work demonstrated that VCD directly was capable of a determination of the supramolecular chiral organization of fibril filaments.

Recently, it has been found that insulin aggregation at pH 2.1 and higher results in the formation of fibrils that show a strong VCD spectrum with peaks near 1554, 1593, 1627, 1647, 1670 cm^{-1} that have (+ + – + +) sign pattern [42]. The fibril VCD spectrum with this sign patters was called "normal VCD." Microscopic examination of these fibrils indicated that a majority of them had a left-handed helical twist [8]. However, if the pH of the aggregation solution is lower than 2.4, the distribution of fibrils shifts to increasingly flat, tape-like, or binary fibrils as the incubation pH continues to be lowered that under microscopic examination show no noticeable chirality or twist on their surface. Nevertheless, these fibrils show a strong, but often somewhat smaller, VCD with a sign pattern (– – + – –) that is nearly the mirror-image of "normal" VCD fibril spectrum and is referred to as the "reversed" polymorph. The fact that flat tape-like fibrils show a strong reversed VCD signal indicates that they must be composed of right-handed filaments, the chirality of which lies below the limit of AFM or SEM detection. The combined VCD-microscopic studies showed that pH determines not only the net handedness of the filaments, precursors of mature fibrils, but also controls their association pathways. Left-handed filaments intertwine, forming left-handed proto-fibrils and mature fibrils that have normal VCD. On the other hand, right-handed filaments associate side-by-side, forming flat, tape-like, or binary fibrils. Thus, pH most likely alters protein-

http://dx.doi.org/10.5772/62672

solvent interactions or causes protonation of some amino acid side chains, which are lying on the surface of the filaments. These changes cause variations in the way these filaments bind together to form mature fibrils that either twist together to form braids or align side-by-side without braiding. In addition, it was discovered that pH not only determines insulin fibril morphology and net chirality at the stage of the protein aggregation, but also may dramatically change the morphology of mature fibrils and overturn their initial chirality.

Most likely, the sensitivity of amino-acid side chains to the aqueous solvent is responsible for this pH sensitivity. Moreover, different ways of constituent side-chains, exposed or not to the solvent, result in different pH sensitivity (high versus low) for the sense of filament chirality observed. This is a long-range fibril property that likely cannot be predicted, even qualitatively, without a realistic model of protein side chain influence on the sense of helical chirality as a function of pH. Moreover, the chirality of individual fibril filaments lies below the sensitivity of AFM or SEM imaging, but can be observed with VCD at the initial and subsequent stages of fibril formation [11].

A growing body of literature indicates that VCD has become a useful tool for the chiral characterization of amyloid aggregates. For example, Measey and Schweitzer-Stenner recently reported a large enhancement of VCD upon aggregation of short polypeptides [73]. They also demonstrated that mature fibrils formed from the N-terminal peptide fragment of the yeast prion protein, Sup35, and the amyloidogenic alanine-rich peptide AKY8 have opposite signed VCD. It has been also demonstrated that opposite signed VCD spectra could be obtained for mature fibrils formed from poly-L or -D glutamic acid [74]. Polyglutamic acid formed spirally twisted aggregates with handedness determined by the amino acid chirality (left-handed for Land right-handed for D).

4. Models of amyloid fibril formation

Accumulated experimental evidence suggested three protein aggregation pathways that lead to the discussed above morphological heterogeneity of amyloid fibrils. According to the first one, fibril polymorphism could be caused by deviations at the stage of monomer-monomer associations, while protein oligomers are formed [75]. Consequently, these structurally different oligomers will lead to structurally and morphologically different fibrils. For example, Srinivasan et al. recently investigated morphologies and structural organization of prefibrilar oligomers and mature fibrils formed from two murine serum amyloid A (SAA) isoforms, named SAA1.1 and SAA2.2 [75]. These two isoforms only have a difference in six amino acids [76]. SAA1.1 had an oligomer-rich fibrillation lag phase of a few days, while SAA2.2 formed small fibrils within a few hours, exhibiting virtually no lag phase [77]. Structural differences of SAA 1.1 and SAA 2.2 resulted in morphological differences of their filaments and consequently fibrils. Specifically, SAA 2.2 formed worm-like filaments that were able to coil and braid. At the same time, the filaments and proto-fibrils of SAA 1.1 had a rod-like supramolecular organization. They were unable to braid and formed thick straight fibrils. Using CD and Raman spectroscopy Srinivasan et al. confirmed structural differences between SAA 1.1 and SAA 2.2 oligomers and fibrils.

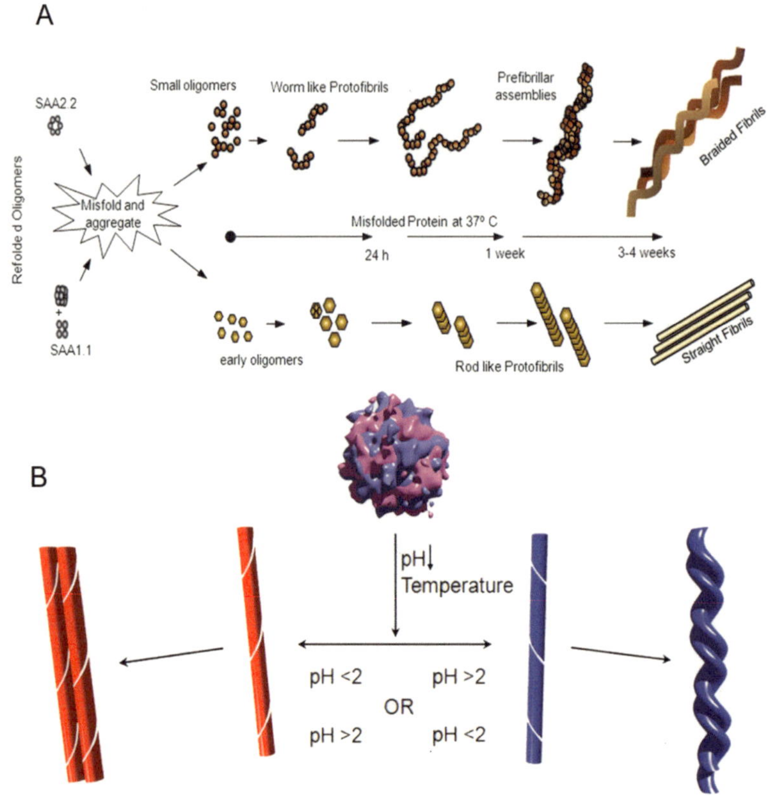

Scheme 1. Models of amyloid fibril formation. Differences in the morphology of mature fibrils can be caused by different ways of protein-protein aggregation on the stage of fibril oligomers' formation (A). Alternatively, protein aggregation leads to the formation of a filament that is able to intertwine forming twisted fibrils, or associate side-by-side (B). In the late case, tape-like fibrils are formed. Adapted from Srinivasan et al. [77] and Kurouski et al. [11].

Alternatively, the heterogeneity of fibril morphologies could be due to different ways of filament associations. Specifically, fibril filaments can either braid and coil or associate side-by-side, forming twisted or tape-like fibrils, respectively (**Scheme 1B**). These morphologically different fibrils will consequently have the same structure [8, 11]. Recently, Kurouski et al. investigated polymorphism of insulin, lysozyme, apo-α-lactalbumin, HET-s (218–289) prion, and a short polypeptide fragment of transtherytin, TTR (105–115). Authors demonstrated that all these proteins form two distinct fibril polymorphs: tape-like and twisted. They have also found that pH directly controls which polymorph will be formed. Using IR and Raman spectroscopy it has been demonstrated that both tape-like and twisted fibril polymorphs have the same secondary structure [11].

Besides braiding and side-by-side association, filament propagation can occur via several alternative pathways. According to Jansen et al. filament fragmentation may result in short filament fragments that serve as templates for lateral rather than axial protein aggregation [62]. As a result, short fibril blocks are formed (**Scheme 2A**). These blocks tend to associate side-by-side forming the fibril that has a right-handed twist upon the microscopic examination.

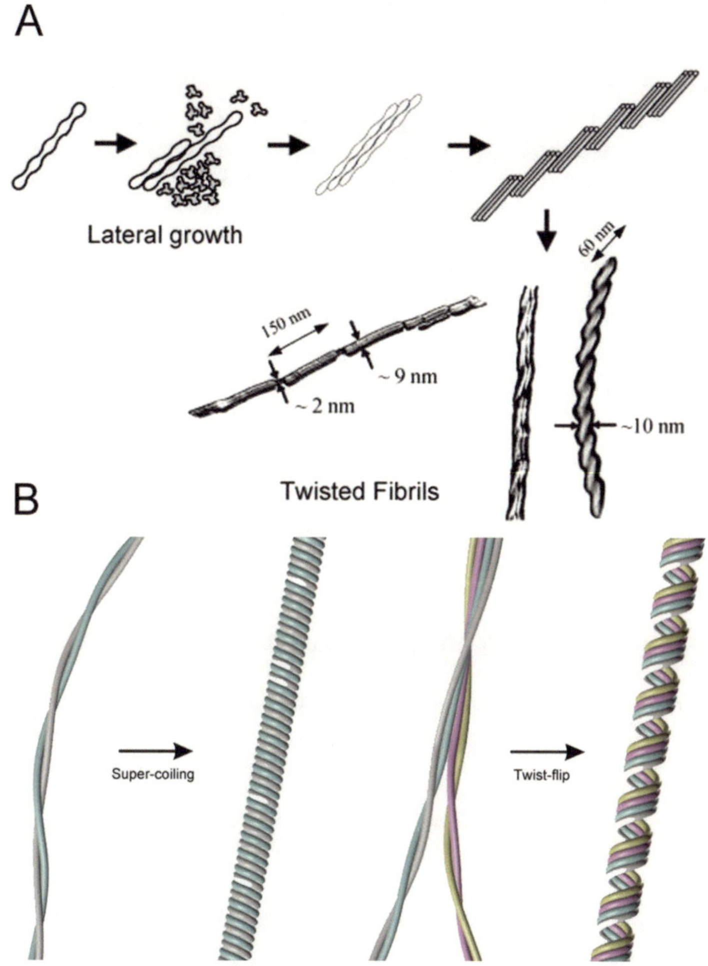

Scheme 2. Models of amyloid filament propagation. Mechanism of side-driven templation (A) and super-coiling of left-twisted fibril filament that leads to the appearance of a right-handed twist on the mature fibril (B). Adapted from R. Jansen et al. [62] and Usov et al. [53].

Separately, Usov et al. proposed two additional mechanisms that resulted in formation of morphologically different fibril polymorphs [53]. According to one, the left-twisted filament may continue twisting along the longitude axis. As a result, a hollow tube-like protein aggregate will be formed. Alternatively, it has been proposed that the left-twisted fibril filament may flip the handedness of its twist, as was discussed in the Section 2.5.

Summarizing, this chapter aimed to demonstrate how microscopy, including electron and probe microscopy, can be utilized to investigate supramolecular organization of amyloid aggregates. It demonstrated that microscopy was capable of elucidating mechanisms of fibril formation and unraveling the origin of fibril polymorphism. It was also shown that using AFM, SEM, and cryo-SEM, chiral nature of fibril supramolecular organization can be determined. The author also wanted to attract reader's attention to VCD. This powerful spectroscopic tool is capable of probing supramolecular chirality of fibril filaments that may to always be accessible for currently available microscopic techniques.

This chapter reviewed supramolecular organization of amyloid fibrils formed by almost all known amyloidogenic proteins, including amyloid β, α-synuclein, tau, insulin, and lysozyme proteins. It demonstrated how physical and chemical factors could change morphology of fibril aggregates at the stage of their formation. It was also shown how these factors, as well as chaperonins, could change the supramolecular organization of already grown fibrils.

One should note that microscopy itself often may not be sufficient for the determination of fibril structure. Therefore, microscopy is often used with numerous spectroscopic techniques, such as ss-NMR, Raman, and IR spectroscopy. These techniques allow for the determination of ψ and φ angles of the peptide backbone, which is necessary to fully elucidate the structure of the fibril cross-β core.

Author details

Dmitry Kurouski*

Address all correspondence to: dkurouski@northwestern.edu

Chemistry Department, Northwestern University, Evanston, IL, USA

References

[1] Dobson CM. Protein folding and misfolding. Nature 2003;426:884–890.

[2] Sipe JD, Cohen AS. Review: history of the amyloid fibril. J. Struct. Biol. 2000;130:88–98.

[3] Kurouski D, Van Duyne RP, Lednev IK. Exploring the structure and formation mechanism of amyloid fibrils by Raman spectroscopy: a review. Analyst 2015;140:4967–4980.

[4] Fandrich M. On the structural definition of amyloid fibrils and other polypeptide aggregates. Cell. Mol. Life Sci. 2007;64:2066–2078.

[5] Dobson CM. Protein aggregation and its consequences for human disease. Prot. Pept. Lett. 2006;13:219–227.

[6] Usov I, Nystrom G, Adamcik J, Handschin S, Schutz C, Fall A, *et al.* Understanding nanocellulose chirality and structure-properties relationship at the single fibril level. Nat. Commun. 2015;6:7564.

[7] Assenza S, Adamcik J, Mezzenga R, De Los Rios P. Universal behavior in the mesoscale properties of amyloid fibrils. Phys. Rev. Lett. 2014;113:268103.

[8] Kurouski D, Dukor RK, Lu X, Nafie LA, Lednev IK. Normal and reversed supramolecular chirality of insulin fibrils probed by vibrational circular dichroism at the protofilament level of fibril structure. Biophys. J. 2012;103:522–531.

[9] Morozova-Roche LA, Zurdo J, Spencer A, Noppe W, Receveur V, Archer DB, et al. Amyloid fibril formation and seeding by wild-type human lysozyme and its disease-related mutational variants. J. Struct. Biol. 2000;130:339–351.

[10] Jimenez JL, Nettleton EJ, Bouchard M, Robinson CV, Dobson CM, Saibil HR. The protofilament structure of insulin amyloid fibrils. Proc. Natl. Acad. Sci. U. S. A. 2002;99:9196–9201.

[11] Kurouski D, Lu X, Popova L, Wan W, Shanmugasundaram M, Stubbs G, et al. Is supramolecular filament chirality the underlying cause of major morphology differences in amyloid fibrils? J. Am. Chem. Soc. 2014;136:2302–2312.

[12] Khurana R, Ionescu-Zanetti C, Pope M, Li J, Nielson L, Ramirez-Alvarado M, et al. A general model for amyloid fibril assembly based on morphological studies using atomic force microscopy. Biophys. J. 2003;85:1135–1144.

[13] Groenning M, Frokjaer S, Vestergaard B. Formation mechanism of insulin fibrils and structural aspects of the insulin fibrillation process. Curr. Protein Pept. Sci. 2009;10:509–528.

[14] Wischik CM, Crowther RA, Stewart M, Roth M. Subunit structure of paired helical filaments in Alzheimer's disease. J. Cell. Biol. 1985;100:1905–1912.

[15] Wischik CM, Novak M, Thogersen HC, Edwards PC, Runswick MJ, Jakes R, et al. Isolation of a fragment of tau derived from the core of the paired helical filament of Alzheimer disease. Proc. Natl. Acad. Sci. U. S. A. 1988;85:4506–4510.

[16] Kurouski D, Luo H, Sereda V, Robb FT, Lednev IK. Deconstruction of stable cross-Beta fibrillar structures into toxic and nontoxic products using a mutated archaeal chaperonin. ACS Chem. Biol. 2013;8:2095–2101.

[17] Paravastu AK, Leapman RD, Yau WM, Tycko R. Molecular structural basis for polymorphism in Alzheimer's beta-amyloid fibrils. Proc. Natl. Acad. Sci. U. S. A. 2008;105:18349–18354.

[18] Sawaya MR, Sambashivan S, Nelson R, Ivanova MI, Sievers SA, Apostol MI, et al. Atomic structures of amyloid cross-b spines reveal varied steric zippers. Nature 2007;447:453–457.

[19] Ma S, Cao X, Mak M, Sadik A, Walkner C, Freedman TB, et al. Vibrational circular dichroism shows unusual sensitivity to protein fibril formation and development in solution. J. Am. Chem. Soc. 2007;129:12364–12365.

[20] Measey TJ, Smith KB, Decatur SM, Zhao L, Yang G, Schweitzer-Stenner R. Self-aggregation of a polyalanine octamer promoted by its C-terminal tyrosine and probed

by a strongly enhanced vibrational circular dichroism signal. J. Am. Chem. Soc. 2009;131:18218–18219.

[21] Lednev LK. Amyloid fibrils: the Eighth Wonder of the world in protein folding and aggregation. Biophys. J. 2014;106:1433–1435.

[22] Betzig E, Patterson GH, Sougrat R, Lindwasser OW, Olenych S, Bonifacino JS, et al. Imaging intracellular fluorescent proteins at nanometer resolution. Science 2006;313:1642–1645.

[23] Hell SW, Wichmann J. Breaking the diffraction resolution limit by stimulated emission: stimulated-emission-depletion fluorescence microscopy. Opt. Lett. 1994;19:780–782.

[24] Heilemann M, van de Linde S, Schuttpelz M, Kasper R, Seefeldt B, Mukherjee A, et al. Subdiffraction-resolution fluorescence imaging with conventional fluorescent probes. Angew. Chem. Int. Ed. Engl. 2008;47:6172–6176.

[25] Kaminski Schierle GS, van de Linde S, Erdelyi M, Esbjorner EK, Klein T, Rees E, et al. In situ measurements of the formation and morphology of intracellular beta-amyloid fibrils by super-resolution fluorescence imaging. J. Am. Chem. Soc. 2011;133:12902–12905.

[26] Tosoni A., Barbiano di Belgiojoso G. and Nebuloni M. (2011). Electron Microscopy in the Diagnosis of Amyloidosis, Amyloidosis - Mechanisms and Prospects for Therapy, Dr. Svetlana Sarantseva (Ed.), ISBN: 978- 953-307-253-1, InTech, Available from: http://www.intechopen.com/books/amyloidosis-mechanisms-andprospects-for-therapy/electron-microscopy-in-the-diagnosis-of-amyloidosis Locatoin: University Campus STeP Ri Slavka Krautzeka 83/A 51000 Rijeka, Croatia

[27] Inoue S, Kuroiwa M, Kisilevsky R. Basement membranes, microfibrils and beta amyloid fibrillogenesis in Alzheimer's disease: high resolution ultrastructural findings. Brain Res. Rev. 1999;29:218–231.

[28] Inoue S, Kuroiwa M, Tan R, Kisilevsky R. A high resolution ultrastructural comparison of isolated and in situ murine AA amyloid fibrils. Amyloid 1998;5:99–110.

[29] Inoue S, Kuroiwa M, Saraiva MJ, Guimaraes A, Kisilevsky R. Ultrastructure of familial amyloid polyneuropathy amyloid fibrils: examination with high-resolution electron microscopy. J. Struct. Biol. 1998;124:1–12.

[30] Kidd M. Paired helical filaments in electron microscopy of Alzheimer's disease. Nature 1963;197:192–193.

[31] Goldsbury CS, Cooper GJ, Goldie KN, Muller SA, Saafi EL, Gruijters WT, et al. Polymorphic fibrillar assembly of human amylin. J. Struct. Biol. 1997;119:17–27.

[32] Goldsbury C, Goldie K, Pellaud J, Seelig J, Frey P, Muller SA, et al. Amyloid fibril formation from full-length and fragments of amylin. J. Struct. Biol. 2000;130:352–362.

[33] Shammas SL, Knowles TP, Baldwin AJ, Macphee CE, Welland ME, Dobson CM, Devlin GL. Perturbation of the stability of amyloid fibrils through alteration of electrostatic interactions. Biophys. J. 2011;100:2783–2791.

[34] Gras SL, Waddington LJ, Goldie KN. Transmission electron microscopy of amyloid fibrils. Methods Mol. Biol. 2011;752:197–214.

[35] Kurouski D, Dukor RK, Lu X, Nafie LA, Lednev IK. Spontaneous inter-conversion of insulin fibril chirality. Chem. Commun. 2012;48:2837–2839.

[36] Petkova AT, Leapman RD, Guo Z, Yau W-M, Mattson MP, Tycko R. Self-propagating, molecular-level polymorphism in Alzheimer's ÃŸ-amyloid fibrils. Science 2005;307:262–265.

[37] Sen A, Baxa U, Simon MN, Wall JS, Sabate R, Saupe SJ, Steven AC. Mass analysis by scanning transmission electron microscopy and electron diffraction validate predictions of stacked beta-solenoid model of HET-s prion fibrils. J. Biol. Chem. 2007;282:5545–5550.

[38] Wasmer C, Lange A, Van Melckebeke H, Siemer AB, Riek R, Meier BH. Amyloid fibrils of the HET-s(218–289) prion form a beta solenoid with a triangular hydrophobic core. Science 2008;319:1523–1526.

[39] Chen B, Thurber KR, Shewmaker F, Wickner RB, Tycko R. Measurement of amyloid fibril mass-per-length by tilted-beam transmission electron microscopy. Proc. Natl. Acad. Sci. U. S. A. 2009;106:14339–14344.

[40] Rubin N, Perugia E, Wolf SG, Klein E, Fridkin M, Addadi L. Relation between serum amyloid A truncated peptides and their suprastructure chirality. J. Am. Chem. Soc. 2010;132:4242–4248.

[41] Rubin N, Perugia E, Goldschmidt M, Fridkin M, Addadi L. Chirality of amyloid suprastructures. J. Am. Chem. Soc. 2008;130:4602–4603.

[42] Kurouski D, Lombardi RA, Dukor RK, Lednev IK, Nafie LA. Direct observation and pH control of reversed supramolecular chirality in insulin fibrils by vibrational circular dichroism. Chem. Commun. 2010;46:7154–7156.

[43] Meinhardt J, Sachse C, Hortschansky P, Grigorieff N, Fandrich M. Abeta(1–40) fibril polymorphism implies diverse interaction patterns in amyloid fibrils. J. Mol. Biol. 2009;386:869–877.

[44] Fandrich M, Meinhardt J, Grigorieff N. Structural polymorphism of Alzheimer Abeta and other amyloid fibrils. Prion 2009;3:89–93.

[45] Antzutkin ON. Amyloidosis of Alzheimer's Abeta peptides: solid-state nuclear magnetic resonance, electron paramagnetic resonance, transmission electron microscopy, scanning transmission electron microscopy and atomic force microscopy studies. Magn. Reson. Chem. 2004;42:231–246.

[46] Klement K, Wieligmann K, Meinhardt J, Hortschansky P, Richter W, Fandrich M. Effect of different salt ions on the propensity of aggregation and on the structure of Alzheimer's abeta(1–40) amyloid fibrils. J. Mol. Biol. 2007;373:1321–1333.

[47] Petkova AT, Leapman RD, Guo Z, Yau WM, Mattson MP, Tycko R. Self-propagating, molecular-level polymorphism in Alzheimer's beta-amyloid fibrils. Science 2005;307:262–265.

[48] Luhrs T, Ritter C, Adrian M, Riek-Loher D, Bohrmann B, Dobeli H, et al. 3D structure of Alzheimer's amyloid-beta(1–42) fibrils. Proc. Natl. Acad. Sci. U. S. A. 2005,102:17342–17347.

[49] Zhang R, Hu X, Khant H, Ludtke SJ, Chiu W, Schmid MF, et al. Interprotofilament interactions between Alzheimer's Abeta1–42 peptides in amyloid fibrils revealed by cryoEM. Proc. Natl. Acad. Sci. U. S. A. 2009;106:4653–4658.

[50] Vilar M, Chou HT, Luhrs T, Maji SK, Riek-Loher D, Verel R, et al. The fold of alpha-synuclein fibrils. Proc. Natl. Acad. Sci. U. S. A. 2008;105:8637–8642.

[51] Crowther RA, Daniel SE, Goedert M. Characterisation of isolated alpha-synuclein filaments from substantia nigra of Parkinson's disease brain. Neurosci. Lett. 2000;292:128–130.

[52] Spillantini MG, Crowther RA, Jakes R, Cairns NJ, Lantos PL, Goedert M. Filamentous alpha-synuclein inclusions link multiple system atrophy with Parkinson's disease and dementia with Lewy bodies. Neurosci. Lett. 1998;251:205–208.

[53] Usov I, Adamcik J, Mezzenga R. Polymorphism complexity and handedness inversion in serum albumin amyloid fibrils. ACS Nano 2013;7:10465–10474.

[54] Adamcik J, Mezzenga R. Adjustable twisting periodic pitch of amyloid fibrils. Soft Matter 2011;7:5437–5443.

[55] Jordens S, Isa L, Usov I, Mezzenga R. Non-equilibrium nature of two-dimensional isotropic and nematic coexistence in amyloid fibrils at liquid interfaces. Nat. Commun. 2013;4:1917.

[56] Jordens S, Ruhs PA, Sieber C, Isa L, Fischer P, Mezzenga R. Bridging the gap between the nanostructural organization and macroscopic interfacial rheology of amyloid fibrils at liquid interfaces. Langmuir 2014;30:10090–10097.

[57] Loksztejn A, Dzwolak W. Chiral bifurcation in aggregating insulin: an induced circular dichroism study. J. Mol. Biol. 2008;379:9–16.

[58] Dzwolak W, Pecul M. Chiral bias of amyloid fibrils revealed by the twisted conformation of Thioflavin T: an induced circular dichroism/DFT study. FEBS Lett. 2005,579:6601–6603.

[59] Dzwolak W. Vortex-induced chiral bifurcation in aggregating insulin. Chirality 2010;22(Suppl. 1):E154–E160.

[60] Campioni S, Carret G, Jordens S, Nicoud L, Mezzenga R, Riek R. The presence of an air-water interface affects formation and elongation of alpha-Synuclein fibrils. J. Am. Chem. Soc. 2014;136:2866–2875.

[61] Qin Z, Hu D, Han S, Hong DP, Fink AL. Role of different regions of alpha-synuclein in the assembly of fibrils. Biochemistry 2007;46:13322–13330.

[62] Jansen R, Dzwolak W, Winter R. Amyloidogenic self-assembly of insulin aggregates probed by high resolution atomic force microscopy. Biophys. J. 2005;88:1344–1353.

[63] Goldsbury C, Kistler J, Aebi U, Arvinte T, Cooper GJ. Watching amyloid fibrils grow by time-lapse atomic force microscopy. J. Mol. Biol. 1999;285:33–39.

[64] Goldsbury C, Baxa U, Simon MN, Steven AC, Engel A, Wall JS, et al. Amyloid structure and assembly: insights from scanning transmission electron microscopy. J. Struct. Biol. 2010;173:1–13.

[65] Lee S, Carson K, Rice-Ficht A, Good T. Small heat shock proteins differentially affect Abeta aggregation and toxicity. Biochem. Biophys. Res. Commun. 2006;347:527–533.

[66] Wilhelmus MM, Boelens WC, Otte-Holler I, Kamps B, de Waal RM, Verbeek MM. Small heat shock proteins inhibit amyloid-beta protein aggregation and cerebrovascular amyloid-beta protein toxicity. Brain. Res. 2006;1089:67–78.

[67] Raman B, Ban T, Sakai M, Pasta SY, Ramakrishna T, Naiki H, et al. AlphaB-crystallin, a small heat-shock protein, prevents the amyloid fibril growth of an amyloid beta-peptide and beta2-microglobulin. Biochem. J. 2005;392:573–581.

[68] Ecroyd H, Carver JA. Crystallin proteins and amyloid fibrils. Cell. Mol. Life Sci. 2009;66:62–81.

[69] Kurouski D, Luo H, Sereda V, Robb FT, Lednev IK. Rapid degradation kinetics of amyloid fibrils under mild conditions by an archaeal chaperonin. Biochem. Biophys. Res. Commun. 2012;422:97–102.

[70] Laksanalamai P, Robb FT. Small heat shock proteins from extremophiles: a review. Extremophiles 2004;8:1–11.

[71] Nafie LA. Vibrational Optical Activity: Principles and Applications. Chichester: Wiley; 2011. 398 p.

[72] Measey TJ, Schweitzer-Stenner R. Vibrational circular dichroism as a probe of fibrillogenesis: the origin of the anomalous intensity enhancement of amyloid-like fibrils. J. Am. Chem. Soc. 2010;133:1066–1076.

[73] Fulara A, Lakhani A, Wojcik S, Nieznanska H, Keiderling TA, Dzwolak W. Spiral superstructures of amyloid-like fibrils of polyglutamic acid: an infrared absorption and vibrational circular dichroism study. J. Phys. Chem. B 2011;115:11010–11016.

[74] Yu J, Zhu H, Guo JT, de Beer FC, Kindy MS. Expression of mouse apolipoprotein SAA1.1 in CE/J mice: isoform-specific effects on amyloidogenesis. Lab. Invest. 2000;80:1797–1806.

[75] Malle E, Sodin-Semrl S, Kovacevic A. Serum amyloid A: an acute-phase protein involved in tumour pathogenesis. Cell. Mol. Life Sci. 2009;66:9–26.

[76] Srinivasan S, Patke S, Wang Y, Ye Z, Litt J, Srivastava SK, et al. Pathogenic serum amyloid A 1.1 shows a long oligomer-rich fibrillation lag phase contrary to the highly amyloidogenic non-pathogenic SAA2.2. J. Biol. Chem. 2013;288:2744–2755.

[77] Kurouski D, Handen JD, Dukor RK, Nafie LA, Lednev IK. Supramolecular chirality in peptide microcrystals. Chem. Commun. 2015;51:89–92.

Chapter 3

Advances in AFM Imaging Applications for Characterizing the Biophysical Properties of Amyloid Fibrils

Wonseok Lee, Hyungbeen Lee, Gyudo Lee and Dae Sung Yoon

Additional information is available at the end of the chapter

http://dx.doi.org/10.5772/63316

Abstract

Although the formation mechanism of amyloid fibrils in bodies is still debated, it has recently been reported how amyloid fibrils can be formed in vitro. Accordingly, we have gained a better understanding of the self-assembly mechanism and intrinsic properties of amyloid fibrils. Because the structure of amyloid fibrils consists of nanoscaled insoluble strands (a few nanometers in diameter and micrometers long), a special tool is needed to study amyloid fibrils at length. Atomic force microscopy (AFM) is supposed to be a versatile toolkit to probe such a tiny biomolecule. The physical/chemical properties of amyloid fibrils have been explored by AFM. In particular, AFM enables the visualization of amyloid fibrillation with different incubation times as well as the concentrations of the formed amyloid fibrils as affected by fibril diameters and lengths. Very recently, the minute structural changes and/or electrical properties of amyloid fibrils have been made by using advanced AFM techniques including dynamic liquid AFM, PeakForce QNM (quantitative nanomechanical mapping), and Kelvin probe force microscopy (KPFM). Herein, we summarize the biophysical properties of amyloid fibrils that are newly discovered with the help of those advanced AFM techniques and suggest our perspectives and future directions for the study of amyloid fibrils.

Keywords: amyloid fibril, biophysical property, atomic force microscopy (AFM), Kelvin probe force microscopy (KPFM), PeakForce QNM (quantitative nanomechanical mapping)

1. Introduction

Proteins and peptides can be transformed under some physiological conditions from their soluble forms into highly ordered fibrous aggregates, which are called "amyloid fibrils" [1–3]. Amyloid fibrils can be deposited in the tissues and organs in the human body, resulting in the generation of degenerative diseases such as Alzheimer's, Parkinson's, Creutzfeldt-Jakob's, and Huntington's diseases depending on specific sequences of proteins or peptides [4, 5]. On the other hand, the amyloid fibrils have often been exploited for functional roles (e.g., extracellular matrix) by living creatures [6–8]. These amyloid fibrils, commonly known as functional amyloid, are found in bacteria, fungi, insects, invertebrates, and humans. Because of their unique mechanical and biological properties, amyloid fibrils had been used in a variety of organisms as a bacterial coatings, scaffolds, biofilm, information storage and transfer, natural adhesives, and structures for the storage of peptide hormones [7–11]. Although the precise formation mechanism of amyloid fibrils and their pathological/functional behaviors in bodies are still controversial, it has been reported how amyloid fibrils can be formed in vitro, allowing us to understand the fibrillation mechanism and/or the intrinsic properties of the fibrils [12]. Because these fibrils have a distinctive structure that consists of β-sheets that are perpendicularly stacked in thousands of units, aggregating to a few nanometers in diameter and several micrometers in length, a special tool is required to study the conformational (structural) changes of amyloid fibrils in various microenvironments. To investigate the structural changes of amyloid fibrils, many technical tools such as fluorescence microscopy with Congo red and thioflavin-T, transmission electron microscopy (TEM), X-ray diffraction, and nuclear magnetic resonance (NMR) have been used [13, 14]. Recently, atomic force microscopy (AFM) is a good candidate for characterizing such a thin fibrous material *via* high-resolution imaging of the molecular structure and interactions. A sharp stylus mounted at the end of a flexible cantilever is used to probe the amyloid fibrils placed on a piezoelectric scanner which controls the cantilever on the sample in the horizontal (x and y) and vertical (z) axis (**Figure 1**). The deflection of the cantilever as a result of the interactions (such as van der Waals forces, capillary forces, chemical bonding, and electrostatic forces) between the tip and the sample on substrate is converted into a laser beam reflected on the back of the cantilever. In this system, laser light from diode reflects off the back of the cantilever, and it is recorded as the amplified signal by a position-sensitive detector (PSD), which reconstructs the molecular structure or interactions of amyloid fibrils. AFM has its advantages, for example, the convenience to prepare a sample, working at room temperature and atmospheric pressure, and high-resolution imaging at the single-molecule level, allowing for measuring the physical/chemical properties of amyloid fibrils. In particular, AFM enables scanning to follow the morphological changes of amyloid fibrils in liquid environments, which is powerful as it permits us to visualize amyloid fibrillation under physiological conditions [15]. Recent in vitro studies of amyloid fibrils have demonstrated time-lapse AFM imaging of amyloid fibrillation with different incubation times and concentrations under physiological conditions [16]. Much more recently, AFM application techniques that lie beyond its primary function (i.e., high-resolution imaging) have shown that abundant information of amyloid fibrils can now be accessible. For instance, PeakForce QNM (quantitative nanomechanical mapping) and KPFM (Kelvin probe force microscopy) are, respectively, beginning to be used to map mechanical properties and to measure the surface charge of amyloid fibrils. Consequently, some unprecedented characteristics (e.g., minute structural changes and/or electrical properties) of amyloid fibrils have been investigated, providing a better understanding of amyloid fibrils [17–23]. In this chapter, we introduce the advanced AFM application methods (i.e., dynamic liquid AFM, PeakForce QNM, and KPFM) for measuring amyloid fibril's features that could not be accessed by conventional AFM technique and summarize the newly discovered biophysical properties of amyloid fibrils with the advanced AFM techniques and suggest our perspectives and future directions for characterizing amyloid fibrils.

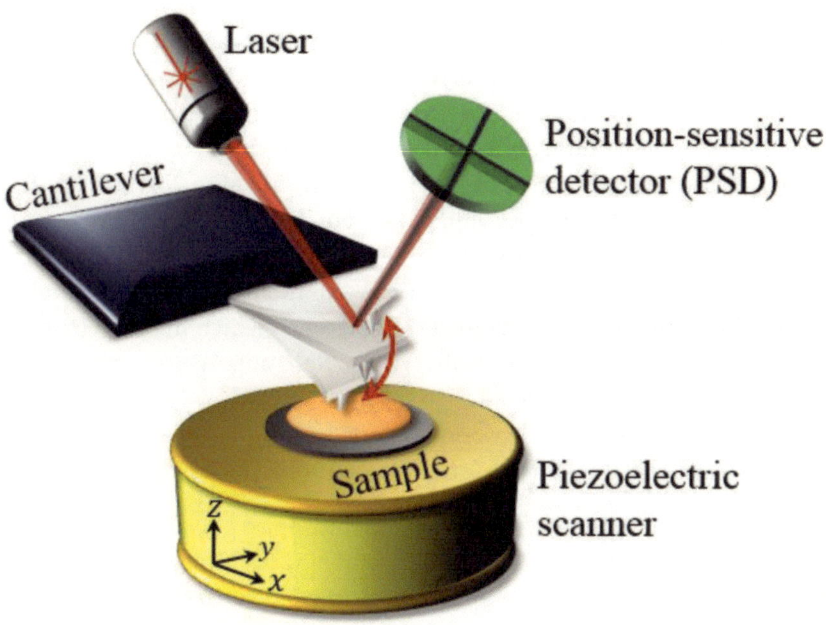

Figure 1. Schematic diagram of the principle of AFM.

2. Imaging of self-assembled amyloid fibrils in liquid environments

Amyloid fibrils are protein aggregates arising from misfolded proteins, transformed to β-sheet-rich and insoluble fibrils, which can be tangled and deposited in tissues and organs [2]. Characterizing the structure of amyloid fibrils can provide some critical clues about the mechanism of fibrogenesis and accordingly the pathological/functional roles of the fibrils. So far a variety of instruments (e.g., light, X-ray scattering, and NMR) [24, 25] and microscopic methods (e.g., fluorescence microscopy with Congo red and thioflavin-T [26, 27], TEM, and scanning electron microscopy (SEM) [14]) had been used to explore the structure of amyloid fibrils. Although many research results about the structure of amyloid fibrils had been reported by using those tools and/or methods, a fully comprehensive investigation of the self-assembly behavior and structure of various amyloid fibrils has not yet been conducted. AFM provides additional capabilities and advantages relative to other microscopic methods. For example, it can directly show and measure the structure of an individual fibril. In addition, it is easy to prepare a sample and to get high-resolution imaging at the single-molecule level, allowing for measuring the physical/chemical properties of amyloid fibrils. Furthermore, AFM can scan the conformational changes of amyloid fibrils in a liquid environment, which is powerful to visualize and measure amyloid fibrillation under physiological conditions.

2.1. Conventional AFM imaging techniques for amyloid fibrils

Since AFM was invented in the 1980s, it has widely been used as a versatile tool for direct imaging of nano/biomolecules and measuring molecular interactions at the single-molecule level [28–33]. In amyloid research, it has been reported that AFM is used to elucidate the fibril formation mechanism and to monitor kinetics and morphology of amyloid fibrils such as α-synuclein, insulin, and the B1 domain of protein G, a base model for immunoglobulin light-chain variable domains related with fibrils [34]. For AFM imaging, the fibrils were deposited on a freshly cleaved mica substrate. AFM images were collected in air under ambient conditions at a scan frequency of 1–2 Hz. From the analysis of AFM images, all fibrils (α-synuclein, insulin, and the B1 domain of protein G) are in correspondence with the general hierarchical assembly model, like amyloid-β (Aβ; 1–40 and 1–42), with which mature amyloid fibrils are formed by the intertwining of protofibrils. When first aggregated into protofibrils, the measured heights (i.e., fibril diameters) range from 1.2 to 3.5 nm. The structural information of the fibrils such as the fibril diameter and contour length depends on the protein species. Several protofibrils can pack together to form a mature fibril (5.2 ± 0.3 nm in height).

It has been reported that different stages of amyloid aggregation (i.e., hierarchy) can be examined by conducting a statistical analysis of acquired high-resolution AFM images [35]. β-Lactoglobulin (β-lg) fibrils are synthesized in vitro by heat denaturation at pH 2. It was shown that the β-lg amyloid-like fibrils are considered to be a semiflexible fibril structure (**Figure 2**). This means that the globular proteins (β-lg monomer) can be transformed into semiflexible fibrillary structures. The average height and contour length of β-lg fibrils were precisely measured by performing a statistical analysis on the AFM images. Each fibril has contour lengths in the range of 50 nm to 10 μm with a persistence length ranging from 16 nm to 1.6 μm. These distinct structural information of fibrils make them ideal model systems for the study of semiflexible polymers [36]. In that study, valuable structural information concerning individual fibrils in AFM images was produced, such as splitting or thinning of fibrils and even periodic height fluctuations of the fibrils. The periodic fluctuations in height provide a highly important clue about the packing of the protofibrils to form mature fibrils. **Figure 2** presents AFM images of fibrils with four different periods ranging from 35 to 135 nm, corresponding to average heights of fibrils ranging from 4 to 10 nm, respectively. Thus, the periodicity is found to increase linearly with the height of the fibrils. These hierarchical structures of β-lg fibrils can be represented from single to five-stranded packed twisted ribbon, helix-like structures, which can be compared with dynamic simulations using a coarse-grain molecular model.

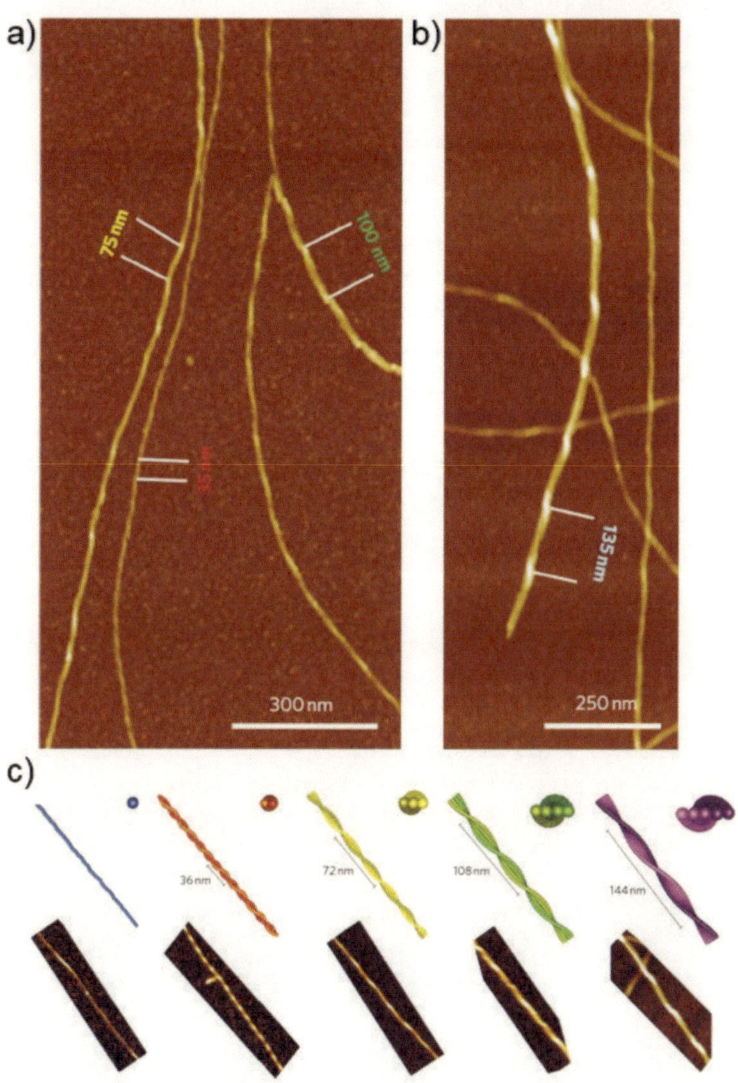

Figure 2. Different periods of β-lactoglobulin fibrils. (a) AFM height image of fibrils with a period of 35 nm (for fibrils with a maximum height of 4 nm), 75 nm (maximum height, 6 nm), and 100 nm (maximum height, 8 nm). (b) Example of a fibril with a period of 135 nm and a maximum height of 10 nm. (c) AFM images and corresponding coarse-grain molecular dynamics reconstructions of left-handed helical fibril formation from the twisting of multistranded ribbons, with the number of filaments ranging between 1 and 5. Figures reproduced with permission from Ref. [35], © 2010 NPG.

It is highly important to study initial fibrillation of amyloid proteins for developing an inhibition method for amyloid fibrils and plaques. Although attempts with many conventional methods such as fluorescent assays with dye and optical spectroscopy had been reported, insight into the mechanisms of formation of initial fibrils at the molecular level has yet to provide clarity. To address that issue, AFM techniques can investigate growing fibrils in greater detail. **Figure 3** shows topological images of the β-lg fibrils acquired after 30 and 45 min incubation [37]. As the incubation time was increased, the contour length of fibrils increased in the range from 520 to 860 nm. The two-filament packed structure was only observed after a heating time of 30 min. But after a heating time of 45 min, fibrils of more than two filaments were observed. From those results, AFM analysis can provide us with some significant structural information not only topological images but also details such as height, contour length, and periodicity from fluctuations along the fibril length. In addition, it can show the formation characteristics of amyloid fibrils, including the critical steps driven by nucleation and growth of individual fibrils. These findings from the use of AFM imaging may help researchers gain understanding of the origin of fibrils and may assist with the development of therapeutic treatments for degenerative diseases that are generated by many different amyloidogenic proteins.

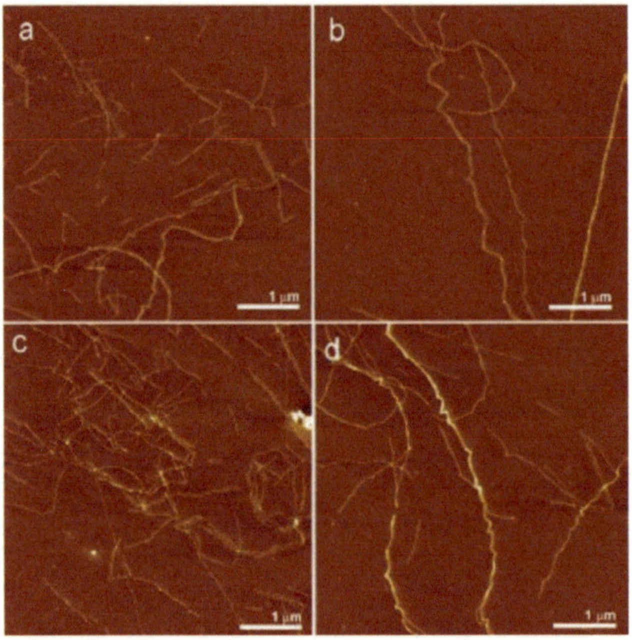

Figure 3. AFM height images of heated β-lactoglobulin at pH 2 and 90°C for the heating time of (a and b) 30 min and (c and d) 45 min. Figures reproduced with permission from Ref. [37], © 2011 The Royal Society of Chemistry.

2.2. Advantages of AFM imaging of amyloid fibrils in liquid environments

As we mentioned above, AFM imaging of amyloid fibrils is strong advantageous not only in the characterization of the structure of amyloid fibrils but also for the observation of initial fibrillation of amyloidogenic proteins. These investigations of amyloid fibrils in ambient atmospheric conditions by AFM imaging yield the basic understandings of the characteristics of amyloid fibrils, but all of these processes (such as fibrillation and conformation changes) actually take place in a liquid environment (i.e., in human body fluid). In addition, the formation of amyloid fibrils continuously occurs in the human body, not discretely, which is why liquid AFM is particularly important to more precisely and continuously observe to fibrils in comparing with conventional AFM.

In the research field of amyloid fibril, real-time monitoring of fibril growth is necessary to investigate the mechanism of amyloid fibril formation. It has been reported that the direct observation of fibrillation of Aβ peptide on different substrates is achieved by using in situ AFM analysis in a liquid environment [15]. They used two types of substrate: hydrophilic mica and hydrophobic graphite. Hydrophilic mica can be considered a model of the hydrophilic components of cell membranes such as anionic phospholipids. The hydrophobic graphite may be used as a model of hydrophobic elements of cell membrane (e.g., lipid bilayers and lipoprotein particles), in which elements Aβ peptide can localize in both plasma and cerebrospinal fluid in vivo. An in situ AFM study of Aβ fibril aggregation was followed by continuous imaging in phosphate-buffered saline (pH 7.4, protein concentration 10–500 mM). Aβ peptides initially were formed with pseudomicellar aggregates and then tend to form linear structures, such as protofibrils, as the Aβ concentration was increased on the hydrophilic mica substrate. However, Aβ peptides were formed with elongated sheets structures on the hydrophobic graphite substrate. This difference by substrates is the distinguishable characteristics between β-sheets and α-helices. These studies show that an in situ AFM study is able to directly observe not only the amyloid aggregation in physiological fluids but also fibrillation driven by interactions at the interface of hydrophilic and hydrophobic substrates. It may be helpful to understand the mechanism of formation of Aβ fibrils in membranes and lipoprotein particles in vivo.

AFM has been employed not only to study the formation of amyloid fibrils in vitro but also to investigate ex vivo amyloid material isolated from organs, specifically hearts, of patients. The AFM analysis of natural amyloid fibrils produced by the Leu174Ser apolipoprotein A-I variant (ApoA-I-LS) has been reported. ApoA-I-LS amyloid fibrils were obtained from two different patients, and conformational changes of the fibrils in both air and liquid environments were measured [38]. The fibrils from both patients were identified by small-angle X-ray diffraction patterns, indicative of residual α-helical structure. In a liquid environment, it was observed that amyloid fibrils show poor adhesion properties on a mica substrate. But, from acquired AFM images, it was found that globular aggregates were easily adsorbed on mica. These results revealed the existence of fibrils as well as pre-fibrillar aggregates, with common morphologies and compatible sizes of fibrils and globules for both patients.

In addition, AFM imaging in a liquid environment is able to reveal unique and intrinsic properties of amyloid fibrils, which cannot be seen by any other method. It has been reported that the conformations of C-terminal tails outside of the α-synuclein amyloid fibrils are variable depending on environmental conditions by using structural information from liquid AFM imaging, as in **Figure 4** [39]. They suggested that the exposed C-terminus is unstructured and looks like a polymer bush and that the strongly negatively charged C-terminus has various functions and conformations with different ion concentrations (i.e., in the range of 0–5 M NaCl). It was also observed that the height of α-synuclein fibrils imaged in air appears to be about 17% lower than those of the same fibrils imaged in a liquid environment. This phenomenon is attributed to the collapse of C-terminus depending on the drying of the fibrils. Measuring the conformational changes of the C-terminus in amyloid fibrils by AFM imaging sheds light on the estimation of the transformation of the exterior structures of amyloid fibrils.

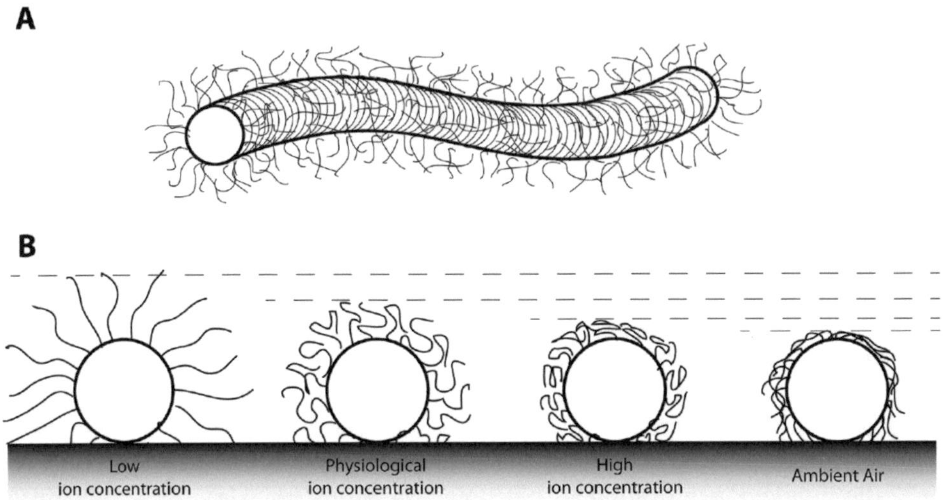

Figure 4. (a) Schematic representation of a fibril with stacked β-sheet folded monomers perpendicular to the fibril axis and an unstructured C-terminus outside the fibril. (b) Different conformations of C-terminal tails outside the fibril core in liquid conditions with different ion concentrations and in ambient air. Figure reproduced with permission Ref. [39], © 2012 American Chemical Society.

3. PeakForce QNM (quantitative nanomechanical mapping) of amyloid fibrils

Amyloid fibrils have been known as β-sheet-rich structures, which are consisted with dense hydrogen-bonding networks [40]. The self-assembly aggregates can be formed with stackings of several hundreds to thousands of cross β-sheet units, a few nanometers in diameter, and several micrometers in length. Such hierarchical structure of fibrils is highly related to pathological meanings as well as to functional features due to their marvelous mechanical properties, which are comparable to those of silk and/or steel [13, 41]. Characterization of biophysical properties of amyloid fibrils has significant implications ranging from application to medicines and engineering for designing amyloid-based nanomaterials. To measure biophysical properties of amyloid fibrils, although in recent decades many research results had been reported that had been obtained by using various techniques such as optical, magnetic tweezer and dynamic mechanical analysis [13], AFM techniques are commonly used for both manipulation at the single-molecule level and force spectroscopy of nanomaterials (i.e., amyloid fibrils). Moreover, AFM nanoindentation has been used to study nanomechanics of amyloid fibrils [42].

AFM nanoindentation is performed by mapping force-distance (F-D) curve on the region of interest in the sample [43, 44]. F-D curve measurement is based on the deflection theory of a cantilever beam and the contact mechanics. The degree of nanomechanical deflection of AFM cantilever originated from the physical interactions between the AFM tip and the sample can be converted to the applied forces to the cantilever. When F-D curve records, the cantilever approaches and indents the sample until a certain predefined force is reached, and then the cantilever is retracted. During the approach and retract cycle, the force is continuously measured, which is a F-D curve for one point of the sample (**Figure 5**). The mechanical properties such as Young's modulus, adhesion force, and deformation energies of amyloid fibrils can be determined directly from the recorded data (F-D curve) by AFM nanoindentation. In particular, to extract the accurate Young's modulus of the sample from F-D curves, contact mechanics theory is used. There are three different types of representative contact mechanics models (Hertz, DMT, and JKR) depending on either the type of sample or the structure of AFM tip [18]. The Hertz model presumes a nonadhesive contact between the tip and the sample, while the Derjaguin-Muller-Toporov (DMT) and Johnson-Kendall-Roberts (JKR) models are considered to be adhesive materials. DMT model further includes the extra constant adhesion term, which indicates the adhesive force outside the contact area. The JKR model demonstrates the adhesion forces inside the contact area between the tip and the sample. Those model equations are as follows:

$$\boldsymbol{Hertz}: F = \frac{4}{3} E^* \sqrt{R}\,\delta^{\frac{3}{2}},$$

$$\boldsymbol{Derjaguin\text{–}Muller\text{–}Toporov\ \ DMT}: F = \frac{4}{3} E^* \sqrt{R}\,\delta^{\frac{3}{2}} - 2\pi R\gamma$$

$$\boldsymbol{Johnson - Kendall - Roberts\ \ JKR}: F = \frac{9}{4} E^* \sqrt{R}\,\delta^{\frac{3}{2}} \cdot \Delta\gamma\pi$$

$$\frac{1}{E^*} = \frac{1 - v_m{}^2}{E_m} + \frac{1 - v_i{}^2}{E_i}$$

where F is the force, δ is the AFM indentation depth (distance), R is the radius of cantilever tip, E^* is the reduced elastic modulus, and γ is the work of adhesion. E^* is calculated by the relationship between the elastic modulus and Poisson ratio of AFM cantilever (E_i, v_i) and sample (E_m, v_m).

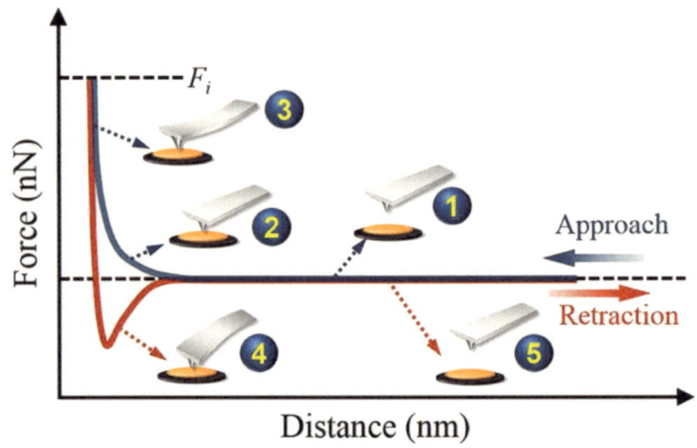

Figure 5. The schematic illustration of F-D curve acquisition process during AFM nanoindentation. Approach (blue) and retraction (red) F-D curves. Illustration depicts the cantilever approaching to and retracting from the sample as follows: (1) approaching, (2) initial contact, and (3) repulsive contact. (4) Adhesion and (5) noncontact regimes recorded upon retracting the cantilever and sample.

In recent decades, to measure the physical properties of amyloid fibrils more precisely and quantitatively, PeakForce QNM technique has been developed. PeakForce QNM is a robust F-D curve mapping technique, which is beneficial for soft delicate biological samples. It is able to map and distinguish between nanomechanical features, including the DMT modulus (1 kPa to 100 GPa), adhesion, energy dissipation, and deformation by utilizing PeakForce tapping technology [45, 46]. It can acquire high-resolution topographic images and simultaneously collect a quantitative mapping of the intrinsic mechanical properties of amyloid fibril.

3.1. Principle of PeakForce QNM

PeakForce tapping is one of the scanning modes, which is especially suited to applications to the measurement of mechanical properties of biological samples [18]. In this mode, the probe is oscillated at a low frequency (1–2 kHz), while capturing a force-distance curve (F-D curve) plots each time the AFM probe taps on the sample by directly controlling the probe-sample interaction. To describe the details, one cycle of the PeakForce tapping trajectory is shown in **Figure 6a** [17]. During the approach to the sample, the probe begins (A) with a noncontact force (i.e., attractive force) until contact on the sample. The Z piezo presses it downward until the probe contacts the sample (B); the probe continuously presses until the probe reaches the setpoint (i.e., maximum force) (C). The setpoint, which is one of the parameters of the probe-sample interaction, is used during AFM topography. After reaching the peak force at point C, the tip is pulled off the surface at point D, which means maximum adhesion. Finally, the curve levels and the probe tip returns to its original position (E).

Accurate controlling of the probe position and feedback permits calculation of several properties from the F-D curve produced by the direct measurements simultaneously at each pixel in **Figure 6b**. From this curve, the peak force is measured at point C, which is used as the imaging feedback signal. As the probe is scanned over the surface, this signal produces a topological image. Adhesion force is measured at D, which is calculated as the force difference between the baseline and the minimum force value of the curve. Simultaneously, Young's modulus is obtained by fitting the DMT contact mechanics model to the retraction curve (at points C to D). The dissipation information is obtained by integrating the area between the extension and retraction curves and the deformation of the sample is calculated as the distance between the contact point on the adhesion curve and the maximum indentation. This unique technique is called PeakForce QNM. Compared to a typical AFM imaging method, PeakForce QNM can simultaneously yield high-resolution AFM imaging with quantitative mechanical property mapping. PeakForce QNM has recently emerged as a means of measuring the intrinsic and biophysical properties of nanomaterials [47], including amyloid fibrils [17, 19]. The following section will discuss the mapping the mechanical properties of amyloid fibrils by PeakForce QNM.

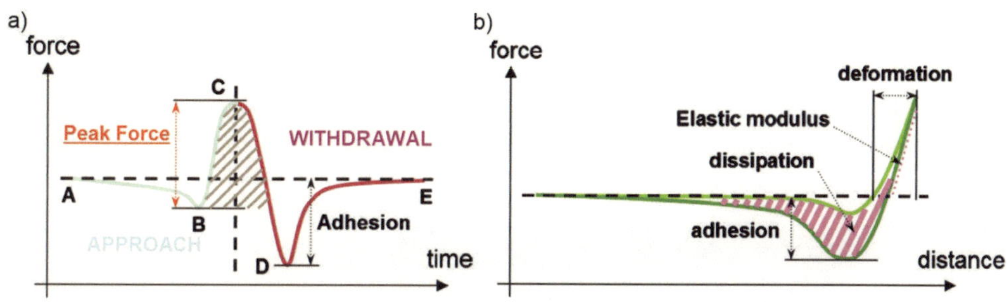

Figure 6. Principle of PeakForce QNM operation. (a) One cycle of the PeakForce tapping curve. (b) Calculation of the different peak force channels. Figure reproduced with permission Ref. [17], © 2011 AIP.

3.2. Mapping the mechanical properties of amyloid fibrils by PeakForce QNM

In the folding process, synthesized peptide chains can be transformed into three-dimensional protein structure, which has diverse functions in biological organism, through intermolecular interactions such as hydrogen and hydrophobic bonding [3, 48]. The proteins have intrinsic mechanical properties depending on the specific amino acid sequence, lengths, and complex environments. Meanwhile, misfolded proteins, commonly known as "amyloid protein," can be transformed into β-sheet-rich fibrillary structure (i.e., amyloid fibril) during fibrillation process. Amyloid fibrils have tremendous mechanical properties (a few GPa), implying a comparatively high stiffness. Moreover, it displays structural polymorphism, including twisted ribbons, helical ribbons, and nanotube structure [19], which is supposed to show a difference in mechanical properties. Amyloid species (amyloid proteins and fibrils) can be accumulated and deposited in the human body, which is associated with proteoglycans, in particular, heparan sulfate proteoglycans [48, 49]. These findings raise the question about the underpinning nature of the correlation between the mechanical properties of amyloid fibrils and its pathological roles in living systems as well as the use of fibrils as nanoscale materials.

PeakForce QNM has emerged as mechanical property mapping variant of AFM nanoindentation that had been used for several decades. PeakForce QNM has been used to measure the Young's modulus of β-lg fibrils deposited on mica [17]. It is of importance to measure the mechanical properties of β-lg fibrils because they have been used to make new nanomaterials by mixing with nanoparticles and nanowires for applications in various research fields. Using PeakForce QNM, the average height of the fibrils was measured to be 2.5 ± 0.5 nm and DMT modulus images were concurrently acquired. The Young's modulus of β-lg fibrils was estimated to be 3.7 ± 1.1 GPa. This result from PeakForce QNM analysis is similar to that of a previously reported Young's modulus of insulin fibrils (~3.3 GPa).

Amyloid fibrils can be generally formed with many different proteins such as Aβ (1–42), α-synuclein, albumin, etc., which have pathological and functional meanings. These fibrils often exhibit structural polymorphism due to interweaving of the several protofibrils. It has been demonstrated that amyloid fibrils appear in various structures such as ribbon-like and nanotube-like packed fibrils. PeakForce can precisely measure the Young's moduli of several amyloid fibrils, assembled from α-synuclein, Aβ (1–42), tau protein, insulin, β-lg, lysozyme, ovalbumin, and bovine serum albumin fibrils, as in **Figure 7** [19]. In addition, it demonstrated that PeakForce QNM can provide us some clues regarding structural polymorphism of amyloid fibrils by the exact estimation of Young's modulus. The measured Young's modulus values are twisted ribbon structure, 2.3 ± 0.6 GPa, and helical ribbon and nanotube structures,

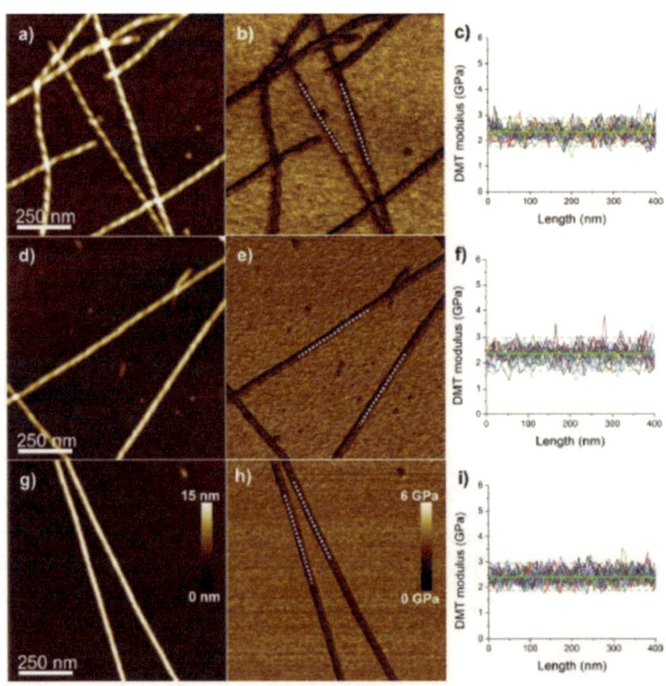

Figure 7. AFM height image of (a) twisted ribbon, (d) helical ribbon, and (g) nanotube-like structures of the end-capped heptapeptide CH_3CONH-βAβAKLVFF-$CONH_2$. AFM DMT modulus image of (b) twisted ribbon, (e) helical ribbon, and (h) nanotube-like structures. The dashed lines mark the positions at which the DMT modulus was analyzed. Profiles of DMT moduli along (c) twisted ribbon, (f) helical ribbon, and (i) nanotube-like structures. The data were obtained by the analysis of 20 fibrils for each type. Figure reproduced with permission Ref. [19], © 2012 The Royal Society of Chemistry.

2.3 ± 0.7 GPa and 2.4 ± 0.5 GPa, respectively. They also measured the value of Young's modulus for insulin amyloid fibrils (3.2 ± 0.6 GPa), which is very similar to that of a previously study of insulin (3.3 ± 0.4 GPa).

Recently, amyloid fibrils have attracted great attention because of outstanding features based on their mechanical properties as nanomaterials. To investigate the potential of amyloid fibrils as biomaterials, it is important to understand the mechanism of the fibrillation process and to quantify the mechanical properties. By performing the PeakForce QNM technique, the mechanical properties of the Aβ-42 fibrils during the fibrillation process have been measured, as in **Figure 8** [21]. The Young's modulus of the oligomers, protofibrils, and mature Aβ-42 fibrils was evaluated. During fibrillation, in which oligomers grow into protofibrils and then finally formed mature fibrils, the mechanical property (i.e., Young's modulus) increased. Hydrogen bonds between β-sheets may need to be reckoned with when one tries to determine the mechanical properties of amyloid fibrils. The changes in β-sheets in oligomers, protofibrils, and mature fibrils may have effects on the mechanical properties during the fibrillation process. These results could be of great significance for the elucidation of the mechanical properties of amyloid fibrils for the planning of new material strategies.

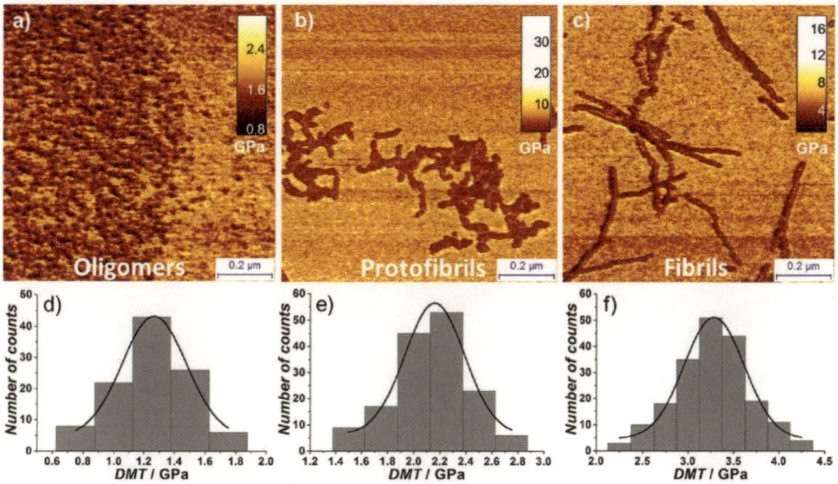

Figure 8. Evolution of the Young's modulus of Aβ-42 during the fibrillation process. DMT modulus AFM images of oligomers at 0 h (a), protofibrils at 48 h (b), and fibrils at 72 h (c). Distribution of the measured Young's modulus for oligomers (d), protofibrils (e), and fibrils (f). Figure reproduced with permission Ref. [21], © 2015 Wiley-VCH Verlag GmbH & Co. KGaA.

4. Kelvin probe force microscopy (KPFM) of amyloid fibrils

The amyloid fibril has been implicated in the various neurodegenerative diseases such as Alzheimer's, Parkinson's, Creutzfeldt-Jakob's, and Huntington's diseases [1–3], but the molecular mechanism of an amyloid toxicity is still debated [49–51]. To address this issue, scientists have investigated different possibilities for molecular behavior of amyloid-forming proteins that are correlated with the amyloid toxicity mechanism [52–54]. The leading proposed mechanism of the amyloid toxicity refers to the electrostatic interactions between the lipid membrane of cells and amyloid oligomers/fibrils (i.e., cytotoxicity) [55–57]. In addition, the electrostatic forces play important roles in the accumulation of proteinaceous aggregates as amyloid plaques or Lewy bodies. Therefore, the measurement of electrical properties of amyloid fibrils offers a new insight into the mechanism of amyloid fibril formation and toxicity.

KPFM has been considered as a powerful instrument for detecting the electrical properties of nano/biomaterials including molecules [58–62] by mapping the surface potential (the work function) of them. KPFM is carried out by a conducting AFM probe, which ascends to lift scan height. While the probe scans a sample surface of interest, a potential offset between the tip and the surface is recorded at each point of the scanned area. Furthermore, a high spatial resolution of KPFM is attributed to highly sharp conducting AFM tip by measuring the local contact potential difference (CPD) between the tip and the sample (**Figure 9**). Accordingly, KPFM has recently been used for characterizing the surface potential of amyloid fibrils [20, 23, 63] to unveil the molecular mechanism governing amyloid fibril formation and toxicities.

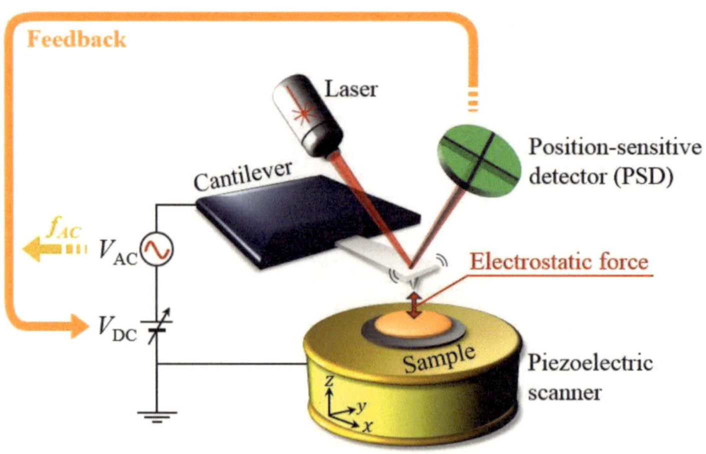

Figure 9. A schematic illustration of Kelvin probe force microscopy (KPFM) method for the measurement of electrical properties of material.

4.1. Principle of KPFM

In KPFM studies of mapping the surface potential, the surface potential of the materials is measured by the CPD between the material surface and the KPFM conducting cantilever tip, where the CPD is the variation in work function between different surfaces (the material surface and the tip) [58]. The CPD of two materials is determined, depending on their electronic/electrical characteristics. The characterization of the CPD is able to use not only for measuring the work function of metallic material and semiconductor surfaces but also for mapping the surface potential of biomolecules such as various proteins [64], DNA molecules [59, 60], and amyloids [20, 23, 63].

The hardware system of KPFM is founded upon the principle of the Kelvin method, which is a standard measurement method of the determination the CPD [65] (this is a reason why KPFM applies the term "Kelvin"). In the Kelvin probe method, the CPD (V_{CPD}) between two different materials is plainly defined as

$$V_{CPD} = \frac{\varphi_1 - \varphi_2}{-e} \tag{1}$$

where φ_1 and φ_2 are the work functions of two different materials (in KPFM, $\varphi_1 = \varphi_{tip}$ and $\varphi_2 = \varphi_{sample}$) and e is the charge of an electron. The probe, which consists of material with a known work function, is aligned to the sample surface for forming a capacitor. The reference electrode probe is vibrated, causing a variation in the capacitance between two plates, resulting in an electric current $i(t)$ and the generated current is given by

$$i(t) = V_{CPD}\omega\Delta C\cos\omega t \tag{2}$$

where ω is the frequency of vibration, ΔC is the change of capacitance, and V_{CPD} is the contact potential between the probe and the sample surface. V_{CPD} is measured by applying an contrasting external DC (direct current) bias voltage (V_{DC}), which is varied until the $i(t)$ is minimized.

The fundamental KPFM system is similar to the Kelvin method [65]. Mapping the surface potential of a material using KPFM, an electrostatic force (F_{ES}) *via* the V_{CPD} between a KPFM conducting tip and a material, is caused by an AC (alternating current) voltage V_{AC} with a DC offset bias V_{DC} which is applied between a tip and a material [66]. The F_{ES} between the tip and sample is defined as

$$F_{ES}(x,t) = -\frac{1}{2}\frac{\partial C(x)}{\partial x}\left[\left(V_{DC} \pm V_{CPD}\right) + V_{AC}\sin\omega t\right]^2 \tag{3}$$

where x is the distance between the KFPM conducting tip and a material. The electrical force component with frequency ω (related to differential value of "($V_{DC} \pm V_{CPD}$) V_{AC} sin ωt") is obtained from the PSD) signals through a lock-in amplifier. A feedback controller applies the V_{DC} to the KPFM system until the electrical force component with frequency ω is minimized. Accordingly, V_{CPD} between a KPFM conducting tip and a material is determined based on altering the DC offset bias V_{DC}.

4.2. Mapping the surface potential of amyloid fibrils

As mentioned above, the evaluation of electrical properties of amyloid fibrils would offer a better understanding of the mechanism of amyloid fibril formation and toxicity. To date, some of researchers have reported KPFM analysis for quantitative estimation of electrical properties of amyloid fibrils. It has been reported that synthesis of the amyloid-β-(25–35) peptide ($A\beta_{25-35}$) (with sequence GSNKGAIIGLM) fibrils and KPFM analysis of them [67]. Although the major components of neurotic plaque found in AD are 10-to-42-residue-long Aβ peptides ($A\beta_{1-40}/A\beta_{1-42}$), shorter fragments of peptides are also involved, such as $A\beta_{25-35}$. It has been reported that $A\beta_{25-35}$ can form readily β-sheet aggregates and is toxic to neurons. The surface potential analysis of $A\beta_{25-35}$ fibrils was performed by KPFM. The samples were prepared for KPFM imaging by depositing the solutions on chemically cleaned silicon (Si) substrates, and KPFM records were made for both the sample topography and the phase shift by using a two-pass method, namely, lift mode KPFM. It was found that the five fibrils have almost the same CPD values, which are about −10~ to −15 mV relative to the Si substrate. By calibrating the work function of cantilever tip, the work function of the $A\beta_{25-35}$ fibril was determined to be about 4.62 eV. However, the main thrust of this study is the surface potential analysis in regards to the interaction of gold nanoparticles (AuNPs) with $A\beta_{25-35}$ peptides, which we shall mention further on.

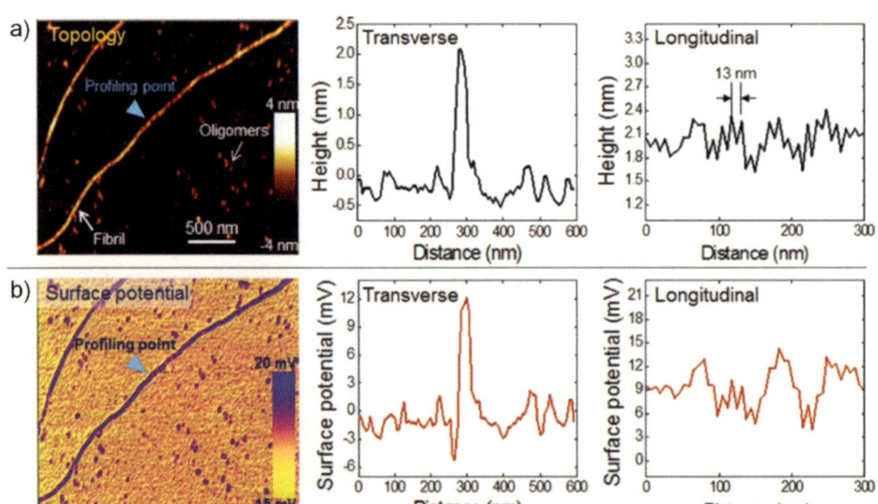

Figure 10. AFM and KPFM images of β-lactoglobulin amyloid fibrils. In each image of AFM topography (panel a) and surface potential (panel b), the white arrow shows a single amyloid fibril. A blue arrow indicates the location of amyloid fibril, at which the transverse profile of surface potential and topography were obtained. In the profiles of both topography and surface potential at longitudinal direction. Figures reproduced with permission from Ref. [20], © 2012 AIP.

Recently, β-lg has attracted much interest as an alternative amyloid precursor to be used to investigate the fibrillation mechanism and to fabricate various composites because of its inexpensive price and easy fabrication. The electrical properties of the β-lg fibrils using KPFM have been studied, which was the first attempt to visualize mapping the surface potential distribution of a single amyloid fibril [20]. As shown in **Figure 10**, the surface potential of the fibril is positive (e.g., ~12 mV) since the pH of a buffer solution is lower than the isoelectric point (pI) of β-lg (p*I* ~ 5.0). Interestingly, it is found that the surface potential profile of the fibril is critically dependent on the fibril diameter and periodicity, which implies that the surface charge distribution of amyloid fibril is closely related to its conformation. This report demonstrated that KPFM is able to accurately obtain the surface potential of the amyloid fibrils with their conformational structures. Moreover, KPFM was shown to have the possibility of being usable as a detection platform for peptide identification of amyloid fibrils because KPFM measurement has proven to be powerful enough to detect a delicate difference of the surface potential.

4.3. Quantifying the electrical properties of amyloid fibrils in different environments

For understanding electrostatic interactions between various nano/biomaterials and amyloid oligomers/fibrils, or the accumulation of proteinaceous aggregates as amyloid fibrils/plaques, many researchers have reported quantifying the electrical properties of amyloid fibrils in different environments. In recent decades, nanomaterials, especially nanoparticles, have been increasingly applied in biomedicine for therapeutic and diagnostic purposes [68–70]. In particular, AuNPs have been widely used in the field of chemistry and biomedical science [71–73] due to their electronic [74] and molecular-recognition properties [75]. Due to the properties of AuNP, it has been found that the AuNPs can either promote or inhibit the aggregation of Aβ proteins, depending on the size and functionality of AuNPs or the pH value of the solution. As mentioned above, the surface potential analysis on the interaction of AuNPs with $A\beta_{25-35}$ peptides has been studied [67]. To investigate the effect of AuNPs on fibrillation, $A\beta_{25-35}$ peptides were incubated with AuNPs at room temperature for 5–12 days. KPFM was used to record both the sample topography and the surface potential of AuNPs with $A\beta_{25-35}$ fibrils. From the KPFM images, it was found that the CPD values of the AuNPs are about −0.7 to −1.1 V, whereas the value for pure $A\beta_{25-35}$ peptide fibrils was about 4.62 eV. *Via* calibration of the work function of cantilever tip, the work function of the AuNPs is obtained as about 4.95–5.20 eV. The work functions of fibrils connected by AuNPs are about 4.78 eV, slightly different from the pure fibrils, which difference may be induced by the local electric fields modified by the presence of AuNPs. From the results, it can be suggested that the presence of AuNPs in $A\beta_{25-35}$ solution has a significant influence on protein aggregation and on their electrical properties. This report demonstrated that it is plausible to suggest that KPFM will be quite useful for monitoring the conformational change and the electrical properties of the amyloid fibrils during self-assembly with nanomaterials.

To precisely investigate the mechanism of amyloid fibril formation, it is necessary to quantify the electrical properties of amyloid fibrils synthesized at different chemical environments. In the fibrillation of amyloid fibrils, the pH condition is one of the most important regulating chemical factors. It has been reported that the surface potential distribution of β-lg fibril is variable as a function of the pH of a buffer solution [20]. As mentioned above, the surface potential of amyloid fibril is critically dependent on the conformation of amyloid fibril. Therefore, the authors have defined the point charge density as related to the surface potential of β-lg fibril per unit fibril thickness: $\alpha(x) \equiv \sigma_{max(x)}/d_{max(x)}$, where $\sigma(x)$ is the measured surface potential and $d(x)$ is the diameter of an amyloid fibril [20]. It is shown that a parameter $\alpha(x)$ is varied with respect to pH and that $\alpha(x)$ becomes zero at pH ~ 4.7, indicating that the p*I* value of β-lg fibril is given by p*I* = 4.7 (**Figure 11a**). The surface potential of amyloid fibrils ranged from 12 mV (pH ~ 2) to −12 mV (pH ~ 7), depending on the pH of the buffer solution. For precise observation of the β-lg fibril's structure, the authors presented high-resolution KPFM images of single amyloid fibril for pH 3 < p*I* (~5.0) and pH 6 > p*I* (**Figure 11b**). With pH 3, they have found pristine β-lg protofilaments; with pH 6, the β-lg fibril had a complex structure of β-lg oligomer-binding protofilaments that had irregular topological height. It was remarkably observed that the pH-dependent electrostatic property of amyloid fibril was responsible for binding affinity between the amyloid small aggregates and the amyloid fibrils.

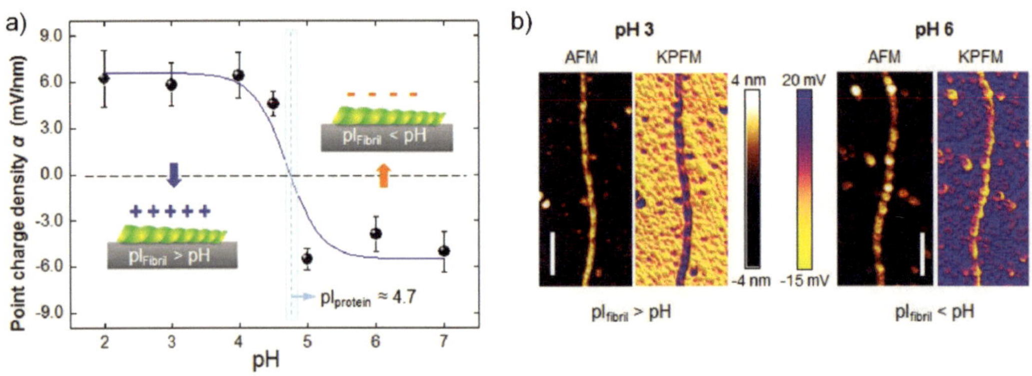

Figure 11. (a) The surface charge distribution of amyloid fibril as a function of the pH of buffer solution in which amyloid fibril is prepared. The isoelectric point (p*I*) value of amyloid fibril is determined in such a way that the pH value, at which surface charge distribution becomes zero, is identical to p*I* value. (b) AFM topography and surface potential images of β-lg amyloid fibrils when they are prepared in buffer solutions, whose pH values are pH 3 and pH 6, respectively. All scale bars are 250 nm. Figures reproduced with permission from Ref. [20], © 2012 AIP.

Moreover, in recent studies of amyloid fibril with AFM, some of scientists have reported about various structural features of amyloid fibrils such as steric zipper pattern [76, 77], helical pattern [48], and length [78], which is a key design parameter that determines the material properties of amyloid fibrils. Nevertheless, it is not quite understood yet how the molecular structures and conformational diversity (heterogeneous conformations) of amyloid fibrils are regulated.

To figure out how amyloid fibrils with heterogeneous conformations are formed, the synthesis of the β-lg fibrils with microwave-assisted chemistry method is considered, which enables the acceleration of biochemical reactions, and performed KPFM analysis of them [63]. It has been reported already that the microwave-assisted chemistry for the synthesis of amyloid fibrils makes the acceleration of fibrillation possible. The mechanism of amyloid fibrillation under microwave irradiation is still debated, but it seems to be related to the enhanced collision frequency due to the microwave-driven temperature changes of the protein solution. The temperature of the β-lg protein solution is rapidly increased by rotating water molecules through microwave irradiation. As such, microwave-assisted chemistry accelerates speed of chemical reactions regarding fibrillations of the β-lg proteins within a few hours (even less than an hour) [79]. It is a remarkable result compared to the classical (conventional) heating method which generally requires long incubation time (several hours) and a large volume of protein solution. However the results of this study show that microwave-assisted chemistry not only allows the acceleration of fibrillation but also enables tuning of the β-lg amyloid fibrils by controlling the microwave irradiation time τ, the time interval for irradiation λ, or the number of irradiations N. It was remarkably observed that a stable protein aggregation is produced in the fibril structure that depends on λ.

Figure 12 represents the topographic and surface potential images of amyloid fibrils that were synthesized based on microwave-assisted chemistry and their conformational heterogeneities. From these results, it is obvious that except for λ = 60 s, the surface potential and the fibril diameter of β-lg amyloid fibrils increase in monotone fashion as λ increases. This result revealed that heterogeneous conformations of β-lg amyloid fibrils are due to the wave-driven change of electrostatic interaction, which has a critical impact on the radial growth mechanisms of amyloid fibrils. As described above, KPFM indeed was a good analytical tool for monitoring the conformational change and the electrical properties of amyloid fibrils with respect to microwave-assisted chemistry.

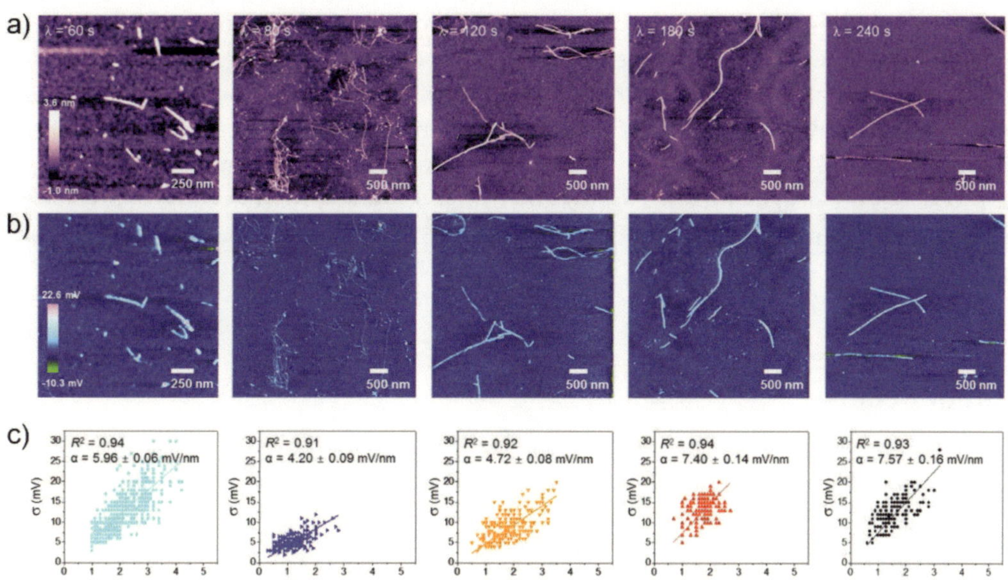

Figure 12. (a) AFM images of amyloid fibrils that are synthesized based on microwave-assisted chemistry using different λ values. (b) KPFM images of the fibrils formed using different λ values. (c) Distribution of surface charges for amyloid fibril as a function of its diameter. The surface potential of an amyloid fibril is almost linearly proportional to its diameter. Figures reprinted with permission from Ref. [63], © 2015 NPG.

5. Conclusion and perspectives

As we surveyed above, because of the marvelous capabilities of the conventional AFM device, it and its extensions as liquid AFM, PeakForce QNM, and KPFM have been widely used to perform accurate measurements of mechanical, electrical, and biophysical properties of various amyloid fibrils. AFM applications can provide researchers with the strong advantage of being able to measure the surface potentials of nanomaterials at the single-molecule level. Moreover, it has been demonstrated that AFM applications enable monitoring the fibrillation behavior of various proteins by measuring morphological properties of amyloid fibrils in air or liquid environments. The changes in morphology of the fibrils indicated that amyloid fibrils can be changed morphologically in liquid environments (e.g., human body) and that implies amyloid fibrils would interact differently with other biomolecules, cells, and tissues in human body. Liquid AFM enables measurement of the characteristics of amyloid fibrils in situ by monitoring the fibrillation and conformation changes of amyloid fibrils. Furthermore, AFM application techniques usually require no labeling with chemical dyes and no chemical reagents for improving the image quality or contrast. Accordingly, AFM is able to get high-resolution images of amyloid fibrils for the detection of conformational changes, by topological imaging in air and liquid environments. We dealt with PeakForce QNM that can simultaneously measure several mechanical properties of amyloid fibrils such as Young's modulus, deformation, and adhesion force by using a precisely operating oscillating probe. With a Kelvin probe, KPFM is highly important for imaging and characterizing the electrical properties (i.e., surface potential and surface potential density of amyloid fibrils) while getting high-resolution topological imaging. Because of these advantages, AFM application is expected to attract much attention as an analytical tool for amyloid research in the future. These AFM-related results shed light on understanding the fibrillation of amyloidogenic proteins and will be the cornerstone for the development of not only the effective prevention methods for amyloidogenic diseases but also therapeutic agents and drugs. These approaches could also contribute to the development of amyloid fibril-based functional nanomaterials such as biocompatible adhesives [80, 81], solar-cell devices [82], and gene delivery systems [83].

Author details

Wonseok Lee[1], Hyungbeen Lee[1], Gyudo Lee[2] and Dae Sung Yoon[3*]

*Address all correspondence to: dsyoon@korea.ac.kr

1 Department of Biomedical Engineering, Yonsei University, Wonju, Korea

2 School of Public Health, Harvard University, Boston, Massachusetts, USA

3 Department of Bio-convergence Engineering, Korea University, Seoul, Korea

References

[1] Chiti F, Dobson CM. Protein misfolding, functional amyloid, and human disease. Annu Rev Biochem. 2006;75(1):333–66.

[2] Dobson CM. Protein misfolding, evolution and disease. Trends Biochem Sci. 1999;24(9): 329–32.

[3] Dobson CM. Protein folding and misfolding. Nature. 2003;426(6968):884–90.

[4] Merlini G, Bellotti V. Molecular mechanisms of amyloidosis. N Engl J Med. 2003;349(6): 583–96.

[5] Selkoe DJ. Folding proteins in fatal ways. Nature. 2003;426(6968):900–4.

[6] Fowler DM, Koulov AV, Balch WE, Kelly JW. Functional amyloid – from bacteria to humans. Trends Biochem Sci. 2007;32(5):217–24.

[7] Fowler DM, Koulov AV, Alory-Jost C, Marks MS, Balch WE, Kelly JW. Functional amyloid formation within mammalian tissue. PLoS Biol. 2005;4(1):e6.

[8] Maji SK, Perrin MH, Sawaya MR, Jessberger S, Vadodaria K, Rissman RA, et al. Functional amyloids as natural storage of peptide hormones in pituitary secretory granules. Science. 2009;325(5938):328–32.

[9] Kelly JW, Balch WE. Amyloid as a natural product. J Cell Biol. 2003;161(3):461–2.

[10] Chapman MR, Robinson LS, Pinkner JS, Roth R, Heuser J, Hammar M, et al. Role of Escherichia coli curli operons in directing amyloid fiber formation. Science. 2002;295(5556):851–5.

[11] Shorter J, Lindquist S. Prions as adaptive conduits of memory and inheritance. Nat Rev Genet. 2005;6(6):435–50.

[12] Jung J-M, Savin G, Pouzot M, Schmitt C, Mezzenga R. Structure of heat-induced β-lactoglobulin aggregates and their complexes with sodium-dodecyl sulfate. Biomacromolecules. 2008;9(9):2477–86.

[13] Knowles TPJ, Buehler MJ. Nanomechanics of functional and pathological amyloid materials. Nat Nanotechnol. 2011;6(8):469–79.

[14] Rubin N, Perugia E, Goldschmidt M, Fridkin M, Addadi L. Chirality of amyloid suprastructures. J Am Chem Soc. 2008;130(14):4602–3.

[15] Kowalewski T, Holtzman DM. In situ atomic force microscopy study of Alzheimer's β-amyloid peptide on different substrates: new insights into mechanism of β-sheet formation. Proc Natl Acad Sci. 1999;96(7):3688–93.

[16] Jeong JS, Ansaloni A, Mezzenga R, Lashuel HA, Dietler G. Novel mechanistic insight into the molecular basis of amyloid polymorphism and secondary nucleation during amyloid formation. J Mol Biol. 2013;425(10):1765–81.

[17] Adamcik J, Berquand A, Mezzenga R. Single-step direct measurement of amyloid fibrils stiffness by peak force quantitative nanomechanical atomic force microscopy. Appl Phys Lett. 2011;98(19):193701.

[18] Sweers K, van der Werf K, Bennink M, Subramaniam V. Nanomechanical properties of α-synuclein amyloid fibrils: a comparative study by nanoindentation, harmonic force microscopy, and Peakforce QNM. Nanoscale Res Lett. 2011;6(1):1–10.

[19] Adamcik J, Lara C, Usov I, Jeong JS, Ruggeri FS, Dietler G, et al. Measurement of intrinsic properties of amyloid fibrils by the peak force QNM method. Nanoscale. 2012;4(15):4426–9.

[20] Lee G, Lee W, Lee H, Lee SW, Yoon DS, Eom K, et al. Mapping the surface charge distribution of amyloid fibril. Appl Phys Lett. 2012;101(4):043703–4.

[21] Ruggeri FS, Adamcik J, Jeong JS, Lashuel HA, Mezzenga R, Dietler G. Influence of the β-sheet content on the mechanical properties of aggregates during amyloid fibrillization. Angew Chem Int Ed. 2015;54(8):2462–6.

[22] Lamour G, Yip CK, Li H, Gsponer J. High intrinsic mechanical flexibility of mouse prion nanofibrils revealed by measurements of axial and radial Young's moduli. ACS Nano. 2014;8(4):3851–61.

[23] Lee W, Jung H, Son M, Lee H, Kwak TJ, Lee G, et al. Characterization of the regrowth behavior of amyloid-like fragmented fibrils decomposed by ultrasonic treatment. RSC Adv 2014;4(100):56561–6.

[24] Jaroniec CP, MacPhee CE, Bajaj VS, McMahon MT, Dobson CM, Griffin RG. High-resolution molecular structure of a peptide in an amyloid fibril determined by magic angle spinning NMR spectroscopy. Proc Natl Acad Sci U S A. 2004;101(3):711–6.

[25] Meersman F, Cabrera RQ, McMillan PF, Dmitriev V. Compressibility of insulin amyloid fibrils determined by X-ray diffraction in a diamond anvil cell. High Pressure Res. 2009;29(4):665–70.

[26] Westermark P, Benson MD, Buxbaum JN, Cohen AS, Frangione B, Ikeda S, et al. Amyloid fibril protein nomenclature—2002. Amyloid. 2002;9(3):197.

[27] Khurana R, Coleman C, Ionescu-Zanetti C, Carter SA, Krishna V, Grover RK, et al. Mechanism of thioflavin T binding to amyloid fibrils. J Struct Biol. 2005;151(3):229–38.

[28] Giessibl FJ. Advances in atomic force microscopy. Rev Mod Phys. 2003;75(3):949.

[29] Binnig G, Quate CF, Gerber C. Atomic force microscope. Phys Rev Lett. 1986;56(9):930.

[30] Muller DJ, Dufrene YF. Atomic force microscopy as a multifunctional molecular toolbox in nanobiotechnology. Nat Nanotechnol. 2008;3(5):261–9.

[31] Custance O, Perez R, Morita S. Atomic force microscopy as a tool for atom manipulation. Nat Nanotechnol. 2009;4(12):803–10.

[32] Nam K, Lee G, Jung H, Park J, Kim CH, Seo J, et al. Single-step electropolymerization patterning of a polypyrrole nanowire by ultra-short pulses via an AFM cantilever. Nanotechnology. 2011;22(22):225303.

[33] Lee G, Jung H, Son J, Nam K, Kwon T, Lee G, et al. Experimental and numerical study of electrochemical nanomachining using an AFM cantilever tip. Nanotechnology. 2010;21(18):185301.

[34] Khurana R, Ionescu-Zanetti C, Pope M, Li J, Nielson L, Ramírez-Alvarado M, et al. A general model for amyloid fibril assembly based on morphological studies using atomic force microscopy. Biophys J. 2003;85(2):1135–44.

[35] Adamcik J, Jung J-M, Flakowski J, De Los Rios P, Dietler G, Mezzenga R. Understanding amyloid aggregation by statistical analysis of atomic force microscopy images. Nat Nanotechnol. 2010;5(6):423–8.

[36] Sagis LMC, Veerman C, van der Linden E. Mesoscopic properties of semiflexible amyloid fibrils. Langmuir. 2004;20(3):924–7.

[37] Bolisetty S, Adamcik J, Mezzenga R. Snapshots of fibrillation and aggregation kinetics in multistranded amyloid [small beta]-lactoglobulin fibrils. Soft Matter. 2011;7(2):493–9.

[38] Relini A, Rolandi R, Bolognesi M, Aboudan M, Merlini G, Bellotti V, et al. Ultrastructural organization of ex vivo amyloid fibrils formed by the apolipoprotein A-I Leu174Ser variant: an atomic force microscopy study. Biochim Biophys Acta. 2004;1690(1):33–41.

[39] Sweers KKM, van der Werf KO, Bennink ML, Subramaniam V. Atomic force microscopy under controlled conditions reveals structure of C-terminal region of α-synuclein in amyloid fibrils. ACS Nano. 2012;6(7):5952–60.

[40] Ahmed M, Davis J, Aucoin D, Sato T, Ahuja S, Aimoto S, et al. Structural conversion of neurotoxic amyloid-[beta]1–42 oligomers to fibrils. Nat Struct Mol Biol. 2010;17(5):561–7.

[41] Cherny I, Gazit E. Amyloids: not only pathological agents but also ordered nanomaterials. Angew Chem Int Ed. 2008;47(22):4062–9.

[42] Smith JF, Knowles TPJ, Dobson CM, MacPhee CE, Welland ME. Characterization of the nanoscale properties of individual amyloid fibrils. Proc Natl Acad Sci. 2006;103(43):15806–11.

[43] Pfreundschuh M, Martinez-Martin D, Mulvihill E, Wegmann S, Muller DJ. Multiparametric high-resolution imaging of native proteins by force-distance curve-based AFM. Nat Protoc. 2014;9(5):1113–30.

[44] Ferencz R, Sanchez J, Blümich B, Herrmann W. AFM nanoindentation to determine Young's modulus for different EPDM elastomers. Polym Test. 2012;31(3):425–32.

[45] Foster B. New atomic force microscopy (AFM) approaches life sciences gently, quantitatively, and correlatively. Am Lab 2012(4):24–8.

[46] Trtik P, Kaufmann J, Volz U. On the use of peak-force tapping atomic force microscopy for quantification of the local elastic modulus in hardened cement paste. Cem Concr Res. 2012;42(1):215–21.

[47] Lee G, Lee H, Nam K, Han J-H, Yang J, Lee SW, et al. Nanomechanical characterization of chemical interaction between gold nanoparticles and chemical functional groups. Nanoscale Res Lett. 2012;7(1):1–11.

[48] Knowles TP, Fitzpatrick AW, Meehan S, Mott HR, Vendruscolo M, Dobson CM, et al. Role of intermolecular forces in defining material properties of protein nanofibrils. Science. 2007;318(5858):1900–3.

[49] Strohman R. Maneuvering in the complex path from genotype to phenotype. Science. 2002;296(5568):701–3.

[50] Verdile G, Fuller S, Atwood CS, Laws SM, Gandy SE, Martins RN. The role of beta amyloid in Alzheimer's disease: still a cause of everything or the only one who got caught? Pharmacol Res. 2004;50(4):397–409.

[51] Drolle E, Hane F, Lee B, Leonenko Z. Atomic force microscopy to study molecular mechanisms of amyloid fibril formation and toxicity in Alzheimer's disease. Drug Metab Rev. 2014;46(2):207–23.

[52] Bucciantini M, Giannoni E, Chiti F, Baroni F, Formigli L, Zurdo J, et al. Inherent toxicity of aggregates implies a common mechanism for protein misfolding diseases. Nature. 2002;416(6880):507–11.

[53] Kayed R, Head E, Thompson JL, McIntire TM, Milton SC, Cotman CW, et al. Common structure of soluble amyloid oligomers implies common mechanism of pathogenesis. Science. 2003;300(5618):486–9.

[54] Glabe CG, Kayed R. Common structure and toxic function of amyloid oligomers implies a common mechanism of pathogenesis. Neurology. 2006;66(1 suppl 1):S74–S8.

[55] Hertel C, Terzi E, Hauser N, Jakob-Røtne R, Seelig J, Kemp J. Inhibition of the electrostatic interaction between β-amyloid peptide and membranes prevents β-amyloid-induced toxicity. Proc Natl Acad Sci. 1997;94(17):9412–6.

[56] Bokvist M, Lindström F, Watts A, Gröbner G. Two types of Alzheimer's β-amyloid (1–40) peptide membrane interactions: aggregation preventing transmembrane anchoring versus accelerated surface fibril formation. J Mol Biol. 2004;335(4):1039–49.

[57] Friedman R, Pellarin R, Caflisch A. Amyloid aggregation on lipid bilayers and its impact on membrane permeability. J Mol Biol. 2009;387(2):407–15.

[58] Nonnenmacher M, o'Boyle M, Wickramasinghe H. Kelvin probe force microscopy. Appl Phys Lett. 1991;58(25):2921–3.

[59] Sinensky AK, Belcher AM. Label-free and high-resolution protein/DNA nanoarray analysis using Kelvin probe force microscopy nature nanotechnology. Nat Nanotechnol. 2007;2(10):653–9.

[60] Leung C, Maradan D, Kramer A, Howorka S, Mesquida P, Hoogenboom BW. Improved Kelvin probe force microscopy for imaging individual DNA molecules on insulating surfaces. Appl Phys Lett. 2010;97(20):203703.

[61] Park J, Yang J, Lee G, Lee CY, Na S, Lee SW, et al. Single-molecule recognition of biomolecular interaction via Kelvin probe force microscopy. ACS Nano. 2011;5(9): 6981–90.

[62] Nam K, Eom K, Yang J, Park J, Lee G, Jang K, et al. Aptamer-functionalized nano-pattern based on carbon nanotube for sensitive, selective protein detection. J Mater Chem. 2012;22(44):23348–56.

[63] Lee G, Lee W, Lee H, Lee CY, Eom K, Kwon T. Self-assembled amyloid fibrils with controllable conformational heterogeneity. Sci Rep 2015;5.

[64] Gao P, Cai Y. Label-free detection of the aptamer binding on protein patterns using Kelvin probe force microscopy (KPFM). Anal Bioanal Chem. 2009;394(1):207–14.

[65] Kelvin LV. Contact electricity of metals. Philos Mag 1898;46(278):82–120.

[66] Melitz W, Shen J, Kummel AC, Lee S. Kelvin probe force microscopy and its application. Surf Sci Rep. 2011;66(1):1–27.

[67] Ma Q, Wei G, Yang X. Influence of Au nanoparticles on the aggregation of amyloid-β-(25–35) peptides. Nanoscale. 2013;5(21):10397–403.

[68] Choi JH, Nguyen FT, Barone PW, Heller DA, Moll AE, Patel D, et al. Multimodal biomedical imaging with asymmetric single-walled carbon nanotube/iron oxide nanoparticle complexes. Nano Lett. 2007;7(4):861–7.

[69] McCarthy JR, Jaffer FA, Weissleder R. A macrophage-targeted theranostic nanoparticle for biomedical applications. Small. 2006;2(8-9):983–7.

[70] Kelley SO, Mirkin CA, Walt DR, Ismagilov RF, Toner M, Sargent EH. Advancing the speed, sensitivity and accuracy of biomolecular detection using multi-length-scale engineering. Nat Nanotechnol. 2014;9(12):969–80.

[71] Lin Y-C, Yu B-Y, Lin W-C, Lee S-H, Kuo C-H, Shyue J-J. Tailoring the surface potential of gold nanoparticles with self-assembled monolayers with mixed functional groups. J Colloid Interface Sci. 2009;340(1):126–30.

[72] Conklin D, Nanayakkara S, Park T-H, Lagadec MF, Stecher JT, Therien MJ, et al. Electronic transport in porphyrin supermolecule-gold nanoparticle assemblies. Nano Lett. 2012;12(5):2414–9.

[73] Stehlik S, Petit T, Girard HA, Kromka A, Arnault J-C, Rezek B. Surface potential of diamond and gold nanoparticles can be locally switched by surrounding materials or applied voltage. J Nanopart Res. 2014;16(4):1–11.

[74] Gutiérrez-Sánchez C, Pita M, Vaz-Domínguez C, Shleev S, De Lacey AL. Gold nanoparticles as electronic bridges for laccase-based biocathodes. J Am Chem Soc. 2012;134(41):17212–20.

[75] Raschke G, Kowarik S, Franzl T, Sönnichsen C, Klar T, Feldmann J, et al. Biomolecular recognition based on single gold nanoparticle light scattering. Nano Lett. 2003;3(7):935–8.

[76] Yoon G, Lee M, Kim JI, Na S, Eom K. Role of sequence and structural polymorphism on the mechanical properties of amyloid fibrils. PLoS one. 2014;9(2):e88502.

[77] Sawaya MR, Sambashivan S, Nelson R, Ivanova MI, Sievers SA, Apostol MI, et al. Atomic structures of amyloid cross-β spines reveal varied steric zippers. Nature. 2007;447(7143):453–7.

[78] Choi B, Yoon G, Lee SW, Eom K. Mechanical deformation mechanisms and properties of amyloid fibrils. Phys Chem Chem Phys. 2015;17(2):1379–89.

[79] Hettiarachchi CA, Melton LD, Gerrard JA, Loveday SM. Formation of β-lactoglobulin nanofibrils by microwave heating gives a peptide composition different from conventional heating. Biomacromolecules. 2012;13(9):2868–80.

[80] Mankar S, Anoop A, Sen S, Maji SK. Nanomaterials: amyloids reflect their brighter side. Nano Rev 2011;2.

[81] Mostaert AS, Higgins MJ, Fukuma T, Rindi F, Jarvis SP. Nanoscale mechanical characterisation of amyloid fibrils discovered in a natural adhesive. J Biol Phys. 2006;32(5):393–401.

[82] Bolisetty S, Adamcik J, Heier J, Mezzenga R. Amyloid directed synthesis of titanium dioxide nanowires and their applications in hybrid photovoltaic devices. Adv Funct Mater. 2012;22(16):3424–28.

[83] Yolamanova M, Meier C, Shaytan AK, Vas V, Bertoncini CW, Arnold F, et al. Peptide nanofibrils boost retroviral gene transfer and provide a rapid means for concentrating viruses. Nat Nanotechnol. 2013;8(2):130–6.

Chapter 4

Effects of Amyloid-β Deposition on Mitochondrial Complex I Activity in Brain: A PET Study in Monkeys

Hideo Tsukada

Additional information is available at the end of the chapter

http://dx.doi.org/10.5772/62901

Abstract

This chapter discusses the capabilities of positron emission tomography (PET) imaging for the diagnosis of Alzheimer's disease (AD) with deposition of amyloid-β (Aβ). We conducted a PET scan using ^{18}F-2-tert-butyl-4-chloro-5-{6-[2-(2-fluoroethoxy)-ethoxy]-pyridin-3-ylmethoxy}-2H-pyridazin-3-one (^{18}F-BCPP-EF), a novel PET probe for mitochondrial complex I (MC-I) activity, in young and aged monkeys to demonstrate the normal aging effects on MC-I activity in the brain. The results revealed an age-related impairment of MC-I activity in the brain. Then, we conducted PET scan using ^{11}C-PIB to detect the Aβ deposition in the some parts, not all, of the brains of some part of aged monkeys. For further assessments, PET scans using ^{11}C-PIB for Aβ, ^{11}C-DPA-713 for inflammation, ^{18}F-fluoro-2-deoxy-D-glucose (^{18}F-FDG) for regional cerebral metabolic rate of glucose (rCMRglc), and ^{18}F-BCPP-EF for MC-I were performed in aged animals. When ^{18}F-BCPP-EF uptake is plotted against ^{11}C-PIB uptake in the cerebral cortical regions, it showed a significant negative correlation between them. Plotting of ^{11}C-DPA-713 uptake against ^{11}C-PIB resulted in a significant positive correlation. In contrast, plotting of rCMRglc against ^{11}C-PIB did not reach a statistically significant level. Taken together, these results strongly suggested that ^{18}F-BCPP-EF could discriminate the neuronally damaged areas with neuroinflammation where ^{18}F-FDG could not, owing to its high uptake into the activated microglia.

Keywords: Alzheimer's disease, aging, brain, mitochondrial complex I, PET

1. Introduction

Alzheimer's disease (AD) is neuropathologically characterized by the presence of neurofibrillary tangles with the deposition of hyperphosphorylated tau protein inside nerve cells and senile plaques with extracellular aggregation of amyloid-β (Aβ) protein, and the imaging of tau and Aβ is expected to provide quantitative information noninvasively for the diagnosis of AD. Pathological aging processes are thought to be a degenerative process caused by accumulated damages, which leads to cellular dysfunction, tissue failure, and death, resulting in detectable changes in brain structure and function. Modern *in vivo* imaging techniques, such as X-ray computed tomography (X-CT), magnetic resonance imaging (MRI), and positron emission tomography (PET), provide useful ways to examine these alterations and to separate normal age-related changes from pathological states. Because functional disturbances precede structural changes determined by X-CT or MRI, the *in vivo* imaging obtained with PET may be abnormal, whereas the brain anatomy appears normal.

One trend is to apply target-specific PET probes for quantitative imaging of the specific neurological target molecules related to diseases, such as the dopaminergic system for schizophrenia [1] and Parkinson's disease (PD) [2], the serotonergic system for depression [3], and the cholinergic system for AD-type dementia [4]. Another trend is to measure more general indices for the pathophysiological abnormalities in diseases. To diagnose these diseases and to assess the treatment efficacy of developing drug candidates noninvasively with PET, we have anticipated PET probes that can provide general indices of brain function, such as regional cerebral blood flow (rCBF) and regional cerebral metabolic rate of oxygen ($rCMRO_2$), both of which have been recognized to be the gold standard indices for cerebral functions [5]. Other useful indicators are the regional cerebral metabolic rate of glucose (rCMRglc) assessed with ^{18}F-fluoro-2-deoxy-D-glucose (^{18}F-FDG; **Figure 1C**) [6]. PET using ^{18}F-FDG is a well-established technique for the quantitative imaging of brain function in the living brain. Some research demonstrated that ^{18}F-FDG could predict an onset of AD. However, as demonstrated in the brains of rat and monkey ischemic models [7, 8], the unexpectedly high uptake of ^{18}F-FDG in damaged areas suggested that ^{18}F-FDG was taken up into not only normal tissues but also inflammatory regions with microglial activation, which hampers the accurate diagnosis of brain function using ^{18}F-FDG.

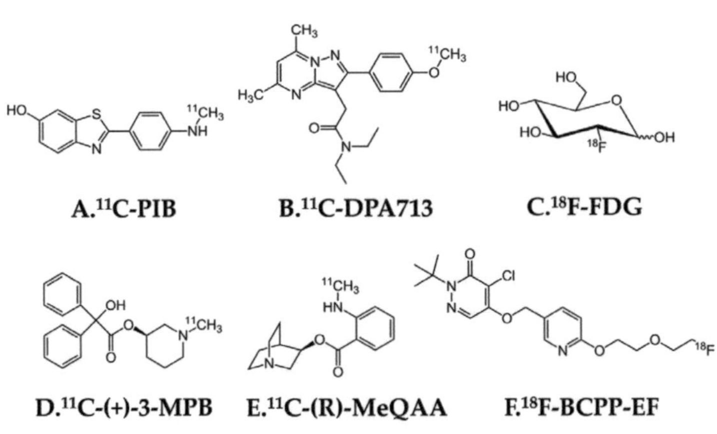

Figure 1. PET probes used: (A) ^{11}C-PIB for Aβ, (B) ^{11}C-DPA-713 for TSPO, (C) ^{18}F-FDG for rCMRglc, (D) ^{11}C-(+)-3-MPB for mAChR, (E) ^{11}C-(*R*)-MeQAA for α7-nAChR, and (F) ^{18}F-BCPP-EF for MC-I.

Several hypotheses of aging at the molecular level, such as shortening of telomerase, DNA methylation, reactive oxygen species (ROS) generation, and mitochondrial abnormalities, have been proposed. Among these, the "mitochondrial free radical theory of aging" has been highlighted [9]. In mammalian cells, the electron transport chain in mitochondria consists of five complexes from I to V, and the main role of mitochondria was recognized to be energy transduction of ATP. Their dysfunction was thought to be limited to ATP deficiency resulting in necrotic cell death; however, the mechanisms of cell death have been found to include mitochondrial contribution to oxidative stress and apoptosis [10]. Previous studies demonstrated an age-related increase in ROS production using rat brain homogenates [11], cortical slices [12], or synaptosomes [13]. Furthermore, mitochondrial dysfunction contributes to the pathophysiology of acute and chronic neurodegenerative disorders [14].

In the present chapter, the capability of assessment of mitochondrial complex I (MC-I) activity is introduced for detection of neurodegenerative damage associated with Aβ deposition. We recently developed and evaluated ^{18}F-2-tert-butyl-4-chloro-5-{6-[2-(2-fluoroethoxy)-ethoxy]-pyridin-3-ylmethoxy}-2H-pyridazin-3-one (^{18}F-BCPP-EF), a novel PET probe for MC-I activity (**Figure 1E**) [15]. The translational research has been conducted using an animal PET to assess the aging as well as Aβ deposition effects on MC-I activity in the living brains of young (3–5 years old, corresponding to high-teens in humans) and aged (20–24 years old, corresponding to 75 years old and more) male monkeys [16, 17].

2. Aging and cholinergic neuronal system

There have been a number of reports on age-related alterations in neurochemical and neurophysiological functions in the brain, associated with changes in the neurotransmitter synthesis in presynaptic neurons, release into synaptic cleft, reuptake availability, binding to receptors, and signal transduction, all of which are related to the declines of specific motor, cognitive and emotional functions in primates. Among the variety of neurotransmitter receptors, we focused on the effects of aging process on cholinergic receptors, which had previously assessed in the postmortem primate brain tissues [18].

2.1. Aging effects on muscarinic cholinergic receptor function

The cholinergic receptor (AChR) population is divided into muscarinic (mAChR) and nicotinic (nAChR) subclasses in the central nervous system (CNS), and the CNS mAChR system plays an important role in memory and cognitive functions. AD is neuropathologically characterized by the presence of neurofibrillary tangles with the deposition of Hyperphosphorylated tau protein inside nerve cells and senile plaques with extracellular aggregation of Aβ protein [19, 20]. Accompanied with tau and Aβ depositions, loss of cholinergic neurons in the forebrain, reduced cholinergic activity in the hippocampus and cortical loss of choline acetyltransferase, and reduced central mAChR binding have been observed in the brain of AD patients [21]. The severity of these cholinergic abnormalities is closely correlated with the degree of memory impairment in aged monkeys [22] and dementia patients [21].

Several antagonist-based ^{11}C-labeled PET probes for imaging mAChR have been developed and attempted to determine quantitatively the age-related alterations of mAChR in the living brain using ^{11}C-benztropine [23], *N*-^{11}C-methyl-4-piperidyl benzilate (^{11}C-4-MPB) [24], and ^{11}C-tropanyl benzilate (TBZ) [25]. These PET probes for mAChR, however, showed relatively low uptake to the brain and also slow dissociation rates from mAChR, which may limit the estimation of the density of binding sites *in vivo* [26]. To solve these problems, we proposed a novel mAChR probe, *N*-^{11}C-methyl-3-piperidyl benzilate (^{11}C-3-MPB) (**Figure 1D**) [27, 28], and assessed the aging effects on mAChR binding in comparison to young and aged monkeys [29].

^{11}C-(+)3-MPB was labeled by *N*-methylation of respective nor-compound with ^{11}C-methyl iodide converted from ^{11}C-CO_2 by $LiAlH_4$ reduction followed by reaction with HI [27, 28]. A monkey (*Macaca mulatta*) was seated on a monkey chair under conscious condition and fixed with stereotactic coordinates under conscious state [30]. For the kinetic analysis of ^{11}C-(+)3-MPB binding, arterial blood sampling was conducted to determine the input function using metabolic profile in plasma. The PET data obtained were reconstructed by the filtered back-projection (FBP) method. Volumes of interest (VOIs) in brain regions were drawn manually on the MRI, and VOIs of MRI were superimposed on the coregistered PET images to measure the time activity curves (TACs) of each PET probe for kinetic analyses using Logan graphical analysis with metabolite-corrected plasma input in the living brain [31].

The TACs of ^{11}C-(+)3-MPB in the frontal, temporal, and occipital cortices reached their peaks 40 min after injection, whereas the striatal and hippocampal regions reached peak values 60

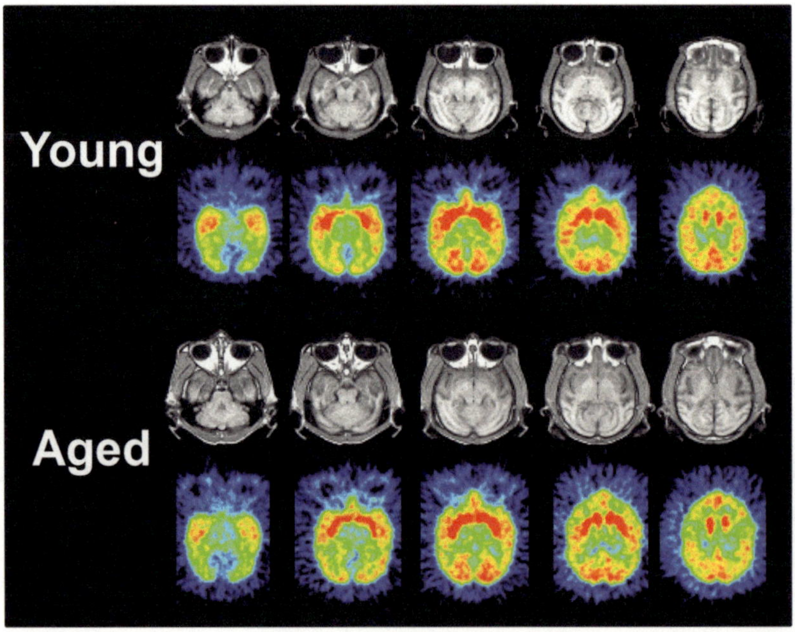

Figure 2. MRI and PET images of ^{11}C-(+)3-MPB in the young and aged monkey brains (*M. mulatta*). PET data were collected in the conscious state with a high-resolution PET scanner. Each PET image was generated by summation of image data from 60 to 91 min post-injection. The stereotactic coordinates of PET and MRI were adjusted based on the orbitomeatal (OM) line.

http://dx.doi.org/10.5772/62901

min after injection [28]. In aged monkeys, the TACs of ^{11}C-(+)3-MPB in regions rich in mAChR peaked at earlier time points, with faster elimination rates than those in young monkeys. As a result of Logan graphical analysis using metabolite-corrected plasma input, significant age-related alterations of the *in vivo* binding of ^{11}C-(+)3-MPB were observed in the temporal and frontal cortices and the striatum (**Figure 2**). Aged animals showed the age-related reduction of the maximum number of binding sites (B_{max}) of mAChR, whereas there were no age-related alterations of the affinity (1/Kd) of mAChR [29].

2.2. Aging effects on nicotinic cholinergic receptor function

The CNS AChR systems, classified into mAChR and nAChR, play an important role in memory and cognitive functions. In the last two decades, 17 different nAChR subunits (α1–α10, β1–β4,γ, δ and ε) have been cloned, and the prominent nAChRs are the α4β2 heteromeric and α7 homomeric subtypes in the brain [32]. Among them, because α7 has high permeability for Ca^{2+}, it can be assumed that, in addition to the ionotropic function induced by membrane depolarization, α7-nAChR is associated with metabotropic activity coupled to Ca^{2+}-regulated second-messenger signaling required for the modulation of neuron excitability, neurotransmitter release, induction of long-term potentiation (LTP), and cognitive-associated processing of learning and memory. In addition, α7-nAChR may contribute to neuroprotection by modulating the neurotrophic system crucial for the maintenance of cholinergic neuron integrity and also by stimulating signal transduction pathways that support neuron survival [32].

A PET study indicated that decreases in ^{11}C-nicotine brain uptake were significantly correlated with cognitive deficits in AD patients [33]; however, nAChR deficits in the different types of dementia are assumed to be reflected by subtype and region specificity. For the noninvasive imaging of α7-nAChR with more subtype specificity, several ^{11}C-labeled PET probes have been developed and evaluated, including ^{11}C-CHIBA-1001, ^{11}C-A-582941, and ^{11}C-A-844606 [34]. However, because of low brain uptake, high nonspecific binding, and/or low selectivity to α7-nAChR against 5-HT_3R, almost none of these PET probes have demonstrated clinically useful specific binding to α7-nAChR in nonhuman primate brain. Because we recently developed novel PET probes for α7-nAChR, (*R*)-2-[^{11}C]methylamino-benzoic acid 1-aza-bicycle[2.2.2]oct-3-yl ester [^{11}C-(*R*)-MeQAA; **Figure 1E**] [35], the aging effects on α7-nAChR binding was assessed using ^{11}C-(*R*)-MeQAA in comparison to young and aged monkeys [36].

^{11}C-(*R*)-MeQAA was labeled by *N*-methylation of respective nor-compounds [(*R*)-BH_3QAA] with ^{11}C-methyl triflate prepared from ^{11}C-methyl iodide through a glass column containing silver triflate [35]. PET measurements of conscious monkeys were conducted as described in Section 2.2 with arterial blood sampling for plasma metabolic analysis followed by PET image reconstruction and TAC acquisition in the VOIs for kinetic analyses. The values of nondisplaceable binding potential (BP_{ND}) were evaluated by two-compartment models (2-TC) analysis using the metabolite-corrected plasma input [37] and simplified reference tissue model (SRTM) analysis using the TAC in the cerebellum as an indirect input function [38].

^{11}C-(*R*)-MeQAA images in the brain of young normal monkeys, showing high and heterogeneous uptake of [^{11}C](*R*)-MeQAA into the brain, were determined between 60 and 90 min after the bolus injection. The uptake of radioactivity was high in the thalamus and striatum, intermediate in the hippocampus, frontal, temporal, and occipital cortices, and low in the cerebellum [35, 36]. The uptake of ^{11}C-(*R*)-MeQAA was significantly higher than that of ^{11}C-(*S*)-MeQAA in the thalamus, hippocampus, and cortical regions, and the specific binding of ^{11}C-(*R*)-MeQAA was inhibited by the preadministration of SSR180711, an α7-nAChR partial agonist [35]. In contrast, the uptake of ^{11}C-(*R*)-MeQAA into the cerebellum of monkeys was not affected by SSR180711 [35], suggesting that the cerebellum could be applicable for the reference region for the quantitative analysis of ^{11}C-(*R*)-MeQAA binding in the living brain. The clearance rate of ^{11}C-(*R*)-MeQAA in plasma was rapid and relatively stable in plasma. To determine the practicality of the simplified analytical method of ^{11}C-(*R*)-MeQAA with SRTM to calculate the BP_{ND} using the TAC in the cerebellum as an indirect input function, we verified it by correlation analyses with 2-TC-BP_{ND} values calculated using the metabolite-corrected plasma input. Because of a good correlation between 2-TC and SRTM analyses, ^{11}C-(*R*)-MeQAA binding to α7-nAChR in young and aged monkey brain was determined as the SRTM-BP_{ND} values without arterial blood sampling to avoid excessive stress on aged animals. When determining the aging effects on ^{11}C-(*R*)-MeQAA binding, all regions, except the occipital cortex, revealed no significant differences in the BP_{ND} values of ^{11}C-(*R*)-MeQAA in the brains of aged and young animals [36]. Although human aging is known to preferentially affect the rCMRglc in the frontal and temporal lobes, our previous studies reported that the occipital cortex showed the most profound reductions of CBF [39], rCMRglc [39], and MC-I [16] in aged monkeys. Because the differences in cortical activity between monkey and human reflect the evolutionary significance of their frontal cortex, the most marked age-related alterations of α7-nAChR activity would be determined in regions such as the frontal cortex, not in the occipital cortex, in humans. These results apparently revealed that aging effects were much less on α7-nAChR compared to mAChR in the living brain.

3. Aging and MC-I activity

Mitochondria are called "cellular power plants" because they generate most of the ATP used as a source of chemical energy. In mammalian cells, the electron transport chain in mitochondria consists of five complexes from I to V, and complex I (MC-I; NADH-ubiquinone oxidoreductase, EC 1.6.5.3) is the first and rate-limiting step of the overall respiratory activity and oxidative phosphorylation under physiological conditions. Glucose is converted to pyruvate followed by transformation into acetyl-CoA by pyruvate dehydrogenase (PDH) in the mitochondria, which is subsequently fed into the tricarboxylic acid (TCA) cycle, ultimately producing ATP via the electron transport system and oxidative phosphorylation (which is indispensable for cell survival). Mitochondrial dysfunction contributes to the pathophysiology of neurodegenerative diseases [40], some part of which has been considered to relate to the fact that mitochondria are the main intracellular source of ROS in cells and also the main target of ROS-mediated damage. Noninvasive assessment of living brain could be useful for the diagnostic, prognostic, and treatment monitoring of neurodegenerative diseases related to impaired MC-I function; however, no proper PET probes for MC-I imaging in the brain have been developed prior to those that we have recently described [15].

3.1. Development of PET probe for MC-I imaging

As PET probe for MC-I imaging, BMS-747158-01 showed inhibitory activity on MC-I function by binding to MC-I, and its F-18 derivative ^{18}F-BMS-747158-01 was originally developed as a myocardial perfusion imaging agent [41]. However, we also realized that ^{18}F-BMS-747158-01 revealed relatively high nonspecific binding in the brain based on the lower degree of inhibition with rotenone, a specific MC-I inhibitor, in both *in vitro* and *in vivo* assessments [7, 8]. To solve the problem, we redesigned to modify the chemical structure of ^{18}F-BMS-747158-01 to induce lower lipophilicity and lower affinity [15, 42]. We recently developed a novel PET probe, ^{18}F-BCPP-EF, and evaluated its properties in the *in vitro* and *in vivo* assessments [7, 8, 15, 16].

For the analysis of the affinity of ^{18}F-BCPP-EF, an *in vitro* binding assay was conducted using ^{3}H-dihydrorotenone and bovine cardiomyocyte submitochondrial particles (SMP) to determine the 50% inhibition (IC_{50}) values, which were converted to the inhibition constant (Ki). ^{18}F-BCPP-EF was radiolabeled by the nucleophilic ^{18}F-fluorination of the corresponding tosylate precursor, toluene-4-sulfonic acid 2-{2-[5-(1-tert-butyl-5-chloro-6-oxo-1,6-dihydro-pyridazin-4-yloxymethyl)-pyridin-2-yloxy]-ethoxy}-ethyl ester [15]. For the assessment of binding specificity of the PET probe to MC-I, vehicle or rotenone, a specific MC-I inhibitor, at a dose of 0.1 mg/kg was infused to anesthetised rats or conscious monkeys through a vein for 1 h, and then ^{18}F-BCPP-EF was injected as a bolus for PET measurement. PET measurements of young monkeys (3–5 years old) were conducted under conscious state as described in Section 2.2 with arterial blood sampling for plasma metabolic analysis followed by PET image reconstruction and TAC acquisition in the VOIs aided by MRI of individual animals for kinetic analyses [16, 17]. The total distribution volume (DV) values were evaluated by Logan plot graphical analysis using the metabolite-corrected plasma input [33].

^{18}F-BCPP-EF showed the lower affinity (Ki=2.31 nM) with lower lipophilicity ($logD_{7.4}$=3.03) for MC-I of bovine cardiomyocytes than that of BMS-747158-01 (Ki=0.95 nM, $logD_{7.4}$=3.69). In PET study in rats, the radioactivity level of ^{18}F-BCPP-EF in the brain showed rapid uptake and gradual decrease with time just after the injection under vehicle condition. In the heart, ^{18}F-BCPP-EF exhibited slow accumulation up to 30 min after the injection followed by a slight washout. With preadministration of rotenone, although a dose escalation study of rotenone was impossible because of its lethal effects on cardiac function, a significant reduction of ^{18}F-BCPP-EF uptake was observed in the brain and heart, even at a relatively low dose of 0.1 mg/kg/h. ^{18}F-BMS-747158-01 showed a tendency of decreased brain uptake with rotenone infusion but was not fully inhibited [7].

In the conscious monkey brain, TACs of ^{18}F-BCPP-EF peaked between 10 and 20 min after the injection, except in the occipital cortex (40 min), followed by the gradual elimination with time. With preadministration of rotenone, a specific MC-I inhibitor, at a dose of 0.1 mg/kg/h, the uptake of ^{18}F-BCPP-EF into the brain, especially in the frontal and temporal cortices and striatum, was significantly facilitated just after the injection followed by faster elimination than normal from the brain regions. The washout and metabolic rates of ^{18}F-BCPP-EF in plasma were rapid; only 10% of nonmetabolized ^{18}F-BCPP-EF was detected 60 min after the injection, which was were nearly identical with that of rotenone-treated animals. The DV values calculated by Logan plot graphical analysis were the highest in the occipital cortex, higher in the striatum, intermediate in the frontal and temporal cortices and cerebellum, and lowest in the hippocampus of young monkey. Rotenone administration resulted in a significant and marked reduction of the binding of ^{18}F-BCPP-EF to MC-I in the living monkey brain [16]. Taken together, these results clearly suggested that ^{18}F-BCPP-EF was a useful PET probe for the quantitative imaging of MC-I activity in the living brain.

3.2. Aging effects on MC-I activity

Several hypotheses of aging have been proposed, and mitochondrial respiratory chain failures have been implicated as factors in the aging process, which was called the "mitochondrial free radical theory of aging" [9–13]. This theory is based on the results that (1) mitochondrial ROS production increases with age, (2) the activity of ROS-scavenging enzymes declines with age, (3) mutations of mitochondrial DNA (mtDNA) accumulate during aging, and (4) somatic mtDNA mutations impair respiratory chain function, which results in a further increase in ROS production [9–13]. Mitochondria are the main intracellular source of ROS and also the main target of oxyradical-mediated damage, and cumulative free radical damage leads to significant changes in brain mitochondrial function.

As described in Section 3.1, because we could confirm the capability of ^{18}F-BCPP-EF as PET probe for the noninvasive assessment of MC-I activity in the living brain, we further explored to see the aging effects on MC-I activity in comparison to young and aged monkeys under conscious condition [16]. All study procedures were identical as described in Section 3.1, except that the subjects were aged male monkeys (20–24 years old).

Aided by MRI of individual monkeys, the VOIs were set on PET images of ^{18}F-BCPP-EF to obtain TACs. The peak of ^{18}F-BCPP-EF slightly shifted to a later time period between 20 and 30 min after the injection and also provided significantly lower levels than those in young animals shown in Section 3.1. The washout and metabolic patterns of ^{18}F-BCPP-EF in plasma of aged monkeys were nearly identical to those in young animals. When determining the effects of aging on ^{18}F-BCPP-EF binding to MC-I assessed by Logan plot graphical analysis, the data revealed significantly lower DV values of ^{18}F-BCPP-EF in every brain region analyzed in aged animals compared to those in young ones [16].

The remarkable finding of the present study was that ^{18}F-BCPP-EF detected the age-related reduction of MC-I activity in the living brain of monkey under conscious conditions with PET (**Figure 3**). It was of interest that the activity of complexes I and IV decreased with age in the brain of humans [43], whereas that of complexes II, III, and V remained mostly unchanged [44]. Because all these findings described above were obtained by the *in vitro* assessments of dissected organ samples, the present data are the first to demonstrate the alterations of MC-I activity in the living brain of a nonhuman primate by a noninvasive method using ^{18}F-BCPP-EF and PET [16].

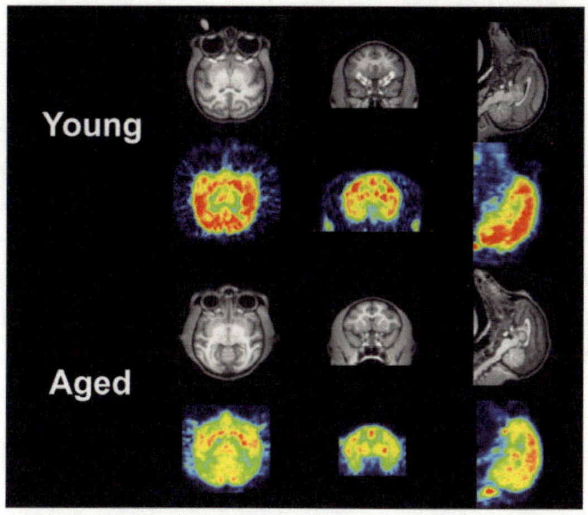

Figure 3. MRI and PET images of ^{18}F-BCPP-EF in young and aged monkeys (*M. mulatta*). PET scans were acquired for 91 min after ^{18}F-BCPP-EF injection with sequential arterial blood sampling. The binding of ^{18}F-BCPP-EF to MC-I was calculated using Logan graphical analysis with metabolite-corrected plasma input.

4. Effects of Aβ deposition on AChR and MC-I

Hallmark pathologies of AD have been assumed to the formation of extracellular aggregation of Aβ protein (senile plaques) [19] and intraneuronal aggregation of phosphorylated tau protein (neurofibrillary tangle) [20], pathogenic microglial activation [45], and oxidative stress reactions [13]. Furthermore, recent reports suggested that nondeposited and nonfibrillar assemblies of Aβ peptides are considered to play a primary role in AD, which might be precursors in fibrillogenesis to mediate the neurotoxicity, including oxidative stress in AD [46]. This session discusses the effects of Aβ-related pathological changes on nAChR binding [36] and also on MC-I activity [17] assessed in aged monkey brain using animal PET.

4.1. Aging effects on Aβ deposition and neuroinflammation

For the quantitative measurements of Aβ deposition in the living brain, ^{11}C-PIB was synthesized by *N*-methylation of nor-compound *N*-desmethyl-PIB with ^{11}C-methyl triflate (**Figure 1A**) [47]. For the assessment of neuroinflammation, ^{11}C-DPA-713 was synthesized by *N*-methylation of nor-compound *N*-desmethyl-DPA with ^{11}C-methyl triflate (**Figure 1B**) [48]. PET measurements with these two PET probes were conducted under conscious state as described in Section 2.2. For the analysis of ^{11}C-PIB uptake, standard uptake value (SUV) images were created, and the VOIs were set on each SUV images with the aid of MRI. For the analysis of ^{11}C-DPA-713 uptake, SUV images were created, and VOIs were set on each SUV images.

We had previously found that some, but not all, of aged monkeys exhibited higher ^{11}C-PIB uptake than young ones, suggesting Aβ deposition even in the brain of monkey [49]. Although the SUVs of ^{11}C-PIB were slightly high in the striatal regions, hippocampus, parietal cortex, and thalamus in aged monkeys, it was reported that aged monkeys did not reveal as high Aβ deposition as determined in AD patients [50] and also that no species besides humans has yet shown drastic neuron loss or cognitive decline approaching clinical-grade AD in humans. The SUVs of ^{11}C-DPA-713 were relatively high in the striatal regions, hippocampus, temporal cortex, and thalamus. The plot of SUV of ^{11}C-DPA-713 against SUV of ^{11}C-PIB revealed significant positive correlation both in the cortical regions. When rCMRglc ratio is plotted against SUV of ^{11}C-DPA-713, the results provided the significant positive correlation in the cortical regions. There results strongly suggest that the Aβ deposition as measured with ^{11}C-PIB induced neuroinflammation with microglial activation as determined with ^{11}C-DPA-713 as well as ^{18}F-FDG (**Figure 4**).

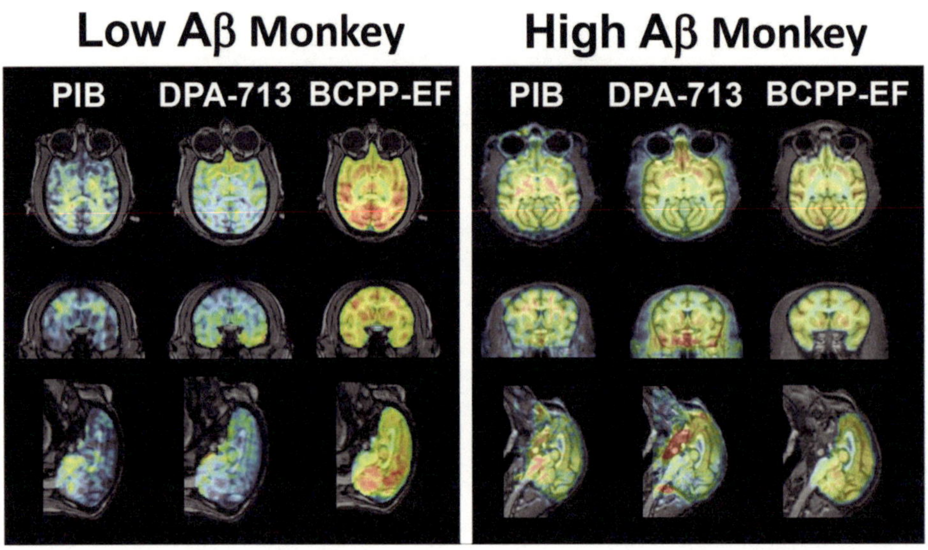

Figure 4. PET/MRI fusion images of ^{11}C-PIB, ^{11}C-DPA-713, and ^{18}F-BCPP-EF uptake in the brains of aged monkeys (*M. mulatta*). ^{18}F-BCPP-EF brain imaging was performed in monkey 1 with the highest binding of all 20 animals in the conscious state and in monkey 2 with the lowest binding.

4.2. Effects of Aβ deposition on nAChR binding

Postmortem studies of human brains have suggested that a deficit of α7-nAChR is related to AD, dementia with Lewy bodies, and schizophrenia [32]. Aβ has a high affinity to α7-nAChR upon being enriched in basal forebrain areas, and initial Aβ deposition in early AD overlaps with α7-nAChR expression in these regions [51]. α7-nAChR facilitates binding, internalization, and accumulation of $A\beta_{1-42}$ and may result in the selective vulnerability of specific cells expressing α7-nAChR [52]. Oligomers of Aβ disrupt synaptic plasticity and cognitive function when administered at nanomolar range concentration through the modulation of NMDA receptor function to depress NMDA-evoked currents [53, 54].

To assess the effect of Aβ deposition on α7-nAChR function, the correlation between ^{11}C-PIB uptake and ^{11}C-(*R*)-MeQAA was analyzed [36]. As described in Section 2.2, all regions, except the occipital cortex, revealed no significant differences in the BP_{ND} values of ^{11}C-(*R*)-MeQAA in the brains of aged and young animals. However, of interest, when the BP_{ND} values of ^{11}C-(*R*)-MeQAA are plotted against the SUVR of ^{11}C-PIB in the corresponding VOIs of aged animals, the results indicated a significant positive correlation between them (**Figure 5**). The α7-nAChR had been assumed to decrease with the aging process; however, the data seem to be controversial because of the dose-dependent interaction aspects between of Aβ and α7-nAChR. In young and normal conditions, there is an equilibrium between production and elimination of Aβ, which maintains Aβ in a steady state to perform physiologic roles by the interaction with α7-nAChR; thus, low (on the order of picomolar) concentrations of $A\beta_{1-42}$ may play a role in modulating synaptic plasticity and enhancing cognitive function in mice via interaction with α7-nAChR, probably in presynaptic neurons [55]. In aging with pathologic conditions, the balance between Aβ formation and clearance is impaired, which leads to Aβ accumulation and α7-nAChR deficit as observed in postmortem brains of AD patients [32]. These results suggest that α7-nAChR-Aβ interaction has dual effects on brain function following aging or injury as well as preserving physiologic roles, causing the controversial results in the aging effects on the α7-nAChR level. One previous study clearly demonstrated the significant reduction of α7-nAChR level in neurons and also Aβ-induced up-regulation of α7-nAChR on astrocytes in postmortem AD brain compared to that in age-matched control [56]. α7-nAChR may be chronically inactivated in an antagonistic fashion through prolonged interaction with increased levels (on the order of nanomolar) of Aβ, resulting in the up-regulation of α7-nAChR.

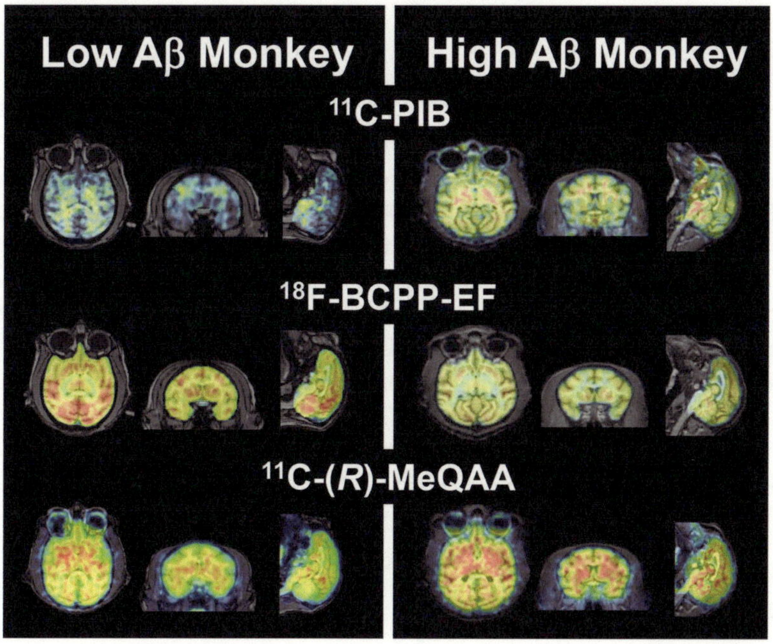

Figure 5. PET/MRI fusion images of ^{11}C-PIB, ^{18}F-BCPP-EF, and ^{11}C-(*R*)-MeQAA in the brains of aged monkeys (*M. mulatta*). PET images of an aged monkey with the lowest and highest ^{11}C-PIB uptake are shown along with ^{18}F-BCPP-EF and ^{11}C-(*R*)-MeQAA.

4.3. Effects of Aβ deposition on MC-I activity

As shown in Section 3.2, ^{18}F-BCPP-EF binding to MC-I in each brain region indicated much larger variation (CV=25.1%) in aged animals than in young ones (7.4%) [16]. Since we had previously found that some of the aged monkeys exhibited high ^{11}C-PIB uptake, suggesting Aβ deposition in the brain [49], the effects of Aβ deposition level assessed in Section 4.1 on MC-I activity evaluated in Section 3.2 were determined. When the ^{18}F-BCPP-EF binding is plotted against the ^{11}C-PIB uptake in the corresponding VOIs of all animals, the results indicated a significant reversal correlation (**Figure 4**). In contrast, no significant relationships were observed in the plot of rCMRglc measured using ^{18}F-FDG against ^{11}C-PIB uptake in the cerebral cortical regions [17]. There results strongly suggest that the Aβ deposition as measured with ^{11}C-PIB induced neuroinflammation with microglial activation as determined with ^{11}C-DPA-713 as well as ^{18}F-FDG. Apart from developed cells such as neurons, activated inflammatory cells produce lactate from glucose, known as the Warburg effect [57] or aerobic glycolysis, accounting for only approximately 5% glucose utilization in oxidative phosphorylation. Because activated inflammatory cells exclusively produce ATP through enhanced glycolysis with a low contribution of the electron transport system, these cells need more glucose to survive than normal neuronal and glial tissues, resulting in the higher ^{18}F-FDG uptake in the neurodegenerative damaged regions. The present results demonstrated that ^{18}F-BCPP-EF could be used to image MC-I activity specifically as well as to detect impaired MC-I activity correlated to Aβ deposition in the living brain of monkeys.

5. Conclusions

In this chapter, the effects of Aβ deposition on α7-nAChR binding, TSPO activity, an established marker of microglial activation, and rCMRglc were assessed simultaneously with MC-I activity. PET using ^{18}F-FDG is a well-established technique for the quantitative imaging of brain function as rCMRglc in the living brain. However, the unexpectedly high uptake of ^{18}F-FDG in damaged brain regions suggested that ^{18}F-FDG was taken up into not only normal tissues but also inflammatory regions with microglial activation, which hampers the accurate diagnosis of brain function using ^{18}F-FDG. Neuroinflammation has recently emerged in several neurodegenerative diseases, including schizophrenia, depression, autism, PD, and AD. PET measurements of MC-I activity using ^{18}F-BCPP-EF will be a superior diagnostic, prognostic, and treatment monitoring tool for AD-type dementia without being affected by inflammation.

Author details

Hideo Tsukada*

Address all correspondence to: tsukada@crl.hpk.co.jp

Central Research Laboratory, Hamamatsu Photonics K.K., Hamamatsu, Japan

References

[1] Patel NH, Vyas NS, Puri BK, Nijran KS, Al-Nahhas A. Positron emission tomography in schizophrenia: A new perspective. J Nucl Med. 2010;51:511–520. DOI: 10.2967/jnumed.109.066076.

[2] Brooke DJ. Imaging approaches to Parkinson disease. J Nucl Med. 2010;51:596–609. DOI: 10.2967/jnumed.108.059998.

[3] Neyer JH. Neuroimaging markers of cellular function in major depressive disorder: Implications for therapeutics, personalized medicine, and prevention. Clin Pharmacol Ther. 2012;91:201–214. DOI: 10.1038/clpt.2011.285.

[4] Kadir A, Nordberg A. Target-specific PET probes for neurodegenerative disorders related to dementia. J Nucl Med. 2010;51:1418–1430. DOI: 10.2967/jnumed.110.077164.

[5] Lammertsma AA, Heather JD, Jones T, Frackowiak RSJ, Lenzi GL. A statistical study of the steady-state technique for measuring regional cerebral blood flow and oxygen utilization using ^{15}0. J Comput Assist Tomogr. 1982;6:566–573.

[6] Phelps ME, Huang SC, Hoffman El, Selin CS, Sokoloff L, Kuhl DE. Tomographic measurement of local cerebral glucose metabolic rate in humans with (F-18) 2-fluoro-2-deoxyglucose: Validation of method. Ann Neurol. 1979;6:371–388. DOI: 10.1002/ana.410060502.

[7] Tsukada H, Nishiyama S, Fukumoto D, Kanazawa M, Harada N. Novel PET probes ^{18}F-BCPP-EF and ^{18}F-BCPP-BF for mitochondrial complex I: A PET study in comparison with ^{18}F-BMS-747158-02 in rat brain. J Nucl Med. 2014;55:473–480. DOI: 10.2967/jnumed.113.125328.

[8] Tsukada H, Ohba H, Nishiyama S, Kanazawa M, Kakiuchi T, Harada N. PET imaging of ischemia-induced impairment of mitochondrial complex I function in monkey brain. J Cereb Blood Flow Metab. 2014;34:708–714. DOI: 10.1038/jcbfm.2014.5.

[9] Bratic A, Larsson NG. The role of mitochondria in aging. J Clin Invest. 2013;123:952–957. DOI: 10.1172/JCI64125.

[10] Ankarcrona M, Dypbukt JM, Bonfoco E, Zhivotovsky B, Orrenius S, Lipton SA, Nicotera P. Glutamate-induced neuronal death: A succession of necrosis or apoptosis depending on mitochondrial function. Neuron. 1995;15:961–973. DOI: 10.1016/0896-6273(95)90186-8.

[11] Baek BS, Kwon HJ, Lee KH, Yoo MA, Kim KW, Ikeno Y, Yu BP, Chung HY. Regional difference of ROS generation, lipid peroxidation, and antioxidant enzyme activity in

rat brain and their dietary modulation. Arch Pharm Res. 1999;22:361–366. DOI: 10.1007/BF02979058.

[12] Kannurpatti SS, Sanganahalli BG, Mishra S, Joshi PG, Joshi NB. Glutamate-induced differential mitochondrial response in young and adult rats. Neurochem Int. 2004;44:361–369. DOI: 10.1007/BF02979058.

[13] Choi BH. Oxidative stress and Alzheimer's disease. Neurobiol Aging. 1995;16:675–678. DOI: 10.1016/0197-4580(95)00065-M.

[14] Schon EA, Przedborski S. Mitochondria: The next (neurode)generation. Neuron. 2011;70:1033–1053. DOI: 10.1016/j.neuron.2011.06.003.

[15] Harada N, Nishiyama S, Kanazawa M, Tsukada H. Development of novel PET probes, [^{18}F]BCPP-EF, [^{18}F]BCPP-BF, and [^{11}C]BCPP-EM for mitochondrial complex I imaging. J Labelled Compd Radiopharm. 2013;56:553–561. DOI: 10.1002/jlcr.3056.

[16] Tsukada H, Ohba H, Kanazawa M, Kakiuchi T, Harada N. Evaluation of ^{18}F-BCPP-EF for mitochondrial complex 1 imaging in conscious monkey brain using PET. Eur J Nucl Med Mol Imaging. 2014;41:755–763. DOI: 10.1007/s00259-014-2821-8.

[17] Tsukada H, Nishiyama S, Ohba H, Kanazawa M, Kakiuchi T, Harada N. Comparing amyloid-β deposition, neuroinflammation, glucose metabolism, and mitochondrial complex I activity in brain: A PET study in aged monkeys. Eur J Nucl Med Mol Imaging. 2014;41:2127–2136. DOI: 10.1007/s00259-013-2628-z.

[18] Court JA, Lloyd S, Johnson M, Griffiths M, Birdsall NJM, Piggott MA, Oakley AE, Ince PG, Perry EK, Perry RH. Nicotinic and muscarinic cholinergic receptor binding in the human hippocampal formation during development and aging. Dev Brain Res. 1997;101:93–105. DOI: 10.1016/S0165-3806(97)00052-7.

[19] Hardy J, Selkoe DJ. The amyloid hypothesis of Alzheimer's disease: Progress and problems on the road to therapeutics. Science. 2002;297:353–356. DOI: 10.1126/science.1072994.

[20] Grundke-Iqbal I, Iqbal K, Tung YC, Quinlan M, Wisniewski HM, Binder LI. Abnormal phosphorylation of the microtubule-associated protein tau (τ) in Alzheimer cytoskeletal pathology. Proc Natl Acad Sci U S A. 1986;83:4913–4917.

[21] Terry AV Jr, Buccafusco JJ. The cholinergic hypothesis of age and Alzheimer's disease-related cognitive deficits: Recent challenges and their implications for novel drug development. J Pharmacol Exp Ther. 2003;306:821–827. DOI: 10.1124/jpet.102.041616.

[22] Tsukada H, Nishiyama S, Fukumoto D, Ohba H, Sato K, Kakiuchi T. Effects of acute acetylcholinesterase inhibition on the cerebral cholinergic neuronal system and cognitive function: Functional imaging of the conscious monkey brain using animal PET in combination with microdialysis. Synapse. 2004;52:1–10. DOI: 10.1002/syn.10310.

[23] Dewey SL, Volkow ND, Logan J, MacGregor RR, Fowler JS, Schlyer DJ, Bendriem B. Age-related decrease in muscarinic cholinergic receptor binding in the human brain

measured with positron emission tomography (PET). J Neurosci Res. 1990;27:569–575. DOI: 10.1002/jnr.490270418.

[24] Zubieta JK, Koeppe RA, Frey KA, Kilbourn MR, Mangner TJ, Foster NL, Kuhl DE. Assessment of muscarinic receptor concentrations in aging and Alzheimer disease with ^{11}C-NMPB and PET. Synapse. 2001;39:275–287. DOI: 10.1002/1098-2396(20010315)39:4<275::AID-SYN1010>3.0.CO;2–3.

[25] Lee KS, Frey KA, Koeppe RA, Buck A, Mulholland GK, David E, Kuhl DE. *In vivo* quantification of cerebral muscarinic receptors in normal human aging using positron emission tomography and [^{11}C]tropanyl benzilate. J Cereb Blood Flow Metab. 1996;16:303–310. DOI: 10.1097/00004647-199603000-00016.

[26] Koeppe RA, Frey KA, Mulholland GK. Kilbourn MR, Buck A, Lee KS, Kuhl DE. [^{11}C]Tropanyl benzilate binding to muscarinic cholinergic receptors: Methodology and kinetic modeling alterations. J Cereb Blood Flow Metab. 1994;14:85–99. DOI: 10.1038/jcbfm.1994.13.

[27] Takahashi K, Murakami M, Miura S, Iida H, Kanno I, Uemura K. Synthesis and autoradiographic localization of muscarinic cholinergic antagonist *N*-^{11}C-methyl-3-piperidyl benzilate as a potent radioligand for positron emission tomography. Appl Radiat Isot. 1999;50:521–525. DOI: 10.1016/S0969-8043(97)10155-5.

[28] Tsukada H, Takahashi K, Miura S, Nishiyama S, Kakiuchi T, Ohba H, Sato K, Hatazawa J, Okudera T. Evaluation of novel PET ligands (+)*N*-[^{11}C]methyl-3-piperidyl benzilate ([^{11}C](+)3-MPB) and its stereoisomer [^{11}C](-)3-MPB for muscarinic cholinergic receptors in the conscious monkey brain: A PET study in comparison with [^{11}C]4-MPB. Synapse. 2001;39:182–192. DOI: 10.1002/1098-2396(200102)39:2<182::AID-SYN10>3.0.CO;2-Q.

[29] Tsukada H, Kakiuchi T, Nishiyama S, Ohba H, Sato K, Harada N, Takahashi K. Age differences in muscarinic cholinergic receptors assayed with (+)*N*-[^{11}C]methyl-3-piperidyl benzilate in the brains of conscious monkeys. Synapse. 2001;41:248–257. DOI: 10.1002/syn.1082.

[30] Tsukada H, Harada N, Nishiyama S, Ohba H, Kakiuchi T, Sato K, Fukumoto D, Kakiuchi T. Ketamine decreased striatal [^{11}C]raclopride binding with no alterations in static dopamine concentrations in the striatal extracellular fluid in the monkey brain: Multiparametric PET studies combined with microdialysis analysis. Synapse. 2000;37:95–103. DOI: 10.1002/1098-2396(200008)37:2<95::AID-SYN3>3.0.CO;2-H.

[31] Logan J, Fowler J, Volkow N, Wolf AP, Dewey SL, Schlyer DJ, MacGregor RR, Hitzemann R, Bendriem B, Gatley SJ, David R, Christman DR. Graphical analysis of reversible radioligand binding from time-activity measurements applied to *N*-^{11}C-methyl-(-)-cocaine PET studies in human subjects. J Cereb Blood Flow Metab. 1990;10:740–747. DOI: 10.1038/jcbfm.1990.127.

[32] Albuquerque EX, Pereira EF, Alkondon M, Rogers SW. Mammalian nicotinic acetylcholine receptors: From structure to function. Physiol Rev. 2009;89:73–120. DOI: 10.1152/physrev.00015.2008.

[33] Kadir A, Almkvist O, Wall A, Långström B, Nordberg A. PET imaging of cortical ^{11}C-nicotine binding correlates with the cognitive function of attention in Alzheimer's disease. Psychopharmacology. 2006;188:509–520. DOI: 10.1007/s00213-006-0447-7.

[34] Wu J, Ishikawa M, Zhang J, Hashimoto K. Brain imaging of nicotinic receptors in Alzheimer's disease. Int J Alzheimer's Dis. 2010;2010:548913. DOI: 10.4061/2010/548913.

[35] Ogawa M, Nishiyama S, Tsukada H, Hatano K, Fuchigami T, Yamaguchi H, Matsushima Y, Ito K, Magata Y. Synthesis and evaluation of new imaging agent for central nicotinic acetylcholine receptor $\alpha 7$ subtype. Nucl Med Biol. 2010;37:347–355. DOI: 10.1016/j.nucmedbio.2009.11.007.

[36] Nishiyama S, Ohba H, Kanazawa M, Kakiuchi T, Tsukada H. Comparing $\alpha 7$ nicotinic acetylcholine receptor binding, amyloid-β deposition, and mitochondria complex-I function in living brain: A PET study in aged monkeys. Synapse. 2015;69:475–483. DOI: 10.1002/syn.21842.

[37] Mintun MA, Raichle ME, Kilbourn MR, Wooten GF, Welch MJ. A quantitative model for the *in vivo* assessment of drug binding sites with positron emission tomography. Ann Neurol. 1984;15:217–227. DOI: 10.1002/ana.410150302.

[38] Innis RB, Cunningham VJ, Delforge J, Fujita M, Gjedde A, Gunn RN, Holden J, Houle S, Huang SC, Ichise M, Iida H, Kimura Y, Koeppe RA, Knudsen GM, Knuuti J, Lammertsma AA, Laruelle M, Logan J, Maguire RP, Mintun MA, Morris ED, Parsey R, Price JC, Slifstein M, Sossi V, Suhara T, Votaw JR, Wong DF, Carson RE. Consensus nomenclature for *in vivo* imaging of reversibly binding radioligands. J Cereb Blood Flow Metab. 2007;27:1533–1539. DOI: 10.1038/sj.jcbfm.9600493.

[39] Noda A, Takamatsu H, Minoshima S, Tsukada H, Nishimura S. Determination of kinetic rate constants for 2-[^{18}F]fluoro-2-deoxy-D-glucose and partition coefficient of water in conscious macaques and alterations in aging or anesthesia examined on parametric images with an anatomic standardization technique. J Cereb Blood Flow Metab. 2003;23:1441–1447.

[40] Schild L, Huppelsberg J, Kahlert S, Keilhoff G, Reiser G. Brain mitochondria are primed by moderate Ca^{2+} rise upon hypoxia/reoxygenation for functional breakdown and morphological disintegration. J Biol Chem. 2003;278:25454–25460. DOI: 10.1074/jbc.M302743200.

[41] Yalamanchili P, Wexler E, Hayes M, Yu M, Bozek J, Kagan M, Radeke HS, Azure M, Purohit A, Casebier DS, Robinson SP. Mechanism of uptake and retention of F-18 BMS-747158-02 in cardiomyocytes: A novel PET myocardial imaging agent. J Nucl Cardiol. 2007;14:782–788. DOI: 10.1016/j.nuclcard.2007.07.009.

[42] Waterhouse RN. Determination of lipophilicity and its use as a predictor of blood-brain barrier penetration of molecular imaging agents. Mol Imaging Biol. 2003;5:376–389. DOI: 10.1016/j.mibio.2003.09.014.

[43] Ojaimi J, Masters CL, Opeskin K, McKelvie P, Byrne E. Mitochondrial respiratory chain activity in the human brain as a function of age. Mech Age Dev. 1999;111:39–47. DOI: 10.1016/S0047-6374(99)00071-8.

[44] Navarro A, Boveris A. The mitochondrial energy transduction system and the aging process. Am J Physiol Cell Physiol. 2007;292:C670–C686. DOI: 10.1152/ajpcell.00213.2006.

[45] Monson NL, Ireland SJ, Ligocki AJ, Chen D, Rounds WH, Li M, Huebinger RM, Cullum CM, Greenberg BM, Stowe AM, Rong Zhang R. Elevated CNS inflammation in patients with preclinical Alzheimer's disease. J Cereb Blood Flow Metab. 2014;34:30–33. DOI: 10.1038/jcbfm.2013.183.

[46] Swomley AM, Förster S, Keeney JT, Triplett J, Zhang Z, Sultana R, Butterfield DA. Aβ, oxidative stress in Alzheimer disease: Evidence based on proteomics studies. Biochim Biophys Acta. 2014;1842:1248–1257. DOI: 10.1016/j.bbadis.2013.09.015.

[47] Klunk WE, Engler H, Nordberg A, Wang Y, Blomqvist G, Holt DP, Bergstrom M, Savitcheva I, Huang GF, Estrada S, Ausen B, Debnath ML, Barletta J, Price JC, Sandell J, Lopresti BJ, Wall A, Koivisto P, Antoni G, Mathis CA, Langstrom B. Imaging brain amyloid in Alzheimer's disease with Pittsburgh Compound-B. Ann Neurol. 2004;55:306–319. DOI: 10.1002/ana.20009.

[48] Boutin H, Chauveau F, Thominiaux C, Gregoire MC, James ML, Trebossen R, Hantraye P, Dolle F, Tavitian B, Kassiou M. Receptor PET ligand for *in vivo* imaging of neuroinflammation. J Nucl Med. 2007;48:573–581. DOI: 10.2967/jnumed.106.036764.

[49] Noda A, Murakami M, Nishiyama S, Fukumoto D, Miyoshi S, Tsukada H, Nishimura S. Amyloid imaging in aged and young macaques with [^{11}C]PIB and [^{18}F]FDDNP. Synapse. 2008;62:472–475. DOI: 10.1002/syn.20508.

[50] Finch CE, Austad SN. Primate aging in the mammalian scheme: The puzzle of extreme variation in brain aging. Age. 2012;34:1075–1091. DOI: 10.1007/s11357-011-9355-9.

[51] Parri HR, Hernandez CM, Dineley KT. Research update: Alpha 7 nicotinic acetylcholine receptor mechanism in Alzheimer's disease. Biochem Pharmacol. 2011;82:931–942. DOI: 10.1016/j.bcp.2011.06.039.

[52] Nagele RG, D'Andrea MR, Anderson WJ, Wang HY. Intracellular accumulation of β-amyloid (1–42) in neurons is facilitated by the $\alpha7$ nicotinic acetylcholine receptor in Alzheimer's disease. Neuroscience. 2002;110:199–211. DOI: 10.1016/S0306-4522(01)00460–2.

[53] Cleary JP, Walsh DM, Hofmeister JJ, Shankar GM, Kuskowski MA, Selkoe DJ, Ashe KH. Natural oligomers of the amyloid-β protein specifically disrupt cognitive function. Nat Neurosci. 2005;8:79–84. DOI: 10.1038/nn1372.

[54] Lesne S, Koh MT, Kotilinek L, Kayed R, Glabe CG, Yang A, Gallagher M, Ashe KH. A specific amyloid-β protein assembly in the brain impairs memory. Nature. 2006;440:352–357. DOI: 10.1038/nature04533.

[55] Puzzo D, Privitera L, Leznik E, Fa M, Staniszewski A, Palmeri A, Arancio O. Picomolar amyloid-β positively modulates synaptic plasticity and memory in hippocampus. J Neurosci. 2008;28:14537–14545. DOI: 10.1523/JNEUROSCI.2692-08.2008.

[56] Yu WF, Guan ZZ, Bogdanovic N, Nordberg A. High selective expression of $\alpha 7$ nicotinic receptors on astrocytes in the brains of patients with sporadic Alzheimer's disease and patients carrying Swedish APP 670/671 mutation: A possible association with neuritic plaques. Exp Neurol. 2005;192:215–225. DOI: 10.1016/j.expneurol.2004.12.015.

[57] Warburg O. On respiratory impairment in cancer cells. Science. 1956;124:267–272. DOI: 10.1126/science.124.3215.267.

Chapter 5

Kinetics of Amyloid Formation by Different Proteins and Peptides: Polymorphism and Sizes of Folding Nuclei of Fibrils

Oxana V. Galzitskaya, Nikita V. Dovidchenko and
Olga M. Selivanova

Additional information is available at the end of the chapter

http://dx.doi.org/10.5772/63359

Abstract

Aggregation of peptides and proteins into amyloid structure is one of the most intensively studied biological phenomena at the moment. To date, there is no developed theory that would allow one to determine what kind of mechanism presents in the given experiment on the basis of aggregation kinetic data. Debates concerning the mechanism of the amyloid fibrils formation and, in particular, the size of the amyloidogenic nucleus are still going on. We created such a theory on the basis of the kinetics of amyloid aggregates formation. In the presented chapter, theoretical and experimental approaches were employed for studding the process of amyloid formation by different proteins and peptides. The current kinetic models described in this chapter adequately describe the key features of amyloid nucleation and growth.

Keywords: amyloidogenic regions, amyloid prediction methods, linear and exponential mechanisms of amyloid growth, polymorphism, prion

1. Introduction

Many studies show that the generation of an amyloid fibril is a fundamental property of all protein molecules, rather than being limited to a narrow range of the so-called amyloid-forming proteins associated with amyloid diseases, as was believed until recently [1, 2]. Normal proteins become toxic upon fibril formation [3]. At the same time, greater cytotoxicity is characteristic of immature water-soluble fibrils compared to mature insoluble amyloid fibrils. It seems that the mechanism of toxicity should be similar to that for fibrils formed by different proteins. The structure of toxic immature fibrils is certainly rich in β-strands and should be universal, because specific antibodies against the precursors of amyloid peptide Aβ, associated with Alzheimer's disease, recognize the precursors of amyloid fibrils formed by other proteins with different amino acid sequences [4]. It was demonstrated that samples of blood serum from patients with Parkinson's disease show an autoimmune response to insulin oligomers and fibrils, which should reveal the presence of insulin aggregates in this disease [5]. Fibril formation depends on the experimental conditions and is expedited by denaturants: to aggregate, proteins should be unfolded, at least partly [6]. Preliminary unfolding is not needed for the aggregation of peptides and proteins associated with amyloidosis such as type II diabetes or Alzheimer's and Parkinson's disease, because these proteins are already unfolded under physiological conditions [7]. However, the majority of natively unfolded proteins do not aggregate in vivo [8] suggesting that unfolding is necessary, but not sufficient for the formation of amyloid fibrils. Most likely, there are specific amino acid motifs that are exposed to the solvent and are more prone to aggregation as compared to other regions of the amino acid sequence. Experimental findings support the hypothesis that small protein regions are responsible for the amyloidogenic behavior [9–11].

2. Identification of aggregation sites in proteins responsible for amyloid formation

We have done comparison of the prediction results for 30 amyloidogenic proteins [12] using seven methods with experimental data: PASTA2 [13], AmylPred2 [12], Tango [14], MetAmyl [15], Waltz [16], FoldAmyloid [17], ArchCandy [18]. More detail comparison with full list of proteins but without new method Archcandy was presented in our recent paper [19]. One can see that FoldAmyloid (which is a relatively old and simple approach) works better than Waltz and Archcandy. PASTA2 is a new more sophisticated approach that performs best among the non-meta-servers. As evident from **Table 1**, the accuracy and sensitivity of PASTA2 predic-

Scoring type	**PASTA2 90% specificity**	**AmylPred2**	**Tango**	**MetAmyl high specificity**	**Waltz best perfo-mance**	**FoldAmy-loid**	**Archcandy default set-tings**
Sensitivity	0.36	0.41	0.19	0.38	0.19	0.28	0.16
Specificity	0.91	0.86	0.95	0.86	0.94	0.92	0.92
False regions predicted as amyloidogen-ic	38	121	37	88	37	31	15
No. correctly predicted re-gions/**total**	33/**46**	42/**46**	17/**46**	33/**46**	22/**46**	29/**46**	8/**46**

Table 1. Averaged results of amyloid predictions for 30 proteins by various algorithms.

tions are only smaller better than those of FoldAmyloid. At the same time, comparison of the overall prediction quality shows only modest improvement, which is due to low sensitivity partly caused by overprediction and partly by the coarseness of the methods.

3. Possible kinetics schemes for amyloid and prion growth

To explain the kinetic features of the aggregation process of protein molecules, a large number of schemes were proposed. There are many approaches for describing the kinetics and mechanism of protein aggregation: kinetic, thermodynamic, and other empirical approaches. The purpose of the first two was the best approximation of the experimental data and obtainment of quantitative values of the rate constants describing such processes as nucleation, growth, and all other parts of the aggregation process. At present, there is no consensus whether a protofilament is formed by joining oligomers or by adding monomers. The following questions can be posed: How many different mechanisms exist in the literature for describing the protein aggregation? What is the essence of each mechanism? What mechanisms or models are used in the literature to describe the experimental kinetic curves? What are the similarities between various mechanisms? The large volume of publications describing the formation of amyloid fibrils allows us to reveal two general mechanisms. There are a mechanism of sequential addition of monomers (linear growth) and a mechanism for describing the aggregation of prions (exponentional growth). Most of these approaches somehow go back to the late fifties [20]. In this study, a kinetic scheme for polymerization of actin was proposed. The experimental data indicated that the polymerization process is very similar to the condensation reaction: The reaction occurs only when the monomer concentration exceeds the critical threshold. The assumption was justified. The cooperative polymerization reaction was confirmed by two facts: (1) The reaction rate in the early stages of the reaction increased upon increasing the concentration of actin; (2) an addition of seed with an already formed unit led to an immediate transition of all free actin to an aggregate. In 1974, Hofrichter et al. [21] used the mechanism of sequential monomer addition to the aggregate to explain the formation of hemoglobin fibrils in sickle cell anemia. To explain the observed effect of "extreme autocatalysis" and strong concentration dependence, Ferrone with the co-authors developed a model of "heterogeneous nucleation" [22]. This model assumes the following sequence of events: First, in the normal course of nucleation, fibrils, and then, subsequent fibrils may form on its surface. This model is included as an equation for the first stage—the homogeneous nucleation, and for the second step—heterogeneous nucleation; the equations were solved numerically. The notion of heterogeneous nucleation was a new and important contribution to the development of the theory of protein aggregation. In 1983, Frieden and Goddette [23] used a model of sequential monomer addition to the unit to describe the process of protein polymerization, with the proviso that each step of monomer addition had its own reaction rate constant. In 1986, Goldstein and Stryer [24] modified the model of sequential addition of monomers to the unit to describe the process of protein polymerization. They identified the nucleus as a "seed" of size s, after the formation of which the kinetic constants are changed. Using protein amylin, it was shown that nucleation can occur in two ways: fibril-independent (or primary nucleation) and fibril-dependent (secondary nucleation) paths. The contribution of each of these processes depends on the external interfaces (or surfaces). In the presence of such a surface, the primary nucleation mechanism is dominating; in the absence of such a surface, the secondary nucleation mechanism is dominating [25]. Heterogeneous nucleation can be seen from another point of view, as an autocatalytic growth in mature seeds. It was not shown experimentally whether seeds are formed on the existing surface of the unit, or the growth simply continues from the surface of the same aggregate. In 1967, Griffith [26] suggested three possible theoretical mechanisms that could explain the self-replication agent causing "scrapie" sheep (scrapie). In 1982, Prusiner [27] was able to provide enough experimental evidence that the "scrapie" infectious agent is the protein called a prion. In 1991, Prusiner suggested the scheme of transfer and development of prion infection [28]. Based on the Prusiner's work, in 1993, Lansbury his work published [29], in which the mechanism of sequential monomer addition to the seed was applied for analysis of kinetic data.

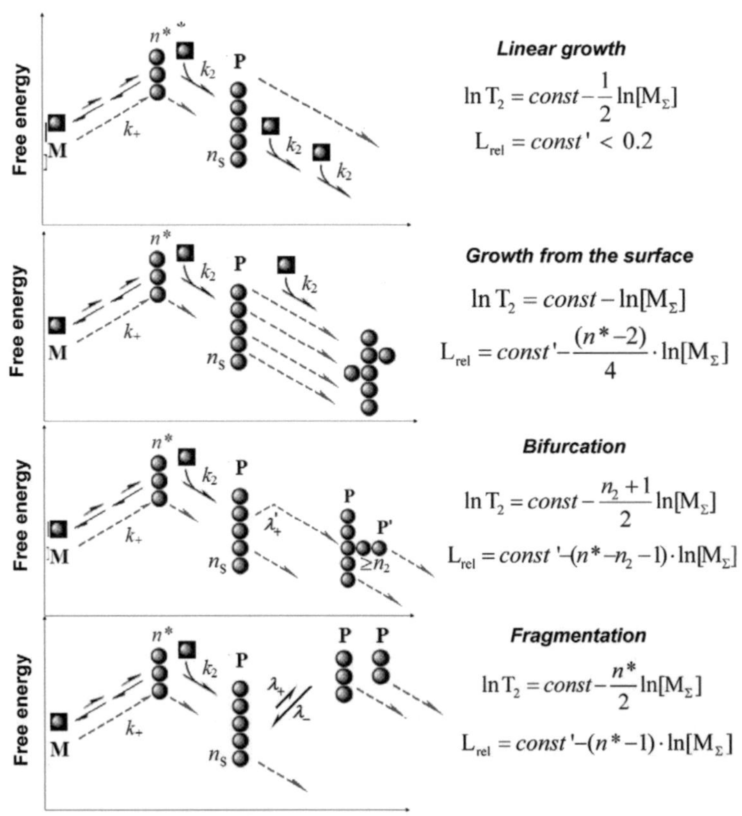

Figure 1. Alternative scenarios for amyloid growth and corresponding kinetic parameters. T_2 is the time of inclusion of all monomers into the aggregate, L_{rel} is the ratio between the duration of the lag phase and the time of inclusion of all monomers into the growing polymer, $[M_\Sigma]$ is the total monomer concentration, n* is the size of the primary nucleus, and n_2 is the size of the secondary nucleus. n_S is the smallest number of monomers in the stable polymer. Modified from [33].

In 2004 in the paper by Collins et al. [30], the formation kinetics of sup35p prion was studied. It was shown that amyloid aggregate growth occurs upon monomer addition to the fiber ends. Also the authors performed experiments with agitation and observed catalysis due to fiber fragmentation, so their kinetic model consisted of three steps: at the first step, oligomers are formed; at the second step, amyloidal seeds are formed through nucleation-conversion, after that the autocatalytic growth occurs where autocatalysis takes place because of fragmentation. Thus, major schemes of amyloid aggregates formation were drawn. In general, schemes can be summed up into the following reaction: out of a pool of monomer nuclei (the most unstable species on the reaction path with the largest free energy) are formed, which then are somehow converted into seed (the smallest stable amyloid aggregate) which is able to attach monomers in a way that monomer free energy only decreases, the result of which is that after some time, all the monomers become associated into fibrils. In some cases, catalysis of reaction occurs through secondary nucleation or fragmentation. In the presence of a catalyst, the amyloidal growth regime can be named "exponential," whereas in the absence of catalysis, the amyloidal growth can be named linear. It should be mentioned that in this general scheme, it is not important what one means by the words "monomer protein"—the monomer itself or some protein aggregate. Despite overall success in the understanding of possible mechanisms hidden beneath amyloidal aggregation, the relation of the kinetic models to the experimentally measurable values was still unclear. Thus, the authors of the paper [31] have shown that despite possible different mechanisms of aggregation, all of the kinetic experimental data could be successfully approximated by a simple sigmoid curve. Fortunately in the same year, the careful introspection of the behavior of the logarithm of lag time versus logarithm of concentration for several amyloidogenic agents by Knowles et al. [32] revealed that different amyloidogenic agents possess a similar linear dependence in those coordinates and such dependence is $T_{lag}/T_{lag_0} \approx (C/C_0)^{-1/2}$, where T_{lag_0} and C_0 are values corresponding to the smallest concentration. In the paper Dovidchenko et al. [33], the authors studied the variance in the mechanisms within scheme monomer ->nucleus->fibril growth with/without catalysis. In the work, the authors were lucky to find bridges between values which can be calculated directly from experimental data—characteristic times such as lag-time T_{lag}, time of inclusion of all monomers into aggregate T_2 and relation $L_{rel} = T_{lag}/T_2$ and mechanism of amyloidogenesis. It turned out that through the study of the concentration dependence of amyloid formation, one can estimate nuclei sizes (the size of the primary nucleus and size of the secondary nucleus if secondary nucleation takes place) and possible mechanisms. For example, linear growth (when no catalysis occurs) has a very narrow range of conditions: L_{rel} should be independent of the logarithm of concentration and its value should not exceed 0.2. In the case of exponential mechanism, one should plot a graph of two dependencies: $\ln T_2$ versus $\ln[M_\Sigma]$ and L_{rel} versus $\ln[M_\Sigma]$, where M_Σ is the initial concentration of monomers. As one can see from **Figure 1**, the dependencies should be linear in those coordinates and thus the calculation of the tangent coefficient of a line drawn through experimental points will point out what mechanism takes place in the given reaction. However, several tangent coefficients (for example, −1/2 which can be either the result of a fragmentation mechanism or a bifurcation mechanism without secondary nucleation) are special cases and can be obtained in different scenarios; for those cases, additional experiments are needed to exclude excess mechanism variants.

4. Polymorphism of amyloid fibrils

The fully matured fibers are not the most toxic species. The importance of intermediate species that define the pathway, toxicity, and even the type of fibers formed at the end should be emphasized. Usually electron microscopy (EM) is used for comprehensive characterization of the amyloid formation and for control of the amyloid morphology. The probes are collected for analyzing periodically over duration of all experiments. The main results of EM experiments at each of the time intervals are the properties of time-dependent structures and their variability (polymorphism). These analyses usually are performed using both commercial and recombinant samples. The use of EM in studying the process of amyloid formation is due to the importance of polymorphism for determining the protein folding pathways. On the other hand, protein folding pathway depends strongly on its amino acid sequence. Further, the resulting protein conformation affects the formation of amyloid fibrils, and the same polypeptide sequence may correspond to the fibrils of different morphologies [34]. The fibril polymorphism is potentially important for the human disease progression, as it may be the reason for natural variability of amyloid-related pathologies such as amyloidosis of light chains of immunoglobulins (AL) and the phenomenon of strain variability of prion infection [34, 35]. The EM images of amyloid fibrils show insignificant morphological differences, and the fibrils are often represented as twisted or parallel clusters of thin protein filaments. One should note also that polymorphism is a serious obstacle in studying fibril structures. A mixture of fibrils of different morphology is always present in solution, and several different types of fibrils can be seen under the same conditions. This creates a problem for image analyses because it requires separation of fibrils by their morphology and performing separate analyses of each type of insulin, Aβ peptide, β_2-microglobulin, glucagon, amylin, calcitonin, etc. It is not completely excluded that different fibril morphologies are due to similar but not identical fibril formation pathways. The differences may be formed at the initial steps of fibril formation including the step of nucleation. The size of the nucleus of a protofibril is still unknown for almost all proteins and peptides. Nucleation is the limiting step of the amyloid fibril formation which can start only when the concentration of amyloid proteins exceeds the critical one. After the nucleation, the fibrils grow rapidly. Proteins may have different sizes of the protofibril nuclei (see the next sections). Also, the conditions at which the fibrils are formed may affect its size. This may result in the formation of the fibrils of different morphologies. In other words, we assume that the fibril formation depends on the nucleation step and goes through different pathways, thus determining the final fibril morphology. Note also that both the morphology and molecular structure are sensitive to small differences under conditions when the fibrils are growing in *de novo* preparations (under fixed pH, temperature, buffer composition, and peptide concentration).

4.1. Polymorphism of Aβ fibrils

It was shown previously that peptide Aβ40 forms fibrils of different morphologies even under the same conditions. For the fibrils formed without mixing, the dominating morphologies are twisted fibrils, while the activated fibrils will be less twisted yet inclined to form lateral associations. The inactivated twisted fibrils are the most toxic for the cells [36]. Therefore, it is important to study all possible formations including oligomers and fibrils, which determine the natural polymorphism. Moreover, it was shown previously that the fibrils associated with diseases have the same nucleation center structure called a β-arcade. The β-strands in these structures are parallel to each other. It is interesting to note that this kind of a nucleus structure is not found in normal proteins and the β-strands are antiparallel to each other [37].

4.1.1. *Morphology of recombinant Aβ40 peptides*

Figure 2 shows the preparation of recombinant Aβ40 peptide after 27 h incubation at 25°C at 50 mM Tris–HCl (pH 7, 5) and C = 0.2 mg/ml. Polymorphism of generated fibrils is seen. In

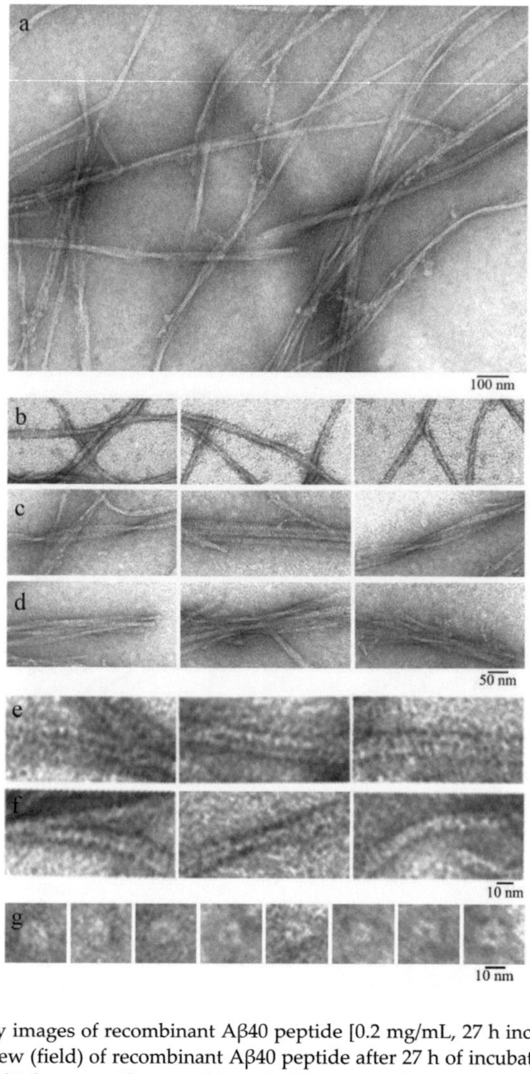

Figure 2. Electron microscopy images of recombinant Aβ40 peptide [0.2 mg/mL, 27 h incubation at 25°C, 50 mM Tris-HCl (pH 7, 5)]. (a) General view (field) of recombinant Aβ40 peptide after 27 h of incubation. (b–d) Gallery of types of Aβ40 peptide fibril images at higher magnification: (b) single fibrils; (c) ribbon-like type of fibrils; (d) bundle-like type of fibrils; (e, f) single fibrils: (e) at horizontal packing; (f) bending sites of the single fibrils. (g) Gallery of ring oligomers.

addition to single fibrils of several microns in length with a diameter of about 8–9 nm, there are also fibrils, forming bands of different widths, and bundles. It seems that single fibrils consist of two filaments. However, under high magnification, it is seen that the fibrils are formed of rounded ring structures. The matter is that upon staining the preparations, the staining agent dyes not only their contours, but also flows into different cavities and openings. This should be taken into account when interpreting EM images; otherwise, a tobacco mosaic virus fibril would consist of two parallel packed short filaments of 300 nm long. In the case of the Aβ40 peptide preparation, under high magnification, it is also seen that the staining agent flows into the openings of ring structures. These ring oligomer structures have a diameter of about 8–9 nm (the width of a single fibril) and a diameter of the internal opening of about 3 nm. Ring structures or Aβ40 oligomers form single fibrils in such a way, that ring oligomers are layered on each other. If a fibril is absorbed on the formvar film sideways, we see a thinner fibril with a diameter of about 4 nm. This size demonstrates an approximate height of a ring-structured oligomer. As a matter of fact, the height is smaller, because the degree of overlapping of ring-structured oligomers should be taken into account. The greater is the overlapping, the larger is the height of such packing of fibrils.

4.1.2. Morphology of synthetic Aβ42 peptide (Invitrogen, lot #73269340A)

The EM image of Aβ42 peptide (Invitrogen, lot #73269340A) (**Figure 3**) shows that after 97 h of incubation at 37°C (water), fibrils of several microns long are formed. Polymorphism of

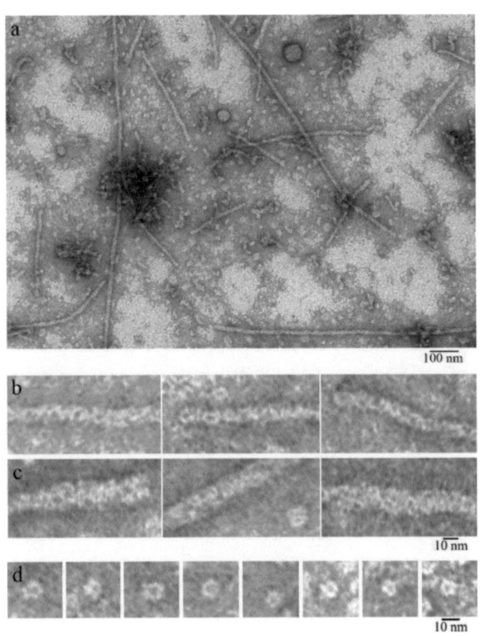

Figure 3. Electron microscopy images of Aβ42 peptide from Invitrogen (lot #73269340A). The sample was incubated at 37°C (water). (a) General view of the sample at 97-h incubation. (b, c) Gallery of types of Aβ42 peptide fibrils at higher magnification: (b) single thin and (c) thick fibrils. (d) Gallery of ring oligomers.

fibrils is observed. Thin fibrils with a diameter of about 7–8 nm and more are seen, and more pronounced polymorphism of the generated fibrils is observed (**Figure 3**). At the same time, fibrils of different diameters are present: thin ones of about 7–8 nm and wider fibrils up to 15 nm. Moreover, rounded ring-structured oligomers of about 8 nm in diameter can be seen; the internal diameter of the ring (the diameter of the hole) is about 3 nm (**Figure 3d**). At magnification, it can be seen that an oligomer consists of 4–6 smaller rounded particles (**Figure 3d**). It is notable that both thin and thick fibrils are formed of such ring-structured oligomers. Thin fibrils are characterized by more ordered interaction of separate oligomers, while thick fibrils are generated due to random sticking of additional oligomers along the fibril axis. Because of this way of generation, fibrils look uneven in EM images with a tendency to branching [38].

Thus, using the EM method, we have demonstrated that fibrils of these peptides are formed by association of rounded ring structures. Negatively stained TEM images of fibrils extracted from AD brain tissues [39] are very similar to our EM results. Moreover, similar structures are observed elsewhere [40].

4.2. Polymorphism of insulin fibrils

Insulin has a high tendency to aggregation and forms fibrils. Insulin fibrils were first described in 1940 by Waugh [41]. At present, the conditions leading to the formation of active insulin fibrils are known [42]. Insulin fibrillation occurs upon various environmental changes (pH, ionic conditions, temperature, organic solvents, and agitation); it also depends on the methods for producing insulin, its delivery, and storage. It should be noted that the human insulin fibrillation is slower than that of the best studied bovine insulin [42–47].

Currently, all insulin preparations for therapeutic purposes are prepared in the form of a Zn-containing hexamer, since in this condition it is more stable and resistant to the formation of fibrils. When treating diabetes, insulin penetrates into muscles by injection, where it typically forms deposits. The large size of the insulin hexamer slows its adsorption, because the hexamer must go through the dimers in the monomeric state and only in this way penetrate into the bloodstream. This leads to slowing down the interaction with insulin receptors and the need to take insulin 1–1.5 h before mealtime.

Despite intensive studies of fibrillogenesis of insulin, there is no generally accepted scheme for the formation of mature fibrils. The main difficulties arise in interpreting the beginning of the fibrillation process. Polymerization of insulin begins from the transition of the monomer protein from the native state to the partially unfolded conformation which can be amyloidogenic. The strong dependence of the reaction of polymerization on various external parameters leads to the formation of insulin fibrils with different morphology, which complicates the analysis of the general scheme of fibril formation.

For electron microscopy (EM) investigations, insulin samples were used at a concentration of 0.2 mg/ml. Zinc-free recombinant human insulin was obtained from "Gerofarm-Bio" (Obolensk, Russia) and was checked by the tandem mass spectrometry technique (LCQ Deca XP, Thermo Finnigan, USA). According to the EM data on polymerization of human insulin, the mature protein fibrils appeared only after 8 h of insulin incubation. Active polymerization of insulin occurs up to 10–11 h of incubation. This is accompanied by the elongation of the fibrils for both samples up to 10–12 μm. The fibrils interact laterally with each other, resulting in the formation of big clusters composed from ribbons, bundles, and twisting bundles (**Figure 4**). Protein aggregation is the result of increasing the incubation time up to 24 h. According to the EM data, the number of large fibril clusters increases in the samples after 24 h, but the length of the fibrils does not change (remains about 10–12 μm) [48].

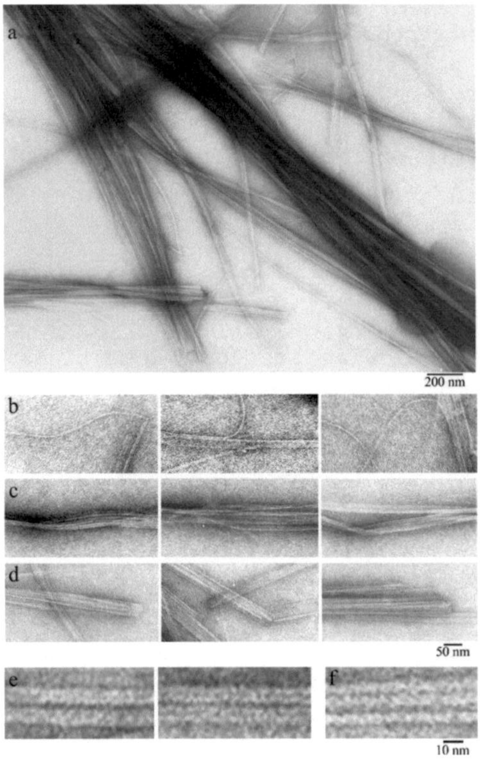

Figure 4. Electron microscopy images of human zinc-free recombinant insulin (0.2 mg/ml, 24 h incubation at 37°C, 20% acetic acid (pH 2.0), 140 mM NaCl). (a) General view (field) of human insulin after 24 h of incubation. (b–d) Gallery of images of types of insulin fibrils at higher magnification: (b) single fibrils; (c) ribbon-like type of fibrils; (d) bundle-type of fibrils. (e, f) The thinnest fibrils: (e) at horizontal packing; (f) at vertical packing of ring oligomers.

5. Example of amyloid growth by the linear nucleation-elongation mechanism (actin, apolipoprotein C-II)

Most quantitative models for linear polymerization stem from the work performed more than half a century ago [20] proposing a kinetic model for actin polymerization. Only two of the proteins (apolipoprotein C-II [49]: $L_{rel} < 0.1$ with the primary nucleus size $n^* \approx 4$–5 and actin with $n^* \approx 3$), studied in our analysis, exhibit linear growth. Formation of actin filaments occurs by linear growth—fibrils increase only due to attachment of monomers to the aggregate ends. This is supported by literature data [50] and by analysis of kinetic data (**Figure 1**). According to the theory advanced in [33] for linear growth (observed in actin), the characteristic time of the relative lag-period L_{rel} does not exceed 0.2 and is independent of $\ln[M_\Sigma]$ as in the case of actin (**Figure 5**) [50]. The size of the primary nucleus was calculated from the slope to be $n = 3.46 \pm 0.28$.

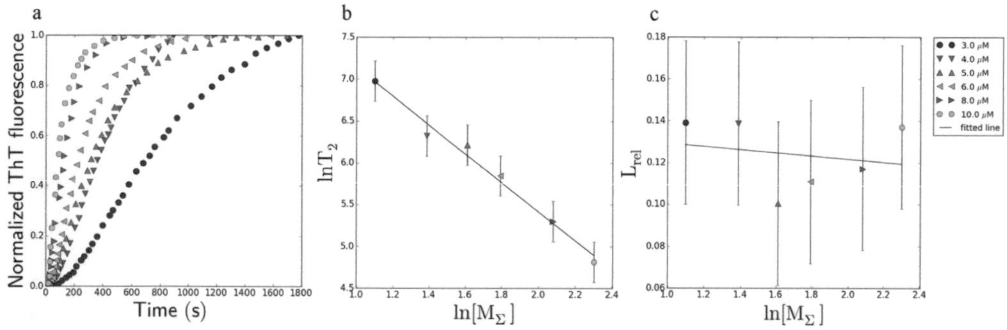

Figure 5. (a) Dependence of normalized ThT fluorescence on time for actin [50]. (b) Dependence of L_{rel} on $\ln T_2$. (c) Dependence of L_{rel} on $\ln[M_\Sigma]$. The slope angle of the fitted line is about −0.01, that is, L_{rel} is independent of $\ln[M_\Sigma]$. All L_{rel} values are also <0.2 which, according to the models of formation of fibrillar aggregates, means that the formation of actin fibrils proceeds by the linear mechanism (see [33]). The errors are computed with the Student's coefficients corresponding to 0.95 confidence level.

6. Examples of amyloid growth by the exponential mechanism and sizes of folding nuclei of fibrils formed by different agents

In order to estimate the size of fibril nucleus (the most unstable state on the monomer to the fibril pathway) and a possible scenario for the formation of aggregates, it is necessary to make a number of kinetic experiments, where the only variable parameter is the monomer concentration. Characteristic times T_{lag} (the lag-period duration), T_2 (the time of transition of all monomers into an aggregate), and L_{rel} (the T_{lag}/T_2 ratio) are calculated for each experimental curve. It was demonstrated that the dependences of $\ln T_2$ and L_{rel} on $\ln[M_\Sigma]$ (the logarithm of the initial concentration of monomers) are linear, with gradients that can be used for the computation of fibril nucleus sizes (including those of non-amyloid type) and for elucidation of the mechanism of aggregate formation.

If $L_{rel} > 0.2$, the linear growth model is excluded, and, independently of $\ln T_2$ and L_{rel} dependence on $\ln[M_\Sigma]$, only the exponential growth scenario remains. The dependences of $\ln T_2$ on $\ln[M_\Sigma]$ and L_{rel} on $\ln[M_\Sigma]$ are formally different for different exponential scenarios (i.e., "growth from the surface," "fragmentation," and "bifurcation"). However, it is impossible, for example, to distinguish the bifurcation from the fragmentation scenario from the kinetics *alone* if the size

n_2 of the secondary nucleus of bifurcation is zero; this implies the need for direct observations of fibril shapes to distinguish these cases (see Refs. [33, 48] for more details).

6.1. Insulin

Now we can present three general schemes of insulin amyloid formation, which differ by the size of folding nuclei of fibrils. For the first type, the size of nucleus is one monomer [44, 51–53]. For the second scheme of fibril formation, the size of nucleus is two monomers and the dimers are precursors of fibrils [5, 54, 55]. For the third scheme of polymerization, oligomers are precursors of fibrils, and the size of oligomer can vary from three to six monomers [42, 43, 56–58].

The basis for choosing between different mechanisms of formation of fibrils is to detect various soluble oligomers. However, at low concentrations and at early times, it is difficult to accomplish accurate detection of the initial aggregates. For this purpose, a variety of optical methods, as well as Cryo-transmission-EM, atom force microscopy, and small-angle X-ray scattering are used [55, 57–59]. However, all these methods are not quantitative, have no reliable standards, do not provide the full size distribution, may yield abnormal results (with microscopic approaches—interaction with the surface during adsorption of samples), and require the analysis of the results of certain programs to prove the statistical significance [52]. Although all these methods provide valuable information, none of them can convincingly demonstrate how an unstable nucleus grows to a stable seed for further growth of protofibrils, and many experimental and theoretical models are based on this assumption.

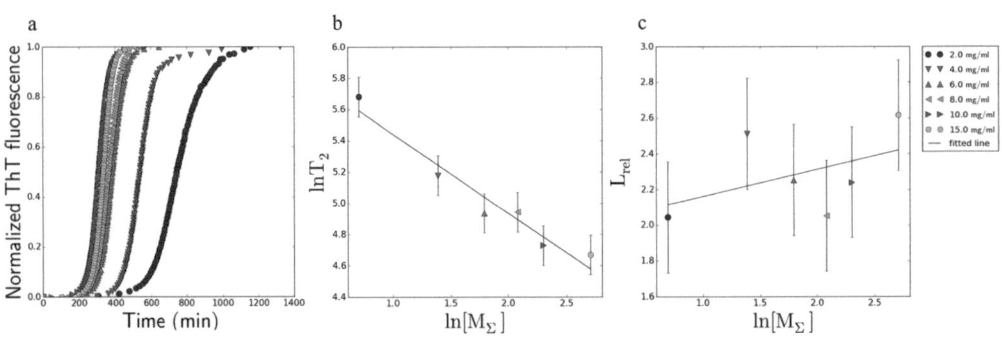

Figure 6. (a) Dependence of normalized ThT fluorescence on time for insulin [48]. The approximation line calculated for insulin amyloid formation with the experimental data from (a) by the least-squares method plotted in coordinates (b): $\{\ln T_2, \ln[M_\Sigma]\}$ and (c): $\{L_{rel}, \ln[M_\Sigma]\}$; $[M_\Sigma]$ is in mg/ml, T_2 in min. The tangent coefficients of the approximation lines are -0.51 ± 0.13 for $d(\ln T_2)/d(\ln[M_\Sigma])$ and 0.15 ± 0.31 for $d(L_{rel})/d(\ln[M_\Sigma])$; the errors are computed with the Student's coefficients corresponding to 0.95 confidence level.

The growth of amyloid fibrils was studied by thioflavin T (ThT) fluorescence, which drastically increases when ThT is bound to fibrils (**Figure 6a**). The renormalized curves, presented in **Figure 6a**, are very similar to one another. They have large lag periods, thus excluding the linear growth scenario. The obtained analytical solution and computer modeling allowed us to determine the size of the nucleus from the experimentally obtained concentration dependences of the relationship between the lag-time duration and the time of growth of amyloid fibrils [33]. **Figure 6b, c** illustrates determination of the fibrillation scenario and the nuclei sizes (n^*, n_2) for human insulin (see **Table 2**) [48]. The value $d(\ln T_2)/d(\ln[M_\Sigma]) \approx -0.5$ is inconsistent with the "growth from the surface" model but consistent with "linear growth" (which, though, should have $L_{rel} < 0.2$, which is inconsistent with L_{rel}), "fragmentation" (which, though, is inconsistent with EM images shown in **Figure 4**), and "bifurcation" (consistent with the EM images), with the secondary nucleus size $n_2 = 0$ calculated as $-1 - d(\ln T_2)/d(\ln[M_\Sigma])$; the primary nucleus size $n^* = 1 + n_2 - d(L_{rel})/d(\ln[M_\Sigma]) = 1$ (see **Table 2**). According to the elaborated theory, it means that the size of the primary nucleus corresponds to one monomer.

Amyloid-forming protein or peptide and a ref. to its experimental study	$[M_\Sigma]$, mg/ml (min–max)	$\ln(T_2/\text{min})$ at various $[M_\Sigma]$ (min–max)	L_{rel} at various $[M_\Sigma]$ (min–max)	$n^* \pm \Delta n^*$, primary nucleus	$n_2 \pm \Delta n_2$, secondary nucleus	Model that follows from the L_{rel} and $\ln T_2$ on $[M_\Sigma]$ dependencies
Human insulin [48] (37°C)	2.0–15	4.71–5.70	1.78–2.48	0.86 ± 0.44	0.01 ± 0.13	Exponential
Human insulin [65] (45°C)	2.5–20	3.60–4.18	5.17–5.56	1.13 ± 0.19	−0.48 ± 0.16	Exponential
LysPro human insulin [48] (37°C)	2.0–15	5.78–4.81	2.04–4.38	0.63 ± 1.04	−0.29 ± 0.24	Exponential

Table 2. The range of L_{rel} and $\ln T_2$ values, the sizes of the primary (n^*) and secondary (n_2) nuclei and the amyloid growth scenarios obtained from experimental kinetic data alone.

6.2. LysPro human analog insulin

We have investigated the kinetics of formation of fibrils by monomeric rapid-acting insulin LysPro [48]. According to our data, fibril formation of the insulin analog at pH 2 proceeds by

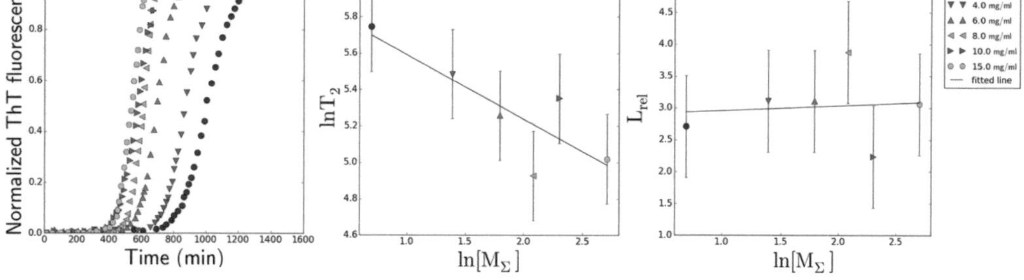

Figure 7. (a) Dependence of normalized ThT fluorescence on time for LysPro insulin [48] The approximation line calculated for LysPro insulin amyloid formation with experimental data from (a) by the least-squares method plotted in coordinates (b): {$\ln T_2$, $\ln[M_\Sigma]$} and (c): {L_{rel}, $\ln[M_\Sigma]$}; $[M_\Sigma]$ is in mg/ml, T_2 in min. The tangent coefficients of the approximation lines are −0.35 ± 0.25 for $d(\ln T_2)/d(\ln[M_\Sigma])$ and 0.07 ± 0. 80 for $d(L_{rel})/d(\ln[M_\Sigma])$; the errors are computed with the Student's coefficients corresponding to 0.95 confidence level.

5 h longer than that of the recombinant human insulin. These data seem to us important because the rate of aggregation of insulin preparations is an important health problem not only in the production and storage of insulin, but also for its frequent injections. In this regard, the process of fibrillation should be analyzed for all developed analogs, already prepared for clinical trials and for mass production. Examination of EM images of growing insulin LysPro fibrils shows that they occurred with a kind of the "bifurcation plus lateral growth" scenario [48]. The growth of amyloid fibrils was studied (**Figure 7**) by thioflavin T (ThT) fluorescence, which drastically increases when ThT is bound to fibrils. The dependence of L_{rel} and $\ln T_2$ on $\ln[M_\Sigma]$ (**Figure 7**) was used to estimate sizes of the primary and secondary nuclei. Similar to insulin fibrils, the size of the first nucleus is one monomer, and the size of the secondary nucleus is zero (see **Table 2**). It should be noted that "one monomer" may correspond to the oligomer structure consisting of 2–6 monomers, if we did not start from the pure monomers in solution.

6.3. Aβ40

The experimental kinetics data on the formation of amyloid aggregates, which we used to calculate the sizes of nuclei of amyloid protofibrils formed by Aβ40, were taken from paper [60]. For all the experimental data, we obtained $L_{rel} >> 0.2$, which means that the process goes by the exponential mechanism of fibril formation (**Figure 8**). For Aβ40, we obtained that the size of the primary nucleus is two monomers, and the secondary nucleus size is one monomer.

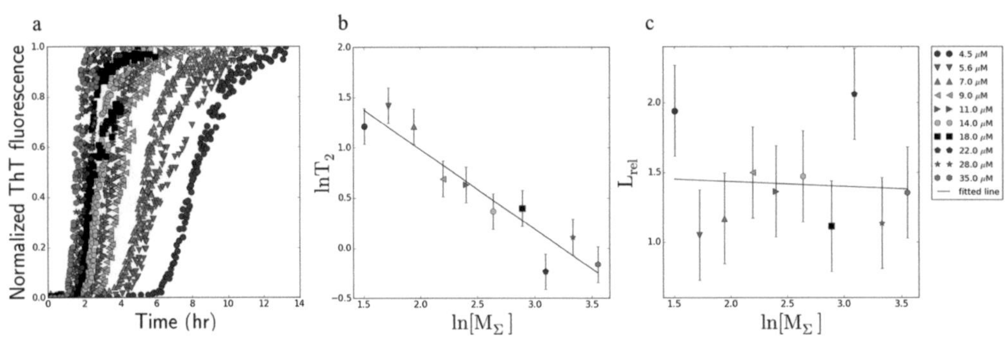

Figure 8. (a) Dependence of normalized ThT fluorescence on time for Aβ40 [60]. The approximation [Insert figure caption here] line calculated for Aβ40 amyloid formation with experimental data from (a) by the least-squares method plotted in coordinates (b): $\{\ln T_2, \ln[M_\Sigma]\}$ and (c): $\{L_{rel}, \ln[M_\Sigma]\}$; $[M_\Sigma]$ is in μM, T_2 in hours. The tangent coefficients of the approximation lines are −0.79 ± 0.18 for $d(\ln T_2)/d(\ln[M_\Sigma])$ and −0.03 ± 0.32 for $d(L_{rel})/d(\ln[M_\Sigma])$; the errors are computed with the Student's coefficients corresponding to 0.95 confidence level.

6.4. Aβ42

The exponential growth with branching takes place for both Aβ40 and Aβ42 peptides (see **Figures 8** and **9**). Interestingly, according to our analysis, for Aβ42, the size of the primary nucleus of the amyloid protofibril is larger than that of Aβ40, although the mechanism of amyloid fibril formation must be similar. This is consistent with the recent data, which compares the behavior of the two peptides during the aggregation process [60]. The primary nucleus size for Aβ42 is three monomers, and the secondary nucleus size is two monomers.

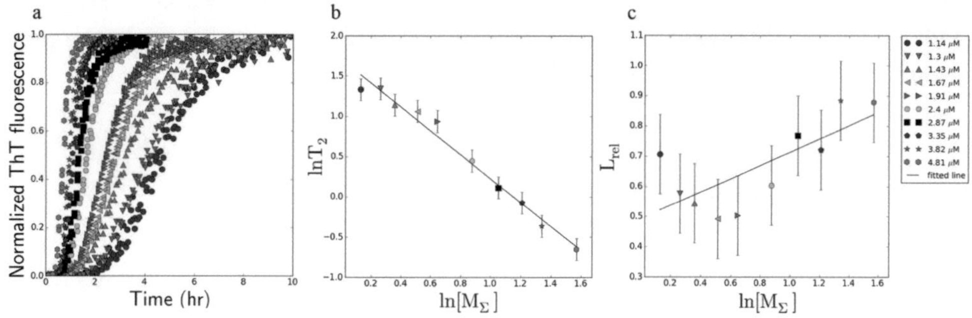

Figure 9. (a) Dependence of normalized ThT fluorescence on time for Aβ42 [61]. The approximation line calculated for Aβ42 amyloid formation with experimental data from (a) by the least-squares method plotted in coordinates (b): {$\ln T_2$, $\ln[M_\Sigma]$} and (c): {L_{rel}, $\ln[M_\Sigma]$}; $[M_\Sigma]$ is in μM, T_2 in hours. The tangent coefficients of the approximation lines are -1.48 ± 0.14 for $d(\ln T_2)/d(\ln[M_\Sigma])$ and 0.22 ± 0.13 for $d(L_{rel})/d(\ln[M_\Sigma])$; the errors are computed with the Student's coefficients corresponding to 0.95 confidence level.

6.5. Human cardiac titin immunoglobulin domain I27 (TI27)

To determine the sizes of folding nuclei for amyloid formation, calculations were done using the data of aggregation kinetics for the I27 immunoglobulin domain from human cardiac titin (TI27) [62]. The set of data was digitized, and in the case of TI27, part of the curve was excluded from the analysis. It was found that the growth of amyloids formed by TI27 is exponential, that is, in addition to the primary core nucleation secondary nucleation by a branching mechanism also takes place, accelerating the formation of new fibrils.

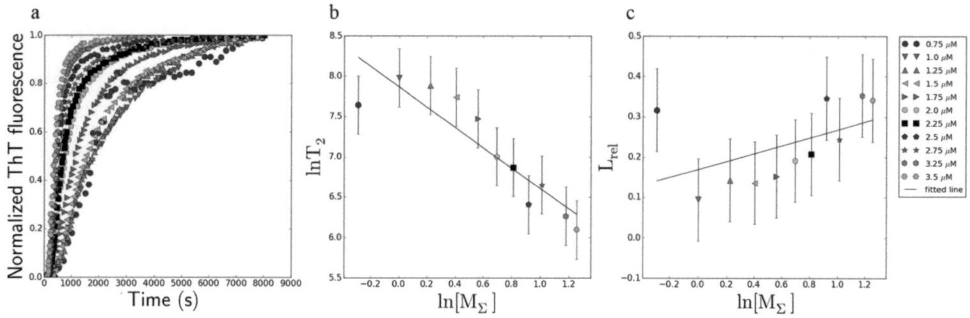

Figure 10. (a) Dependence of normalized ThT fluorescence on time for TI27 [62]. (b) Dependence of $\ln T_2$ on $\ln[M_\Sigma]$ for TI27. This was used to calculate the size of the secondary nucleus. The slope of the fitted line is about −1.26 which, according to formulas from [33], indicates that the size of the secondary nucleus is $n_2 = 1.52 \pm 0.36$. (c) Dependence of L_{rel} on $\ln[M_\Sigma]$ for TI27. The slope of the fitted line is −0.1, that is, L_{rel} is dependent on $\ln[M_\Sigma]$. Some L_{rel} values exceed 0.2 and, according to [33], cannot be explained by the linear model. The size of the primary nucleus was calculated based on the size of the secondary nucleus, and the slope of the straight line is 2.42 ± 0.46. The errors are computed with the Student's coefficients corresponding to 0.95 confidence level.

It is seen from **Figure 10c** that though the values of L_{rel} for TI27 do not exceed 0.2, L_{rel} depends on $\ln[M_\Sigma]$ and so, as mentioned above, cannot occur by the linear mechanism. This effect can be explained by the presence of second nucleation cores with $n_2 = 1.52 \pm 0.36$ (**Figure 10b**). It is interesting that in spite of the difference in the aggregation mechanism, the size of the primary nucleation core for TI27 was 2.42 ± 0.46 (**Figure 10c**) similar (within error) to the primary nucleation core, 3.46 ± 0.28 (**Figure 5**), calculated for actin [50].

7. Concluding remarks

Amyloid fibril polymorphism suggests various ways of their formation from monomers through different oligomers (intermediates of various sizes and shapes) to mature fibrils of different morphology. It is very likely that the surface of the formed fibrils can serve as a matrix for lateral polymerization of monomers/oligomers on it, as reported in the literature [47, 63, 64]. The above complicates the explanation of the mechanism of formation of fibrils and the proposal of a single scheme of polymerization for many proteins. It should be noted that a combination of several mechanisms is quite possible and can be observed sometimes in experiments.

Thus, despite some common features of formation of fibrils of different proteins, each of them has its own specific route for fibrillogenesis, which is originally determined by the amino acid sequence of the protein and is strongly dependent on environmental conditions and seed addition. It is clear that there is need for a serious analysis of data on various proteins to explain various routes for fibril formation that will help identify conditions that affect the initial formation paths (lag time) and find ways to block the entire process, which is an important task in the prevention and treatment of diseases associated with amyloid deposits.

A detailed study of molecular and cellular processes underlying the development of protein-opathy, search for targets for drug development and the use of the obtained data in the development of methods for early diagnosis are essential for the successful treatment and prevention of common diseases. Due to the new generation of neuroprotective drugs acting directly on the pathogenesis of the disease, all components of the cascade of pathological key protein aggregation proteinopathy can be regarded as potential targets. We believe that the combination of theoretical and experimental approaches employed throughout our research is particularly useful and productive for obtaining new important results.

Acknowledgements

We thank T.B. Kuvshinkina, E.I. Grigorashvili, M. Yu. Suvorina, A.V. Finkelstein, and A.K. Surin for assistance in the manuscript preparation. This study was supported by the Russian Science Foundation No. 14-14-00536.

Author details

Oxana V. Galzitskaya*, Nikita V. Dovidchenko and Olga M. Selivanova

*Address all correspondence to: ogalzit@vega.protres.ru

Institute of Protein Research, Russian Academy of Sciences, Pushchino, Moscow Region, Russia

References

[1] Chiti F, Webster P, Taddei N, Clark A, Stefani M, Ramponi G, et al. Designing conditions for in vitro formation of amyloid protofilaments and fibrils. Proc. Natl. Acad. Sci. U. S. A. 1999;96:3590–4.

[2] Fändrich M, Fletcher MA, Dobson CM. Amyloid fibrils from muscle myoglobin. Nature. 2001;410:165–6.

[3] Bucciantini M, Calloni G, Chiti F, Formigli L, Nosi D, Dobson CM, et al. Prefibrillar amyloid protein aggregates share common features of cytotoxicity. J. Biol. Chem. 2004;279:31374–82.

[4] Kayed R, Head E, Thompson JL, McIntire TM, Milton SC, Cotman CW, et al. Common structure of soluble amyloid oligomers implies common mechanism of pathogenesis. Science. 2003;300:486–9.

[5] Ivanova MI, Sievers SA, Sawaya MR, Wall JS, Eisenberg D. Molecular basis for insulin fibril assembly. Proc. Natl. Acad. Sci. U. S. A. 2009;106:18990–5.

[6] Dobson CM. Protein misfolding, evolution and disease. Trends Biochem. Sci. 1999;24:329–32.

[7] Rochet JC, Lansbury PT. Amyloid fibrillogenesis: themes and variations. Curr. Opin. Struct. Biol. 2000;10:60–8.

[8] Uversky VN, Gillespie JR, Fink AL. Why are "natively unfolded" proteins unstructured under physiologic conditions? Proteins. 2000;41:415–27.

[9] Tenidis K, Waldner M, Bernhagen J, Fischle W, Bergmann M, Weber M, et al. Identification of a penta- and hexapeptide of islet amyloid polypeptide (IAPP) with amyloidogenic and cytotoxic properties. J. Mol. Biol. 2000;295:1055–71.

[10] von Bergen M, Friedhoff P, Biernat J, Heberle J, Mandelkow EM, Mandelkow E. Assembly of tau protein into Alzheimer paired helical filaments depends on a local sequence motif ((306)VQIVYK(311)) forming beta structure. Proc. Natl. Acad. Sci. U. S. A. 2000;97:5129–34.

[11] Ivanova MI, Sawaya MR, Gingery M, Attinger A, Eisenberg D. An amyloid-forming segment of beta2-microglobulin suggests a molecular model for the fibril. Proc. Natl. Acad. Sci. U. S. A. 2004;101:10584–9.

[12] Tsolis AC, Papandreou NC, Iconomidou VA, Hamodrakas SJ. A consensus method for the prediction of "aggregation-prone" peptides in globular proteins. Plos One. 2013;8:e54175.

[13] Walsh I, Seno F, Tosatto SCE, Trovato A. PASTA 2.0: an improved server for protein aggregation prediction. Nucleic Acids Res. 2014;42:W301–7.

[14] Fernandez-Escamilla A-M, Rousseau F, Schymkowitz J, Serrano L. Prediction of sequence-dependent and mutational effects on the aggregation of peptides and proteins. Nat. Biotechnol. 2004;22:1302–6.

[15] Emily M, Talvas A, Delamarche C. MetAmyl: a METa-predictor for AMYLoid proteins. Plos One. 2013;8:e79722.

[16] Maurer-Stroh S, Debulpaep M, Kuemmerer N, Lopez de la Paz M, Martins IC, Reumers J, et al. Exploring the sequence determinants of amyloid structure using position-specific scoring matrices. Nat. Methods. 2010;7:237–42.

[17] Garbuzynskiy SO, Lobanov MY, Galzitskaya OV. FoldAmyloid: a method of prediction of amyloidogenic regions from protein sequence. Bioinform. Oxf. Engl. 2010;26:326–32.

[18] Ahmed AB, Znassi N, Château M-T, Kajava AV. A structure-based approach to predict predisposition to amyloidosis. Alzheimers Dement. J. Alzheimers Assoc. 2015;11:681–90.

[19] Dovidchenko NV, Galzitskaya OV. Computational approaches to identification of aggregation sites and the mechanism of amyloid growth. Adv. Exp. Med. Biol. 2015;855:213–39.

[20] Oosawa F, Asakura S, Hotta K, Imai N, Ooi T. G–F transformation of actin as a fibrous condensation. J. Polym. Sci. 1959;37:323–36.

[21] Hofrichter J, Ross PD, Eaton WA. Kinetics and mechanism of deoxyhemoglobin S gelation: a new approach to understanding sickle cell disease. Proc. Natl. Acad. Sci. U. S. A. 1974;71:4864–8.

[22] Ferrone FA, Hofrichter J, Sunshine HR, Eaton WA. Kinetic studies on photolysis-induced gelation of sickle cell hemoglobin suggest a new mechanism. Biophys. J. 1980;32:361–80.

[23] Frieden C, Goddette DW. Polymerization of actin and actin-like systems: evaluation of the time course of polymerization in relation to the mechanism. Biochemistry. 1983;22:5836–43.

[24] Goldstein RF, Stryer L. Cooperative polymerization reactions. Analytical approximations, numerical examples, and experimental strategy. Biophys. J. 1986;50:583–99.

[25] Ruschak AM, Miranker AD. Fiber-dependent amyloid formation as catalysis of an existing reaction pathway. Proc. Natl. Acad. Sci. U. S. A. 2007;104:12341–6.

[26] Griffith JS. Self-replication and scrapie. Nature. 1967;215:1043–4.

[27] Prusiner SB. Novel proteinaceous infectious particles cause scrapie. Science. 1982;216:136–44.

[28] Prusiner SB. Molecular biology of prion diseases. Science. 1991;252:1515–22.

[29] Jarrett JT, Lansbury PT. Seeding "one-dimensional crystallization" of amyloid: a pathogenic mechanism in Alzheimer's disease and scrapie? Cell. 1993;73:1055–8.

[30] Collins SR, Douglass A, Vale RD, Weissman JS. Mechanism of prion propagation: amyloid growth occurs by monomer addition. Plos Biol. 2004;2:e321.

[31] Morris AM, Watzky MA, Agar JN, Finke RG. Fitting neurological protein aggregation kinetic data via a 2-step, minimal/"Ockham's Razor" model: the Finke–Watzky mechanism of nucleation followed by autocatalytic surface growth. Biochemistry. 2008;47:2413–27.

[32] Knowles TPJ, Waudby CA, Devlin GL, Cohen SIA, Aguzzi A, Vendruscolo M, et al. An analytical solution to the kinetics of breakable filament assembly. Science. 2009;326:1533–7.

[33] Dovidchenko NV, Finkelstein AV, Galzitskaya OV. How to determine the size of folding nuclei of protofibrils from the concentration dependence of the rate and lag-time of aggregation. I. Modeling the amyloid protofibril formation. J. Phys. Chem. B. 2014;118:1189–97.

[34] Fändrich M, Schmidt M, Grigorieff N. Recent progress in understanding Alzheimer's β-amyloid structures. Trends Biochem. Sci. 2011;36:338–45.

[35] Fändrich M, Meinhardt J, Grigorieff N. Structural polymorphism of Alzheimer Abeta and other amyloid fibrils. Prion. 2009;3:89–93.

[36] Petkova AT, Leapman RD, Guo Z, Yau W-M, Mattson MP, Tycko R. Self-propagating, molecular-level polymorphism in Alzheimer's beta-amyloid fibrils. Science. 2005;307:262–5.

[37] Kajava AV, Baxa U, Steven AC. Beta arcades: recurring motifs in naturally occurring and disease-related amyloid fibrils. FASEB J. 2010;24:1311–9.

[38] Suvorina MY, Selivanova OM, Grigorashvili EI, Nikulin AD, Marchenkov VV, Surin AK, et al. Studies of polymorphism of amyloid-β 42 peptide from different suppliers. J. Alzheimers Dis. 2015;47:583–93.

[39] Paravastu AK, Qahwash I, Leapman RD, Meredith SC, Tycko R. Seeded growth of beta-amyloid fibrils from Alzheimer's brain-derived fibrils produces a distinct fibril structure. Proc. Natl. Acad. Sci. U. S. A. 2009;106:7443–8.

[40] Lashuel HA, Hartley DM, Petre BM, Wall JS, Simon MN, Walz T, et al. Mixtures of wild-type and a pathogenic (E22G) form of Abeta40 in vitro accumulate protofibrils, including amyloid pores. J. Mol. Biol. 2003;332:795–808.

[41] Waugh DF. Regeneration of insulin from insulin fibrils by the action of alkali. J. Am. Chem. Soc. 1948;70:1850–7.

[42] Nielsen L, Khurana R, Coats A, Frokjaer S, Brange J, Vyas S, et al. Effect of environmental factors on the kinetics of insulin fibril formation: elucidation of the molecular mechanism. Biochemistry. 2001;40:6036–46.

[43] Nielsen L, Frokjaer S, Brange J, Uversky VN, Fink AL. Probing the mechanism of insulin fibril formation with insulin mutants. Biochemistry. 2001;40:8397–409.

[44] Nielsen L, Frokjaer S, Carpenter JF, Brange J. Studies of the structure of insulin fibrils by Fourier transform infrared (FTIR) spectroscopy and electron microscopy. J. Pharm. Sci. 2001;90:29–37.

[45] Dzwolak W, Ravindra R, Lendermann J, Winter R. Aggregation of bovine insulin probed by DSC/PPC calorimetry and FTIR spectroscopy. Biochemistry. 2003;42:11347–55.

[46] Jansen R, Grudzielanek S, Dzwolak W, Winter R. High pressure promotes circularly shaped insulin amyloid. J. Mol. Biol. 2004;338:203–6.

[47] Jansen R, Dzwolak W, Winter R. Amyloidogenic self-assembly of insulin aggregates probed by high resolution atomic force microscopy. Biophys. J. 2005;88:1344–53.

[48] Selivanova OM, Suvorina MY, Dovidchenko NV, Eliseeva IA, Surin AK, Finkelstein AV, et al. How to determine the size of folding nuclei of protofibrils from the concentration dependence of the rate and lag-time of aggregation. II. Experimental application for insulin and LysPro insulin: aggregation morphology, kinetics, and sizes of nuclei. J. Phys. Chem. B. 2014;118:1198–206.

[49] Binger KJ, Pham CLL, Wilson LM, Bailey MF, Lawrence LJ, Schuck P, et al. Apolipoprotein C-II amyloid fibrils assemble via a reversible pathway that includes fibril breaking and rejoining. J. Mol. Biol. 2008;376:1116–29.

[50] Sept D, McCammon JA. Thermodynamics and kinetics of actin filament nucleation. Biophys. J. 2001;81:667–74.

[51] Brange J, Dodson GG, Edwards DJ, Holden PH, Whittingham JL. A model of insulin fibrils derived from the X-ray crystal structure of a monomeric insulin (despentapeptide insulin). Proteins. 1997;27:507–16.

[52] Pease LF, Sorci M, Guha S, Tsai D-H, Zachariah MR, Tarlov MJ, et al. Probing the nucleus model for oligomer formation during insulin amyloid fibrillogenesis. Biophys. J. 2010;99:3979–85.

[53] Brange J, Andersen L, Laursen ED, Meyn G, Rasmussen E. Toward understanding insulin fibrillation. J. Pharm. Sci. 1997;86:517–25.

[54] Turnell WG, Finch JT. Binding of the dye congo red to the amyloid protein pig insulin reveals a novel homology amongst amyloid-forming peptide sequences. J. Mol. Biol. 1992;227:1205–23.

[55] Nayak A, Sorci M, Krueger S, Belfort G. A universal pathway for amyloid nucleus and precursor formation for insulin. Proteins. 2009;74:556–65.

[56] Ahmad A, Millett IS, Doniach S, Uversky VN, Fink AL. Partially folded intermediates in insulin fibrillation. Biochemistry. 2003;42:11404–16.

[57] Ahmad A, Uversky VN, Hong D, Fink AL. Early events in the fibrillation of monomeric insulin. J. Biol. Chem. 2005;280:42669–75.

[58] Vestergaard B, Groenning M, Roessle M, Kastrup JS, van de Weert M, Flink JM, et al. A helical structural nucleus is the primary elongating unit of insulin amyloid fibrils. Plos Biol. 2007;5:e134.

[59] Podestà A, Tiana G, Milani P, Manno M. Early events in insulin fibrillization studied by time-lapse atomic force microscopy. Biophys. J. 2006;90:589–97.

[60] Meisl G, Yang X, Hellstrand E, Frohm B, Kirkegaard JB, Cohen SIA, et al. Differences in nucleation behavior underlie the contrasting aggregation kinetics of the Aβ40 and Aβ42 peptides. Proc. Natl. Acad. Sci. U. S. A. 2014;111:9384–9.

[61] Cohen SIA, Linse S, Luheshi LM, Hellstrand E, White DA, Rajah L, et al. Proliferation of amyloid-β42 aggregates occurs through a secondary nucleation mechanism. Proc. Natl. Acad. Sci. U. S. A. 2013;110:9758–63.

[62] Wright CF, Teichmann SA, Clarke J, Dobson CM. The importance of sequence diversity in the aggregation and evolution of proteins. Nature. 2005;438:878–81.

[63] Manno M, Mauro M, Craparo EF, Podestà A, Bulone D, Carrotta R, et al. Kinetics of different processes in human insulin amyloid formation. J. Mol. Biol. 2007;366:258–74.

[64] Loksztejn A, Dzwolak W. Vortex-induced formation of insulin amyloid superstructures probed by time-lapse atomic force microscopy and circular dichroism spectroscopy. J. Mol. Biol. 2010;395:643–55.

[65] Fodera V, Librizzi F, Groenning M, van de Weert M, Leone M. Secondary Nucleation and Accessible Surface in Insulin Amyloid Fibril Formation. J. Phys. Chem. B 2008, 112, 3853–3858.

Chapter 6

Role of Glycation in Amyloid: Effect on the Aggregation Process and Cytotoxicity

Clara Iannuzzi, Gaetano Irace and Ivana Sirangelo

Additional information is available at the end of the chapter

http://dx.doi.org/10.5772/62995

Abstract

Although the aggregation process of amyloidogenic proteins has been widely studied in vitro and many physiological factors have been identified, the molecular mechanisms underlying the formation of aggregates in vivo and under pathological conditions are still poorly understood. Post-translational modifications are known to affect protein structure and function. Some of these modifications might affect proteins in detrimental ways and lead to their misfolding and accumulation. Reducing sugars play an important role in modifying proteins, forming advanced glycation end-products (AGEs) in a nonenzymatic process, called glycation. Recently, much attention has been devoted to the role played by glycation in stimulating amyloid aggregation and cellular toxicity. Proteins in amyloid deposits are often found glycated, suggesting a direct correlation between protein glycation and amyloidosis.

AGE products increase in aging and are considered a marker for several diseases such as Alzheimer disease and diabetes. In addition to directly affecting the protein structure and function, AGEs also induce cellular toxicity.

This chapter focuses on the molecular effects induced by glycation in the amyloid aggregation of several protein models. In particular, both the structural effects induced by glycation and their consequence on cellular toxicity will be extensively described.

Keywords: amyloid aggregation, protein glycation, AGEs, cellular toxicity

1. Introduction

Reducing sugars play an important role in modifying proteins, forming advanced glycation end-products (AGEs) in a nonenzymatic process, called glycation. This process is different from glycosylation; indeed, these two post-translational modifications affect the structure of the target protein in a different way. Glycosylation is a selective protein modification, driven by specific enzymes, that is generally associated with a gain of function (or stabilization) of the target protein. Nonenzymatic glycation is a nonselective modification, and it is generally associated with a loss of function of the target protein due to modifications of its native structure. While glycosylation is a well-controlled cellular mechanism, nonenzymatic glycation depends on the exposure of free amino groups in the polypeptide chain, concentration of the sugar, and oxidative conditions. Glycation is a pathological process that is highly relevant in diabetes patients, as it plays a crucial role not only in diabetic complications but also in the normal aging process. Increasing evidence suggests a link between diabetes and neurodegenerative processes such as Alzheimer and Parkinson diseases [1]. In this respect, much attention has been recently devoted to the role played by nonenzymatic glycation of proteins in stimulating amyloid aggregation and toxicity. The observation that proteins in amyloid deposits, such as β-amyloid, tau, prions, transthyretin, and β_2-microglobulin, are often found glycated in patients suggests a direct correlation between protein glycation and amyloid formation [2–8]. This is thought to be associated with the formation of cross-links that stabilize protein aggregates. Indeed, AGEs formation can not only interfere with the regular functioning of the proteins to which they are attached but also induce the formation of covalent cross-links with close proteins. In addition, glycation can affect the protein degradation process [9], and, being an abnormal modification, it has been found to induce some proteins to misfold and, thus, promote protein aggregation [10–12].

Moreover, the AGE-modified proteins are tightly involved in physiopathological cellular mechanisms. Once formed, AGEs interact with specific cellular receptors leading to the activation of different signaling pathways. The most studied AGE-receptor, known as RAGE, is a multiligand receptor belonging to the immunoglobulin superfamily [13, 14]. The activation of RAGE regulates key cellular processes such as inflammation, apoptosis, proliferation, autophagy, and recently it has been associated with the pathogenesis of amyloidosis [15, 16]. In neurons, glia, and endothelial cells, RAGE is also the binding site for Aβ peptide on the cell surface and mediates Alzheimer's disease pathology [15, 17, 18].

2. Protein glycation

The nonenzymatic glycation of protein amino groups by reducing sugars (also called Maillard reaction) is a chemical reaction common to all cell types: glycated products slowly accumulate in vivo, leading to several different protein dysfunctions caused by alterations of their integrity [19, 20]. The process begins with a nucleophilic addition reaction between a free amino group of a protein and a carbonyl group of a reducing sugar, forming a reversible intermediate product (Schiff's base). Side-chains of arginine and lysine residues and the N-terminal amino group of proteins are the main targets of protein glycation. The process depends on several conditions, such as the concentration and reactivity of the glycation agent, the presence of catalytic factors (metals, buffer ions, and oxygen), the physiological pH, temperature, and the half-life of each protein. All reducing sugars can participate in glycation reactions and, among them, D-ribose is the most active form, and its intracellular level can be quite high. D-glucose is the less reactive form and its intracellular concentration is negligible, while dicarbonyl compounds, such as methylglyoxal and glyoxal, are far more reactive. These compounds are intermediates of glycation reaction, but can also be generated by various oxidative processes and be formed through other metabolic pathways such as glycolysis and catabolism of threonine and ketone bodies. The levels of D-ribose in the blood are estimated around 20 mg/L in healthy individuals, while that of D-glucose are around 6–10 g/L. Once formed, the Schiff's base can convert into a stable ketoamine by Amadori rearrangement (**Figure 1**). This reaction is reversible, depending on the concentration of the reactants. The late stage of the process is an irreversible cascade of reactions involving enolization, dehydration, condensation, oxidation, fragmentation, and other rearrangements, leading to the formation of AGEs [21]. Glucose, Schiff's base, and Amadori product, can also exhibit auto-oxidation reactions that are responsible for free radicals and highly reactive carbonyl compound production. These compounds can react with other amino acid side-chains and further contribute to post-translational modifications. Unlike organic syntheses, AGEs formation does not produce well-defined products but a large number of structures. The pathways leading to several AGEs are extensively outlined in [22]. Glycation reaction produces very reactive intermediates that can promote the formation of intramolecular and intermolecular cross-links within AGE-modified protein monomers. However, the reaction can also evolve into AGE protein adducts unable to form covalent cross-links (**Figure 1**).

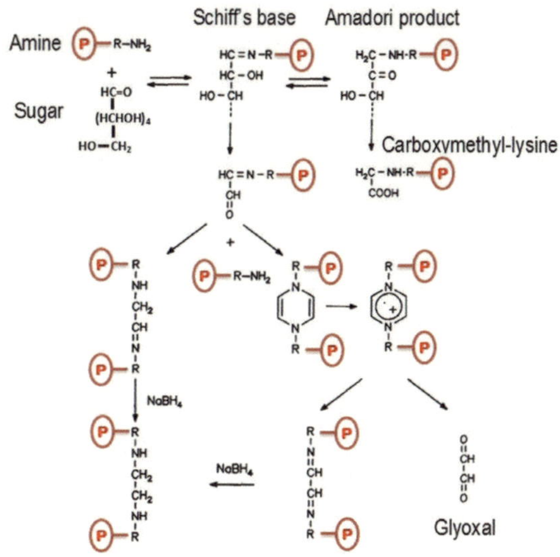

Figure 1. Simplified reaction scheme of some chemical processes involved in AGE formation. The reaction between a free amino group of a protein and the carbonyl group of a reducing sugar leads to the production of the Schiff's base that can turn into a stable ketoamine by Amadori rearrangement. Glycation reaction can evolve to AGE derivatives, forming, that is, di-aminoethyl bridge, or not forming, that is, carboxymethyl-lysine, intramolecular and intermolecular protein cross-links. Adapted from Glomb and Monnier [23].

3. Differential effects of glycation on protein aggregation and cytotoxicity

Several proteins related and not related to misfolding diseases have been so far examined to investigate the effect of glycation on their propensity to aggregate and form amyloid structure.

3.1. Proteins related to misfolding diseases

3.1.1. Aβ-peptide

Aβ-peptide is crucially involved in Alzheimer's disease as the main component of the amyloid plaques found in the brains of Alzheimer patients. This peptide results from the amyloid precursor protein (APP), which is cleaved by beta-secretase and gamma-secretase. Although carbohydrates are directly involved in the formation of neurofibrillary tangles and senile plaques in the brains of the patients with Alzheimer disease (AD) [24–26], their influence on the mechanism of Aβ peptide aggregation and induced cell toxicity is still controversial. Vitek et al. [10] reported, for the first time, that plaque fractions of AD brains contained about threefold more AGE adducts than preparations from healthy, age-matched controls. This observation was further corroborated by immunohistochemical studies on postmortem tissues that identified AGEs as major components of amyloid plaques [27]. Studies in vitro have shown that AGE-modified Aβ peptide-nucleation seeds induce fast aggregation of the soluble Aβ peptide compared to nonmodified seed material [10]. Aggregation of the Aβ peptide follows a nucleation-dependent polymerization process, consisting of two steps, an initial slow nucleus formation, followed by a rapid growth phase. The formation of a nucleus is a reversible process dependent on the concentration of the peptide monomer; thus, it is likely that the initiation of the process at a subthreshold concentration may be started by irreversible covalent cross-linking of the glycated monomers [10]. The AGEs species that enhance nucleation were suggested to be the relatively early glycation products as evidenced by the time course over which glucose accelerated the formation of Aβ peptide aggregates. Successively, it has been reported that glycation by fructose also promotes amyloid aggregation in vitro of Aβ peptide. During the aggregation process, both nucleus formation and aggregates' growth were accelerated by AGE-mediated cross-linking [28, 29]. Specifically, an increased content of oligomeric forms at the expense of fibrillar species was detected when Aβ peptide was incubated in the presence of glucose or fructose [29]. These species resulted to improve cell viability probably due to the stabilization of the oligomeric forms. Indeed, the mechanism by which Aβ induces toxicity is intimately associated to the conformational state of the peptide, the fibrillar forms rather than the soluble oligomers result more toxic to cells [30]. However, increasing evidence has recently shown that soluble oligomers are also cytotoxic, both in vitro and in vivo [31, 32]. The idea that all amyloid oligomers are intrinsically toxic has recently been questioned by a number of evidence showing that, depending on the growth conditions, the same protein/peptide can generate structurally different oligomers endowed with different stability, hydrophobic exposure, compactness, and cytotoxicity [33]. Aβ oligomers display a high degree of polymorphism with different structural, biophysical, and cytotoxic properties. In particular, Aβ oligomers have been classified as A+ and A-, with A+ more toxic than A- oligomers, possibly as a consequence of the increased exposure of hydrophobic residues

http://dx.doi.org/10.5772/62995

that would favor their interaction with the plasma membrane [34, 35]. In this respect, glycation could affect the structural and physicochemical features of amyloid oligomers as well as their interaction to the cell membrane and, consequentially, induce different cytotoxicities. Also, glycation by methylglyoxal promotes the formation of β-sheets, oligomers, and protofibrils in Aβ peptide as well as the increase in size of the oligomers, suggesting an enhancement of intermolecular and intramolecular interactions which stabilizes the aggregate species [36].

Aβ peptide has been identified as a ligand of RAGE, and the Aβ–RAGE interaction triggers the activation of different signaling pathways responsible for the neuronal cell death [37]. RAGE is overexpressed in the AD brains, and its upregulation has been shown to mediate Aβ-induced oxidative stress, activation of transcription factor Nf-κB, and apoptosis [38, 39]. Recently, Li et al. [40] have reported that fully glycated Aβ peptide (long incubation with methylglyoxal) exacerbates the neuronal toxicity by the upregulation of RAGE and subsequent activation of death-signaling pathways. These apparently contrasting effects of the cytotoxic properties of the glycated Aβ could be explained, assuming that glycation induces two different mechanisms in time: an immediate cytoprotective effect, likely associated with the structural properties of the oligomers, and a toxic effect at longer times associated to AGE formation.

3.1.2. β_2-Microglobulin

β_2 microglobulin (β_2M) is a major constituent of amyloid fibrils deposited in patients with hemodialysis-associated amyloidosis. This type of amyloidosis is a common and serious complication in patients on long-term hemodialysis.

Glycation seems to promote amyloid aggregation in β_2M. In particular, D-ribose has been shown to rapidly induce human β_2M to generate AGEs and form aggregates in a time-dependent manner [41]. The process takes few days in vitro and proceeds through the formation of covalent cross-links that are likely to favor protein aggregation. Ribosylated β_2M was highly oligomerized compared to unglycated protein, and had a granular morphology [41]. Furthermore, once ribosylated β_2M aggregates have been formed, they are difficult to be degraded by proteases and can persist in human tissues for a long period. These oligomeric aggregates show significant cytotoxicity to human neuroblastoma and fibroblast cells. Indeed, the exposure of cells to ribosylated β_2M aggregates resulted in a significant increase of intracellular reactive oxygen species (ROS), and thereby induced apoptosis [41]. Inhibition of fibril extension in vitro was reported for β_2M also upon glycation with D-glucose [42]. As glycated β_2M is found as a major component of the amyloid deposits in hemodialysis-associated amyloidosis [2], these findings suggest that glycation could promote the formation of stable β_2-microglobulin aggregates in vivo that contribute to the cell dysfunction and death, thus playing an important role in the pathogenesis of β_2M-associated diseases.

3.1.3. Insulin

Insulin is a small protein hormone that is crucial for the control of glucose metabolism. Monomeric insulin undergoes amyloid aggregation in vivo, and insulin amyloid-like fibrils are the hallmark of a clinical condition observed in insulin-dependent diabetic patients, called insulin injection amyloidosis.

Glycation of insulin has been reported to differentially affect protein structure, stability, and aggregation, depending on the glycating agent and/or environmental conditions. This protein is intimately associated with glycemia and is vulnerable to glycation by glucose and other highly reactive carbonyls, especially in diabetic conditions [43]. Glycated insulin is unable to regulate glucose homeostasis in vivo and to stimulate glucose transport and adipose tissue lipogenesis [44].

In vitro experiments have shown that insulin can be glycated by glucose to be able to react with Lys29 in the C-terminal region of chain B and with N-terminus of chains A and B [45, 46]. Glucose induces the formation of glycated insulin adducts having different structural features, depending on the experimental conditions used. In particular, glycation in reducing conditions is able to induce insulin oligomerization, thus accelerating amyloid formation. On the contrary, glycation in nonreducing conditions strongly inhibit amyloid formation in a way proportional to the glycation extent [47]. Probably, under the latter conditions, insulin adducts possess a higher internal dynamics that prevent formation of the rigid cross-β core structure, thus reducing the ability to form fibrils. Human insulin can also be glycated by methylglyoxal able to react with a single site, that is, Arg22 of the B-chain. This modification promotes the formation of native-like aggregates and reduces the ability of human insulin to form fibrils by impairing the formation of the seeding nuclei. These aggregates are small, soluble, nonfibrillar, and retain a native-like structure. The lag-phase of the nucleation-dependent polymerization process increased as a function of methylglyoxal concentration [48]. Also, using ribose as the glycating agent, the insulin's native conformation is preserved and does not evolve in amyloid aggregates, because ribosylation impairs the α-helix to β-sheet transition, maintaining the protein in a soluble monomeric state [49]. Again, the effects may be ascribed to a higher dynamics in glycated insulin leading to impairment in the formation of the rigid cross-β structure. However, ribose-glycated insulin strongly affects the cell viability, triggering a death pathway involving the activation of apoptotic signaling, intracellular reactive oxygen species (ROS) production, and activation of the transcription factor Nf-κB [49].

3.1.4. α-Synuclein

α-Synuclein is a natively unfolded protein which is found in the typical amyloid fibrillar form in the intraneuronal Lewy bodies (LBs) in Parkinson's disease (PD). Several factors such as metals, oxidative stress, failure of proper protein degradation, and mutations are associated to the altered protein conformation and function [50, 51]. Post-translational modifications like phosphorylation and glycation are known to affect the α-synuclein aggregation process [52]. Glycation was first reported to be present in the substantia nigra and locus coeruleus of peripheral LBs [53]. Increased accumulation of AGEs was detected in neuronal LBs and glial cells in the frontal cortex of early-stage PD brains, suggesting a role for AGEs in the disease

[54]. Moreover, AGEs and α-synuclein were found similarly distributed and colocalized in early LBs in the brains of PD patients [6, 55]. Intracellular accumulation of AGEs precedes α-synuclein-positive inclusion body formation, and extracellular AGEs accelerate the process of intracellular α-synuclein-positive inclusion body formation [56].

In vitro studies showed that AGEs promote cross-linking of α-synuclein. The protein contains 15 lysine residues making it a target for glycation at multiple sites. Glycation with both methylglyoxal and glyoxal induces oligomerization of α-synuclein and inhibits the formation of amyloid fibrils [57, 58]. Under aggregation conditions, glycated α-synuclein promoted the β-sheet conversion and the formation of spherical aggregates which were similar to oligomeric intermediates in their size and morphology, but no further elongation to fibrils was observed. Moreover, protein fibrillization was significantly suppressed by the seeding of modified α-synuclein species [57]. However, AGEs formation did not alter the secondary structure: the glycated α-synuclein showed similar random coil conformation as the native protein [57, 58]. Similar results were obtained with D-ribose: ribosylation of α-synuclein promotes the formation of molten globule-like aggregates and not fibrils. Moreover, these aggregates induce oxidative stress in cell models and result in high cytotoxicity. Changes in secondary structure upon ribosylation were not detected in α-synuclein. However, conformational changes in the tertiary structure occurred as suggested by change in intrinsic fluorescence and exposure of hydrophobic patches [59]. The glycation-induced folding alterations might affect the aggregation kinetics of α-synuclein inducing oligomerization and stabilize oligomeric aggregates.

Choi and Lim [60] reported, in a mouse model of parkinsonism, that α-synuclein is modified by AGEs in vivo. The authors showed that an oligomeric form of α-synuclein is linked to Nε-(carboxymethyl)lysine (CML) and Nε-(carboxyethyl)lysine (CEL) suggesting that the AGEs modification is involved in the aggregation of the α-synuclein in vivo.

These results indicate that glycation of α-synuclein results in the formation of oligomeric or globular structures that are the more toxic aggregate forms. Thus, it is likely that, in a glycation-prone environment, more cytotoxic α-synuclein aggregates or oligomers are formed contributing to the pathogenesis of PD.

3.1.5. Lysozime

Hen egg white lysozyme (HEWL) has also been used to study the impact of glycation on protein structure and aggregation. HEWL is a structural homolog of human lysozyme, responsible for systemic amyloidosis disease and, for this reason, it is considered a very good model for amyloid aggregation studies. HEWL undergoes glycation in vitro, and potential glycation sites are considered to be the N-terminal α-amino group, ε-amino group of lysine residues, and guanidino group of arginine residues [61]. Glycation of HEWL has been tested over a prolonged period in the presence of D-glucose, D-fructose, and D-ribose [62, 63]. Among the tested sugars, D-ribose resulted to be the most effective one, and glycation has been found to promote formation of cross-linked oligomers but no fibrillar species in HEWL. More recently, ribosylation of HEWL in the early phase of the process has been studied by complementary high-resolution techniques [64]. These studies indicate that ribosylation modifies the protein surface in HEWL without altering the overall structure but affecting its hydrophobic surface. Such modifications lead to the formation of native-like spherical oligomers, able to affect cell viability, which further evolve into insoluble native-like protofibrils [64].

3.2. Proteins not related to misfolding diseases

3.2.1. Albumin

Human serum albumin (HSA) is the most abundant protein in human plasma or serum (around 60% of total proteins). Serum albumin is known to be capable of self-assembling in amyloidogenic aggregates under particular experimental conditions (pH, temperature, concentration, and isoelectric point) and is a widely used model for the study of amyloid aggregation. Both HSA and bovine serum albumin (BSA) have been shown to be efficiently glycated in vitro by different glycating agents. Glycation and AGE modifications of serum albumin induce structural changes that depend on the chemical reactivity of the modifying reagent and the concentration used for in vitro glycation. However, glycation has been shown to promote strong conformational changes affecting both secondary and tertiary structures. Such modifications in tertiary structure have been revealed by complementary spectroscopical techniques: circular dichroism (CD), Fourier transform infrared (FTIR), nuclear magnetic resonance (NMR), and fluorescence spectroscopy [65–69]. In particular, the microenvironment of Trp214 seems to be strongly affected by glycation as indicated by fluorescence and NMR spectroscopy [66, 69]. Such conformational changes in the tertiary structure could be a consequence of molecular rearrangements after the formation of AGE products. Indeed, some of these AGEs forming covalent cross-links within adjacent protein strands require conformational changes which produce more apolar and tight molecules with respect to the native protein. Besides, the accessibility of the hydrophobic regions in the protein has been shown to increase with glycation [67, 68]. Modification at the secondary structure level can be detected only at longer times of incubation with glycating agents. This could be due to the fact that glycation is likely to induce loss of tertiary structure before that of secondary structure, as suggested by comparing intrinsic fluorescence and far-UV CD results in glycated albumin [65, 66, 70].

Glycation-induced protein misfolding promotes the formation of amyloid-like aggregates in serum albumin [12, 71, 72]. These amyloid-like deposits appear as densely staining granules under atomic force microscopy and are able to bind the amyloid-specific dye thioflavin T. Also, they were shown to induce high cytotoxicity that triggers cell death by activation of cellular signaling cascades. In fact, independent experiments have shown that aggregates of glycated BSA are able to induce ROS-mediated oxidative stress and apoptosis in both neurotypic SH-SY5Y and MCF-7 cells. These results indicate that glycation of serum albumin results in the formation of oligomeric or globular structures that are the more toxic aggregate forms [68, 72].

These observations could have important implications, as serum albumin, being a circulating protein, is likely undergoing glycative alteration in the case of diabetes pathology and hyperglycemia. For instance, antioxidant activities of serum albumin were impaired in patients with diabetes.

3.2.2. Apomyoglobin

Apomyoglobin (i.e., heme-free myoglobin) is a small, soluble α-helical protein able to form amyloid fibrils under particular experimental conditions. In addition, an apomyoglobin mutant, that is, W7FW14F, is able to form amyloid fibrils in physiological conditions of pH and temperature, and for this reason this protein is a good model for the study of amyloidosis [73–78].

Wild-type apomyoglobin is rapidly glycated in vitro by different glycating agents, and glycation has been shown to induce strong conformational changes, affecting both secondary and tertiary structures. In particular, glycation induces partial loss of the helical content in apomyoglobin without promoting an α to β transition, typical of the amyloid aggregates. Glycation induces strong modifications in the tridimensional organization, as suggested by the loss of ability of the glycated protein to bind the prosthetic group [79]. Such modifications eventually lead to the formation of oligomeric species, stabilized by intermolecular cross-links, able to affect cell viability as observed for amyloid prefibrillar oligomeric aggregates, specifically, cell exposure to fully glycated wild-type apomyoglobin-induced ROS-mediated apoptosis [79].

At the same time, glycation has been shown to affect the aggregation kinetics in the W7FW14F apomyoglobin mutant, able to form amyloid fibrils in physiological conditions [73–78]. In particular, glycation accelerates the formation of harmless amyloid fibrils in the apomyoglobin this amyloidogenic mutant [76]. A plausible explanation for such faster kinetics could be related to a higher tendency of the mutant to form intermolecular links upon glycation able to reduce the flexibility of aggregation-prone regions and thus favor the subsequent step of fibril elongation.

Although apomyoglobin is not related to any amyloidogenic diseases, it represents a suitable model for studying the role of glycation in amyloid aggregation. Indeed, due to the different aggregation propensities of the native protein and the W7FW14F mutant in physiological conditions, this protein model allows to dissect the effect of glycation in promoting amyloid aggregation and contributes to the aggregation kinetics. The above results indicate that glycation can be considered not only a triggering factor in amyloidosis but also a player in later stages of the aggregation process.

4. Molecular effects of glycation on amyloid aggregation process

The overall evidences on several model proteins indicate that AGE modifications may alter the folding state of proteins and their solubility, thereby influencing protein aggregation. The main outcome of this study is that the effect of glycation on amyloid aggregation cannot be generalized. Indeed, being a post-translational modification, it differentially affects the aggregation process in proteins by promoting, accelerating, and/or stabilizing on-pathway and off-pathway species (**Figure 2**). Molecular basis of such modulation are still poorly understood. Most of the evidence indicate that glycation strongly affects the tertiary structure of the target protein promoting the formation of globular amyloid-like deposits [62, 72]. Depending on the protein involved, glycation induces chemical modifications of the positively charged side chains (mostly lysine, arginine, and N-terminus), thus affecting the protein charge and favoring the exposure of its hydrophobic surface. This effect could trigger native-like aggregation favoring the formation of small oligomers that, being stabilized by the AGE-derived covalent cross-links, do not evolve into amyloid fibrils. Recent evidence indicates that glycation promotes the formation of the amyloid oligomeric species in several model proteins (**Figure 2B**). However, glycation does not necessarily induce protein oligomerization. Due to the complexity of the glycation reaction, some AGE adducts might not evolve to the formation of protein cross-links. In this case, glycation seems to stabilize the monomeric form thus inhibiting the amyloid aggregation process as observed for ribosylated human insulin (**Figure 2C**). Moreover, the cross-links of AGE-derived oligomers do not necessarily show amyloid properties (**Figure 2D**). However, AGEs-modified proteins are always able to affect cell viability, irrespective of amyloid properties.

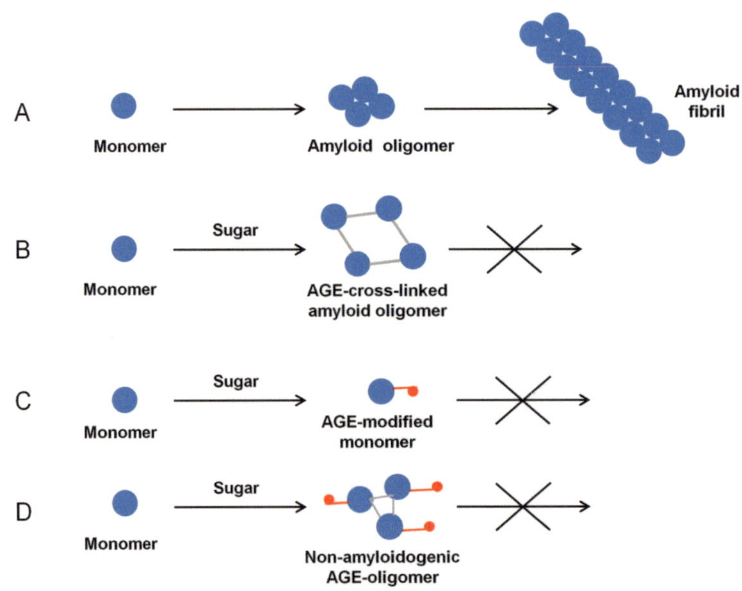

Figure 2. Effects of glycation in amyloid aggregation. Protein monomers are shown as blue dots, AGE-derived cross-links are shown in gray, and AGE modification are shown in red. (A) Typical amyloid aggregation pathway. Possible effects induced by glycation: (B) promote the formation of amyloid oligomeric species stabilized by covalent cross-links; (C) stabilize the monomeric form thus inhibiting amyloid aggregation; (D) promote the formation of cross-linked nonamyloidogenic oligomers.

5. Role of glycation in the amyloid-induced cell toxicity

The effect of glycation on the aggregation process has important implications in the pathological mechanisms involved in amyloid diseases. In most proteins, glycation has been shown

http://dx.doi.org/10.5772/62995

to stabilize the aggregates in the oligomeric forms. This modification has important pathological implications as oligomeric species are known to be far more toxic than the fibrillar aggregates [80, 81]. The oligomeric species may interact with the cell membrane, altering its permeability and leading to cell homeostasis imbalance and neuronal cell dysfunction [82]. Recent evidence indicates that the amyloid oligomer toxicity is not strictly related to the oligomer properties, but rather a behavior that results from a complex interplay between the structural properties of both oligomers and cell membrane taken as a whole. Indeed, oligomers of comparable size but different structure and biophysical properties can display different toxicities, possibly as a consequence of the increased exposure of hydrophobic residues that would destabilize them and favor the interaction with the plasma membrane [83]. In this respect, glycation could affect structural and physicochemical features of amyloid oligomers as well as their interaction to the cell membrane and subsequently modulate and/or induce the cell toxicity. Also, the glycated oligomeric species can induce formation of reactive oxygen species, worsening the oxidative stress in the cell and further promoting protein glycation. Moreover, protein glycation leads to the formation of AGEs which have a pathological role in several diseases [84–86]. AGE adducts may therefore activate, through interaction with RAGE receptor, inflammatory response generally associated to amyloid toxicity [13]. The AGE–RAGE binding results in the activation of NADPH-oxidases that leads to an increased production of ROS. A key downstream target of RAGE is the proinflammatory Nf-κB pathway, which in turn leads to high RAGE expression, producing a feedback loop in which continuous activation of RAGE keeps the cellular inflammatory state activated [14, 87].

Glycated proteins are also resistant to proteasomal degradation; once proteins become glycated at their exposed lysine residues, clearance by the ubiquitin–proteasome system would be impaired, because ubiquitination at lysine residues, a modification that targets proteins to the proteasome for degradation, might be impeded. Thus, accumulation of proteins as aggregates or as depositions or inclusions in tissues might be favored after glycation.

Taking into account the above considerations, protein glycation can be considered a key dynamic contributor to these multifactorial diseases. In fact, it can both promote the formation of pathological oligomeric species and directly trigger cell dysfunction, damage, and death through the AGEs formation. For these reasons, AGEs are considered key therapeutic targets in amyloidosis, and anti-AGEs drugs are objects of intense ongoing research. Specifically, three main strategies have been developed to counteract the AGEs' effects: (i) to prevent the formation of AGEs; (ii) to break cross-links after their formation; (iii) to prevent AGEs' negative effects.

In vitro and in vivo experiments have shown that many compounds including aminoguanidine, antioxidants such as vitamin C and vitamin E, pyridoxamine, thiamine and its synthetic derivative benfotiamine, alpha-lipoic acid, taurine, pimagedine, aspirin, carnosine, metformin, pioglitazone, and pentoxifylline are able to inhibit AGE formation. Some of these compounds have already been used in clinical practice and some others are under clinical trials. Compounds that have been shown to break existing AGE cross-links mainly include alagebrium (and related ALT-462, ALT-486, and ALT-946) and N-phenacylthiazolium bromide. Studies with the aim to counteract the negative effects of the AGEs mainly involve the use of natural products as polyphenols, such as resveratrol and curcumin and some flavonoids [88–90].

However, although in vitro and in vivo studies have shown the beneficial effects of various coumpounds, the potential clinical value of these interventions remains to be established. In fact, it seems that safety and/or efficacy in clinical studies with these compounds are still a concern.

Author details

Clara Iannuzzi, Gaetano Irace and Ivana Sirangelo*

*Address all correspondence to: ivana.sirangelo@unina2.it

Department of Biochemistry, Biophysics and General Pathology, Second University of Naples, Naples, Italy

References

[1] Hassan M, Sehgal SA, Rashid S. Regulatory cascade of neuronal loss and glucose metabolism. CNS Neurol Disord Drug Targets. 2014; 13(7), 1232–45.

[2] Miyata T, Oda O, Inagi R, Iida Y, Araki N, Yamada N, Horiuchi S, Taniguchi N, Maeda K, Kinoshita T. Beta 2-microglobulin modified with advanced glycation end products is a major component of hemodialysis-associated amyloidosis. J Clin Invest. 1993; 92, 1243–52.

[3] Ledesma MD, Bonay P, Colaco C, Avila J. Analysis of microtubule-associated protein tau glycation in paired helical filaments. J Biol Chem. 1994; 269(34), 21614–19.

[4] Sasaki N, Fukatsu R, Tsuzuki K, Hayashi Y, Yoshida T, Fujii N, Koike T, Wakayama I, Yanagihara R, Garruto R, Amano N, Makita Z. Advanced glycation end products in Alzheimer's disease and other neurodegenerative diseases. Am J Pathol. 1998; 153, 1149–55.

[5] Kikuchi S, Ogata A, Shinpo K, Moriwaka F, Fujii F, Taniguchi N, Tashiro K. Detection of an Amadori product, 1-hexitol-lysine, in the anterior horn of the amyotrophic lateral sclerosis and spinobulbar muscular atrophy spinal cord: evidence for early involvement of glycation in motoneuron diseases. Acta Neuropathol. 2000; 99, 63–6. doi: 10.1007/PL00007407.

[6] Munch G, Luth HJ, Wong A, Arendt T, Hirsch E, Ravid R, Riederer P. Crosslinking of alpha-synuclein by advanced glycation endproducts–an early pathophysiological step in Lewy body formation? J Chem Neuroanat. 2000; 20, 253–7.

[7] Dukic-Stefanovic S, Schinzel R, Riederer P, Munch G. AGES in brainageing: AGE-inhibitors as neuroprotective and anti-dementia drugs? Biogerontology. 2001; 2, 19–34. doi: 10.1023/A:1010052800347.

[8] Gomes R, Sousa Silva M, Quintas A, Cordeiro C, Freire A, Pereira P, Martins A, Monteiro E, Barroso E, Ponces Freire A. Argpyrimidine, a methylglyoxal-derived advanced glycation end-product in familial amyloidotic polyneuropathy. Biochem J. 2005; 385, 339–45.

[9] Höhn A, Jung T, Grune T. Pathophysiological importance of aggregated damaged proteins. Free Radic Biol Med. 2014; 71, 70–89. doi: 10.1016/j.freeradbiomed.2014.02.028.

[10] Vitek MP, Bhattacharya K, Glendening JM, Stopa E, Vlassara H, Bucala R, Manogue K, Cerami A. Advanced glycation end products contribute to amyloidosis in Alzheimer disease. Proc Natl Acad Sci USA. 1994; 91, 4766–70. doi: 10.1073/pnas.91.11.4766.

[11] Chellan P, Nagaraj RH. Protein crosslinking by the Maillard reaction: dicarbonyl-derived imidazolium crosslinks in aging and diabetes. Arch Biochem Biophys. 1999; 368, 98–104. doi: 10.1006/abbi.1999.1291.

[12] Bouma B, Kroon-Batenburg LM, Wu YP, Brunjes B, Posthuma G, Kranenburg O, De Groot PG, Voest EE, Gebbink MF. Glycation induces formation of amyloid cross-beta structure in albumin. J Biol Chem. 2003; 278, 41810–9. doi: 10.1074/jbc.M303925200.

[13] Xie J, Méndez JD, Méndez-Valenzuela V, Aguilar-Hernández MM. Cellular signalling of the receptor for advanced glycation end products (RAGE). Cell Signal. 2013; 25(11), 2185–97. doi: 10.1016/j.cellsig.2013.06.013.

[14] Ott C, Jacobs K, Haucke E, Santos AN, Grune N, Simm A. Role of advanced glycation end products in cellular signaling. Redox Biol. 2014; 2, 411–29. doi: 10.1016/j.redox.2013.12.016.

[15] Lue LF, Yan SD, Stern DM, Walker DG. Preventing activation of receptor for advanced glycation endproducts in Alzheimer's disease. Curr Drug Targets CNS Neurol Disord. 2005; 4(3), 249–66.

[16] Vicente Miranda H, Outeiro TF. The sour side of neurodegenerative disorders: the effects of protein glycation. J Pathol. 2010; 221(1), 13–25. doi: 10.1002/path.2682.

[17] Wan W, Chen H, Li Y. The potential mechanisms of Aβ-receptor for advanced glycation end-products interaction disrupting tight junctions of the blood-brain barrier in Alzheimer's disease. Int J Neurosci. 2014; 124(2), 75–81. doi: 10.3109/00207454.2013.825258.

[18] Galasko D, Bell J, Mancuso JY, Kupiec JW, Sabbagh MN, van Dyck C, Thomas RG, Aisen PS; Alzheimer's Disease Cooperative Study. Clinical trial of an inhibitor of RAGE-Aβ interactions in Alzheimer disease. Neurology. 2014; 82(17), 1536–42. doi: 10.1212/WNL.0000000000000364.

[19] Miyata T, van Ypersele de Strihou C, Kurokawa K, Baynes JW. Alterations in nonenzymatic biochemistry in uremia: origin and significance of "carbonyl stress" in long-term uremic complications. Kidney Int. 1999; 55, 389–99. doi: 10.1046/j.1523-1755.1999.00302.x.

[20] Gul A, Rahman MA, Salim A, Simjee SU. Advanced glycation end products in senile diabetic and nondiabetic patients with cataract. J Diabetes Complications. 2009; 23, 343–8. doi: 10.1016/j.jdiacomp.2008.04.001.

[21] Ulrich P, Cerami A. Protein glycation, diabetes, and aging. Recent Prog Horm Res. 2001; 56, 1–2.

[22] Cho SJ, Roman G, Yeboah F, Konishi Y. The road to advanced glycation end products: a mechanistic perspective. Curr Med Chem. 2007; 14(15), 1653–71.

[23] Glomb MA, Monnier VM. Mechanism of protein modification by glyoxal and glycolaldehyde reactive intermediates of the Maillard reaction. J Biol Chem. 1995; 270, 10017–26.

[24] Münch G, Thome J, Foley P, Schinzel R, Riederer P. Advanced glycation end products in ageing and Alzheimer's disease. Brain Res Brain Res Rev. 1997; 23, 134–143.

[25] Münch G, Schinzel R, Loske C, Wong A, Durany N, Li JJ, Vlassara H, Smith MA, Perry G, Riederer P. Alzheimer's disease—synergistic effects of glucose deficit, oxidative stress and advanced glycation endproducts. J Neural Transm. 1998; 105, 439–461.

[26] Münch G, Deuther-Conrad W, Gasic-Milenkovic J. Glycoxidative stress creates a vicious cycle of neurodegeneration in Alzheimer's disease—a target for neuroprotective treatment strategies? J Neural Transm Suppl. 2002; 62, 303–307.

[27] Smith MA, Taneda S, Richey PL, Miyata S, Yan SD, Stern D, Sayre LM, Monnier VM, Perry G. Advanced Maillard reaction end products are associated with Alzheimer disease pathology. Proc Natl Acad Sci USA. 1994; 91(12), 5710–4.

[28] Münch G, Mayer S, Michaelis J, Hipkiss AR, Riederer P, Müller R, Neumann A, Schinzel R, Cunningham AM. Influence of advanced glycation end-products and AGEinhibitors on nucleation-dependent polymerization of β-amyloid peptide. Biochim Biophys Acta. 1997; 1360, 17–29.

[29] Fernandez-Busquets X, Ponce J, Bravo R, Arimon M, Martianez T, Gella A, Cladera J, Durany N. Modulation of amylois β peptide 1-42 cytotoxicity and aggregation in vitro by glucose and chondroitin sulfate. Curr Alzheimer Res. 2010; 7, 428–38. doi: 10.2174/156720510791383787.

[30] Pike CJ, Burdick D, Walencewicz AJ, Glabe CG, Cotman CW. Neurodegeneration induced by beta-amyloid peptides in vitro: the role of peptide assembly state. J Neurosci. 1993; 13, 1676–87.

[31] Dahlgren KN, Manelli AM, Stine WB Jr, Baker LK, Krafft GA, LaDu MJ. Oligomeric and fibrillar species of amyloid-beta peptides differentially affect neuronal viability. J Biol Chem. 2002; 277(35), 32046–53.

[32] Chromy BA, Nowak RJ, Lambert MP, Viola KL, Chang L, Velasco PT, Jones BW, Fernandez SJ, Lacor PN, Horowitz P, Finch CE, Krafft GA, Klein WL. Self-assembly of Abeta(1-42) into globular neurotoxins. Biochemistry. 2003; 42(44), 12749–60.

[33] Sakono M, Zako T. Amyloid oligomers: formation and toxicity of Abeta oligomers. FEBS J. 2010; 277(6), 1348–58. doi: 10.1111/j.1742-4658.2010.07568.x.

[34] Ladiwala AR, Litt J, Kane RS, Aucoin DS, Smith SO, Ranjan S, Davis J, Van Nostrand WE, Tessier PM. Conformational differences between two amyloid β oligomers of similar size and dissimilar toxicity. J Biol Chem. 2012; 287(29), 24765–73. doi: 10.1074/jbc.M111.329763.

[35] Stefani M. Structural polymorphism of amyloid oligomers and fibrils underlies different fibrillization pathways: immunogenicity and cytotoxicity. Curr Protein Pept Sci. 2010; 11(5), 343–54.

[36] Chen K, Maley J, Yu PH. Potential implications of endogenous aldehydes in beta-amyloid misfolding, oligomerization and fibrillogenesis. J Neurochem. 2006; 99, 1413–24. doi: 10.1111/j.1471-4159.2006.04181.x.

[37] Yan SD, Chen X, Fu J, Chen M, Zhu H, Roher A Slattery T, Zhao L, Nagashima M, Morser J, Migheli A, Nawroth P, Stern D, Schmidt AM. RAGE and amyloid-beta peptide neurotoxicity in Alzheimer's disease. Nature. 1996; 382, 685–91.

[38] Takuma K, Fang F, Zhang W, Yan S, Fukuzaki E, Du H Sosunov A, McKhann G, Funatsu Y, Nakamichi N, Nagai T, Mizoguchi H, Ibi D, Hori O, Ogawa S, Stern DM, Yamada K, Yan SS. RAGE-mediated signaling contributes to intraneuronal transport of amyloid-beta and neuronal dysfunction. Proc Natl Acad Sci USA. 2009; 106, 20021–6.

[39] Hadding A, Kaltschmidt B, Kaltschmidt C. Overexpression of receptor of advanced glycation end products hypersensitizes cells for amyloid beta peptide-induced cell death. Biochimica et Biophysica Acta. 2004; 1691, 67–72.

[40] Li XH, Du LL, Cheng XS, Jiang X, Zhang Y, Lv BL, Liu R, Wang JZ, Zhou XW. Glycation exacerbates the neuronal toxicity of β-amyloid. Cell Death Dis. 2013; 4, e673. doi: 10.1038/cddis.2013.180.

[41] Kong FL, Cheng W, Chen J, Liang Y. D-Ribose glycates b2-microglobulin to form aggregates with high cytotoxicity through a ROS-mediated pathway. Chem Biol Interact. 2011; 194, 69–78. doi: 10.1016/j.cbi.2011.08.003.

[42] Hashimoto N, Naiki H, Gejyo F. Modification of beta 2-microglobulin with D-glucose or 3-deoxyglucosone inhibits A beta 2M amyloid fibril extension in vitro. Amyloid. 1999; 6, 256–64. doi: 10.3109/13506129909007337.

[43] Brange J, Andersen L, Laursen ED, Meyn G, Rasmussen E. Toward understanding insulin fibrillation. J Pharm Sci. 1997; 86, 517–25. doi: 10.1021/js960297s.

[44] Boyd AC, Abdel-Wahab YH, McKillop AM, McNulty H, Barnett CR, O'Harte FP, Flatt PR. Impaired ability of glycated insulin to regulate plasma glucose and stimulate glucose transport and metabolism in mouse abdominal muscle. Biochim Biophys Acta. 2000; 1523(1), 128–34.

[45] O'Harte FPM, Højrup P, Barnett CR, Flatt PR. Identification of the site of glycation of human insulin. Peptides. 1996; 17, 1323–30.

[46] Guedes S, Vitorino R, Domingues MR, Amado F, Domingues P. Mass spectrometry characterization of the glycation sites of bovine insulin by tandem mass spectrometry. J Am Soc Mass Spectrom. 2009; 20, 1319–26. doi: 10.1016/j.jasms.2009.03.004.

[47] Alavi P, Yousefi R, Amirghofran S, Karbalaei-Heidari HR, Moosavi-Movahedi AA. Structural analysis and aggregation propensity of reduced and nonreduced glycated insulin adducts. Appl Biochem Biotechnol. 2013; 170, 623–38. doi: 10.1016/j.ijbiomac. 2012.05.021.

[48] Oliveira LM, Lages A, Gomes RA, Neves H, Família C, Coelho AV, Quintas A. Insulin glycation by methylglyoxal results in native-like aggregation and inhibition of fibril formation. BMC Biochem. 2011; 12, 41. doi: 10.1186/1471-2091-12-41.

[49] Iannuzzi C, Borriello M, Carafa V, Altucci L, Vitiello M, Balestrieri ML, Ricci G, Irace G, Sirangelo I. D-ribose-glycation of insulin prevents amyloid aggregation and produces cytotoxic adducts. Biochim Biophys Acta. 2016; 1862(1), 93–104. doi: 10.1016/ j.bbadis.2015.10.021.

[50] Hashimoto M, Hsu LJ, Xia Y, Takeda A, Sisk A, Sundsmo M, Masliah E. Oxidative stress induces amyloid-like aggregate formation of NACP/α-synuclein in vitro. Neuro Report. 1999; 10, 717–21.

[51] Paik SR, Shin HJ, Lee JH. Metal catalyzed oxidation of α-synuclein in the presence of copper (II) and hydrogen peroxide. Arch Biochem Biophys. 2000; 378, 269–77.

[52] Guerrero E, Vasudevaraju P, Hegde ML, Britton GB, Rao KS. Recent advances in α-synuclein functions, advanced glycation, and toxicity: implications for Parkinson's disease. Mol Neurobiol. 2013: 47(2), 525–36.

[53] Castellani R, Smith MA, Richey PL, Perry G. Glycoxidation and oxidative stress in Parkinson disease and diffuse Lewy body disease. Brain Res. 1996; 737: 195–200.

[54] Dalfo E, Portero-Otin M, Ayala V, Martinez A, Pamplona R, Ferrer I. Evidence of oxidative stress in the neocortex in incidental Lewy body disease. J Neuropathol Exp Neurol. 2005; 64: 816–30.

[55] Castellani RJ, Perry G, Siedlak SL, Nunomura A, Shimohama S, Zhang J, Montine T, Sayre LM, Smith MA. Hydroxynonenal adducts indicate a role for lipid peroxidation in neocortical and brainstem Lewy bodies in humans. Neurosci Lett. 2002; 319, 25e28.

[56] Shaikh S, Nicholson LF. Advanced glycation end products induce in vitro cross-linking of alpha-synuclein and accelerate the process of intracellular inclusion body formation. J Neurosci Res. 2008; 86, 2071–82.

[57] Lee D, Park CW, Paik SR, Choi KY. The modification of alpha-synuclein by dicarbonyl compounds inhibits its fibril-forming process. Biochim Biophys Acta. 2009; 1794, 421–30. doi: 10.1016/j.bbapap.2008.

[58] Padmaraju V, Bhaskar JJ, Prasada RUJ, Salimath PV, Rao KS. Role of advanced glycation on aggregation and DNA binding properties of alpha-synuclein. J Alzheimers Dis. 2011; 24, 211–21. doi: 10.1007/s13105-011-0091-5.

[59] Chen L, Wei Y, Wang X, He R. Ribosylation rapidly induces alpha-synuclein to form highly cytotoxic molten globules of advanced glycation end products. PLoS One 2010; 5: e9052. doi: 10.1371/journal.pone.0009052.

[60] Choi YG, Lim S. N(Varepsilon)-(carboxymethyl)lysine linkage to alpha-synuclein and involvement of advanced glycation end products in alpha-synuclein deposits in an MPTP-intoxicated mouse model. Biochimie. 2010; 92(10), 1379–86. doi: 10.1016/j.biochi.2010.06.025.

[61] Tagami U, Akashi S, Mizukoshi T, Suzuki E, Hirayama K. Structural studies of the Maillard reaction products of a protein using ion trap mass spectrometry. J Mass Spectrom. 2000; 35, 131–8. doi: 10.1002/(SICI)1096-9888(200002)35:2.

[62] Fazili NA, Naeem A. In vitro hyperglycemic condition facilitated the aggregation of lysozyme via the passage through a molten globule state. Cell Biochem Biophys. 2013; 66, 265–75. doi: 10.1007/s12013-012-9479-2.

[63] Ghosh S, Pandey NK, Singha Roy A, Tripathy DR, Dinda AK, Dasgupta S. Prolonged glycation of hen egg white lysozyme generates non amyloidal structures. PLoS One 2013; 8, e74336. doi: 10.1371/journal.pone.0074336.

[64] Adrover M, Mariño L, Sanchis P, Pauwels K, Kraan Y, Lebrun P, Vilanova B, Muñoz F, Broersen K, Donoso J. Mechanistic insights in glycation-induced protein aggregation. Biomacromolecules. 2014; 15(9), 3449–62. doi: 10.1021/bm501077j.

[65] Mendez DL, Jensen RA, McElroy LA, Pena JM, Esquerra RM. The effect of non-enzymatic glycation on the unfolding of human serum albumin. Arch Biochem Biophys. 2005; 444, 92–99. doi: 10.1016/j.abb.2005.10.019.

[66] Sattarahmady N, Moosavi-Movahedi AA, Ahmad F, Hakimelahi GH, Habibi-Rezaei M, Saboury AA, Sheibani N. Formation of the molten globule-like state during prolonged glycation of human serum albumin. Biochim Biophys Acta. 2007; 1770, 933–42. doi: 10.1016/j.bbagen.2007.02.001.

[67] Rondeau P, Navarra G, Cacciabaudo F, Leone M, Bourdon E, Militello V. Thermal aggregation of glycated bovine serum albumin. Biochim Biophys Acta. 2010; 1804, 789–98. doi: 10.1016/j.bbapap.2009.12.003.

[68] Khan MS, Dwivedi S, Priyadarshini M, Tabrez S, Siddiqui MA, Jagirdar H, Al-Senaidy AM, Al-Khedhairy AA, Musarrat J. Ribosylation of bovine serum albumin induces ROS accumulation and cell death in cancer line (MCF-7). Eur Biophys J. 2013; 42, 811–18. doi: 10.1007/s00249-013-0929-6.

[69] Szkudlarek A, Sułkowska A, Maciążek-Jurczyk M, Chudzik M, Równicka-Zubik J. Effects of non-enzymatic glycation in human serum albumin. Spectroscopic analysis. Spectrochim Acta A Mol Biomol Spectrosc. 2016; 152, 645–53. doi: 10.1016/j.saa.2015.01.120.

[70] Vetter SW, Indurthi VS. Moderate glycation of serum albumin affects folding, stability, and ligand binding. Clin Chim Acta. 2011; 412, 2105–16. doi: 10.1016/j.cca.2011.07.022.

[71] Sattarahmady N, Moosavi-Movahedi AA, Habibi-Rezaei M, Ahmadian S, Saboury AA, Heli H, Sheibani N. Detergency effects of nanofibrillar amyloid formation on glycation of human serum albumin. Carbohydr Res. 2008; 343, 2229–34. doi: 10.1016/j.carres.2008.04.036.

[72] Wei Y, Chen L, Chen J, Ge L, He R Q. Rapid glycation with D-ribose induces globular amyloid-like aggregations of BSA with high cytotoxicity to SH-SY5Y cells. BMC Cell Biol. 2009; 10, 10. doi: 10.1186/1471-2121-10-10.

[73] Infusini G, Iannuzzi C, Vilasi S, Maritato R, Birolo L, Pagnozzi D, Pucci P, Irace G, Sirangelo I. W-F substitutions in apomyoglobin increase the local flexibility of the N-terminal region causing amyloid aggregation: a H/D exchange study. Protein Pept Lett. 2013; 20(8), 898–904.

[74] Vilasi A, Vilasi S, Romano R, Acernese F, Barone F, Balestrieri ML, Maritato R, Irace G, Sirangelo I. Unraveling amyloid toxicity pathway in NIH3T3 cells by a combined proteomic and 1 H-NMR metabonomic approach. J Cell Physiol. 2013; 228(6), 1359–67. doi: 10.1002/jcp.24294.

[75] Sirangelo I, Giovane A, Maritato R, D'Onofrio N, Iannuzzi C, Giordano A, Irace G, Balestrieri ML. Platelet-activating factor mediates the cytotoxicity induced by W7FW14F apomyoglobin amyloid aggregates in neuroblastoma cells. J Cell Biochem. 2014; 115(12), 2116–22. doi: 10.1002/jcb.24888.

[76] Iannuzzi C, Maritato R, Irace G, Sirangelo I. Glycation accelerates fibrillization of the amyloidogenic W7FW14F apomyoglobin. PLoS One. 2013; 8(12), e80768. doi: 10.1371/journal.pone.0080768.

[77] Iannuzzi C, Maritato R, Irace G, Sirangelo I. Misfolding and amyloid aggregation of apomyoglobin. Int J Mol Sci. 2013; 14(7), 14287–300. doi: 10.3390/ijms140714287.

[78] Iannuzzi C, Irace G, Sirangelo I. Differential effects of glycation on protein aggregation and amyloid formation. Front Mol Biosci. 2014; 1, 9. doi: 10.3389/fmolb.2014.00009.

[79] Iannuzzi C, Carafa V, Altucci L, Irace G, Borriello M, Vinciguerra R, Sirangelo I. Glycation of wild-type apomyoglobin induces formation of highly cytotoxic oligomeric species. J Cell Physiol. 2015; 230(11), 2807–20. doi:10.1002/jcp.25011.

[80] Stefani M. Protein aggregation diseases: toxicity of soluble prefibrillar aggregates and their clinical significance. Methods Mol Biol. 2010; 648, 25–41. doi: 10.1007/978-1-60761-756-3_2.

[81] Stefani M. Structural features and cytotoxicity of amyloid oligomers: implications in Alzheimer's disease and other diseases with amyloid deposits. Prog Neurobiol. 2012; 99(3), 226–45. doi: 10.1016/j.pneurobio.2012.03.002.

[82] Cecchi C, Stefani M. The amyloid-cell membrane system. The interplay between the biophysical features of oligomers/fibrils and cell membrane defines amyloid toxicity. Biophys Chem. 2013; 182, 30–43. doi: 10.1016/j.bpc.2013.06.003.

[83] Calamai M, Evangelisti E, Cascella R, Parenti N, Cecchi C, Stefani M, Pavone F. Single molecule experiments emphasize GM1 as a key player of the different cytotoxicity of structurally distinct Aβ1-42 oligomers. Biochim Biophys Acta. 2016; 1858(2), 386–92. doi: 10.1016/j.bbamem.2015.12.009.

[84] Salahuddin P, Rabbani G, Khan RH. The role of advanced glycation end products in various types of neurodegenerative disease: a therapeutic approach. Cell Mol Biol Lett. 2014; 19(3), 407–37. doi: 10.2478/s11658-014-0205-5.

[85] Münch G, Westcott B, Menini T, Gugliucci A. Advanced glycation endproducts and their pathogenic roles in neurological disorders. Amino Acids. 2012; 42(4), 1221–36. doi: 10.1007/s00726-010-0777-y.

[86] Takeuchi M, Yamagishi S. TAGE (toxic AGEs) hypothesis in various chronic diseases. Med Hypotheses. 2004; 63(3), 449–52.

[87] Nass N, Bartling B, Navarrete Santos A, Scheubel RJ, Börgermann J, Silber RE, Simm A. Advanced glycation end products, diabetes and ageing. Z Gerontol Geriatr. 2007; 40(5), 349–56.

[88] Engelen L, Stehouwer CD, Schalkwijk CG. Current therapeutic interventions in the glycation pathway: evidence from clinical studies. Diabetes Obes Metab. 2013; 15(8), 677–89. doi: 10.1111/dom.12058.

[89] Nagai R, Shirakawa J, Ohno R, Moroishi N, Nagai M. Inhibition of AGEs formation by natural products. Amino Acids. 2014; 46(2), 261–6. doi: 10.1007/s00726-013-1487-z.

[90] Sadowska-Bartosz I, Bartosz G. Prevention of protein glycation by natural compounds. Molecules. 2015; 20(2), 3309–34. doi: 10.3390/molecules20023309.

Chapter 7

Is Alzheimer's Associated Amyloid Beta an Innate Immune Protein

Ruth Kandel, Mitchell R White, I-Ni Hsieh and
Kevan L. Hartshorn

Additional information is available at the end of the chapter

http://dx.doi.org/10.5772/63021

Abstract

There is now abundant evidence that chronic inflammation in the brain is central to the pathogenesis of Alzheimer's disease (AD) and that this is precipitated through accumulation of amyloid beta (Aβ) peptides. In this review, we first outline this evidence and how specific receptors on microglia and monocyte/macrophages determine whether extracellular Aβ peptides can be cleared through non-inflammatory phagocytosis or instead result in pro-inflammatory cytokine generation. Most efforts of treatment for AD so far have focused on reduction of Aβ levels (in particular neurotoxic oligomers of Aβ1-42) in the brain. Recent findings suggest an alternative approach in which pro-inflammatory responses to Aβ peptides are targeted to reduce injury. Most recently evidence has come to light that Aβ peptides resemble antimicrobial peptides which are part of the innate defense system against infection. Such peptides act both by directly inactivating pathogens, but also by modulating responses of innate immune cells, including phagocytes. Indeed, Aβ peptides, particularly Aβ1-42, do inhibit a range of potential pathogens, including bacteria, fungi, and viruses. Coupling this with evidence linking chronic viral, bacteria, or fungal infection to AD suggests that production of Aβ peptides in the brain is part of an innate immune response which might normally be beneficial, but which leads to harm when it is chronic or uncontrolled. This suggests that discovery of the original possibly infectious (or other inflammatory) stimulus for Aβ production would allow early intervention to prevent development of AD.

Keywords: Inflammasome, TREM2, Microglia, antimicrobial peptide

1. Introduction

Aβ accumulation is believed to contribute strongly to the pathogenesis of AD, although the actual physiological function and reason for accumulation of Aβ in the brain are not known. Aβ is a fragment of the larger β amyloid precursor protein (APP) which is a transmembrane protein which can be broken down by various proteases into a variety of fragments, including extracellular and intracellular fragments and the peptide fragments Aβ1-42 and Aβ1-40 which are composed partly of the extracellular and partly of the transmembrane domain of APP. Aβ1-40 is more abundant than Aβ1-42, but Aβ1-42 is the more amyloidogenic and neurotoxic species [1–3]. The neurotoxicity of Aβ1-42 has been shown to depend on the ability of this peptide to form unstable oligomers (pentamers mainly), whereas the protofibrils or fibrils formed from the peptide are less neurotoxic. Recent studies are at last starting to elucidate why accumulation of Aβ, especially the 1–42 form leads to brain injury. These studies focus on the role of Aβ as a trigger of inflammation and emphasize its interaction with glial cells in the brain. A vicious cycle appears to occur in which Aβ peptides activate glial and other phagocytic cells which in turn impairs the ability of these cells to clear Aβ peptides and plaques from the brain. The reasons for production of Aβ in the brain in the first place are less clear. Recent findings that Aβ peptides function as antibacterial and antimicrobial peptides have given rise to the hypothesis that production of Aβ peptides may have evolved as part of the innate host defense system.

I. Evidence for a link between chronic inflammation and AD—At the outset, it is important to distinguish between early onset AD and late onset AD. Both forms of AD are strongly linked to excess accumulation of Aβ in plaques in the brain; however, the causes of Aβ accumulation may differ. In the case of early onset disease, there is a link to actual mutations in the Aβ gene or in genes involved in proteolytic processing of the precursor protein to form Aβ peptides. The most commonly used mouse model, the APP-PS1 model, of AD is based on over-expression of Aβ peptides in the brain in a similar manner. Late onset AD appears mainly to result from impaired clearance of Aβ peptides (rather than increased production per se) and is linked to polymorphisms of several genes as outlined below. There is strong and growing evidence for a link between chronic inflammation and the development of both forms of AD and some other dementing illnesses. We refer the reader to several recent excellent reviews for in depth consideration this topic [4–6]. A link between inflammation and AD has long been suspected in part based on clinical findings (e.g., the apparent protective effect of long-term non-steroidal anti-inflammatory use against development of sporadic AD) [7, 8]. In addition, pathological studies have shown evidence of inflammation surrounding neuritic plaques in AD. Complement factors, clusters of activated microglia and cytokines has been found in and near Aβ plaques [5, 9]. These findings of inflammation were also noted as early events in the brains of patients with AD. Expression of genes associated with inflammation in brain is increased in aging, and this effect is accentuated in patients with AD [10, 11].

II. Microglia and monocyte/macrophages as pivotal cells in mediating clearance or inflammatory responses to Aβ peptides—Microglia are resident phagocytic cells in the brain that plays a key role in maintaining the health of neurons and responding to sterile or infectious injury. Evidence is now converging from genome-wide association studies (GWAS), in vitro cell biologic experiments and mouse models of excess Aβ accumulation, that microglia and to an extent recruited blood monocyte macrophages, are critical in mediating either protective clearance of Aβ or damage through inflammatory activation by Aβ peptides.

A. GWAS studies—The first gene to show strong linkage to development of AD was the ε4 variant of apolipoprotein E (APOE). Although APOE is mainly known for its ability to regulate cholesterol and lipid transport, the APOEε4 allele is linked to accumulation of Aβ in plaques in humans and mouse models [12]. In addition, there is evidence that APOEε4 may be linked to inflammatory responses in the brain through interaction with receptors on microglia [13]. For instance, crossing APOEε4 over-expressing mice with APP/PS1 mice results in worsening inflammatory responses to lipopolysaccharide (LPS) as compared to APP/PS1 mice over-expressing APOEε3 [7]. Other proteins which modulate lipid metabolism, for instance surfactant protein D, have innate immune activity as well [14]. Of interest, surfactant protein D has also been linked to dementia [15]. Several other gene variants which are primarily expressed on microglia or other myeloid cells have been linked to AD. The most prominent of these is the triggering receptor expressed on myeloid cells 2 (TREM2) [6, 16–18]. This receptor mediates phagocytic activity and cytokine responses of myeloid cells and polymorphic forms of this receptor are linked to development of late onset AD with an effect size similar to APOEε4. Similar polymorphisms of the complement receptor CR-1 and an additional myeloid cell receptor, CD33, have been linked to development of AD [19, 20]. The contributions of these and other myeloid receptors to accumulation of Aβ and neuronal injury are now being elucidated through in vivo and in vitro studies.

B. Cell biology and mouse model studies—There is abundant evidence that accumulation of Aβ1-42 itself activates microglia and monocyte macrophages through binding to various receptors on these cells, either directly or through binding to other proteins (e.g., complement). A key hypothesis which brings together the various studies is that the ability of microglia to ingest Aβ1-42, or to degrade it through proteolysis is protective, whereas production of pro-inflammatory cytokines (e.g., TNF, IL-1 or IL-18) in response to Aβ1-42 is harmful. Microglia and macrophages can have a variety of phenotypes, with two major categories being the MI and M2 phenotypes. The MI phenotype is associated with pro-inflammatory cytokine generation as well as production of nitric oxide or superoxide radicals. In contrast, the M2 phenotype (presumably the more beneficial phenotype in the context of Aβ accumulation) is associated with enhanced phagocytosis and reduced pro-inflammatory signaling. Given the sensitive nature of the brains and neurons, clearance of pathogens, harmful proteins, or cellular debris ideally would proceed with minimal inflammation. The beneficial or harmful effects of various myeloid receptors have been categorized according to whether they mediate either M1 or M2 like activities [5, 21].

Microglial scavenger receptors—Receptors shown to promote phagocytosis and non-inflammatory clearance of Aβ1-42 include the scavenger receptors SR-A or Scara-A [22, 23]. In contrast, CD36, which is another scavenger receptor, appears to mediate pro-inflammatory responses to Aβ1-42 [24, 25]. Crossing of APP/PS1 with mice-lacking SR-A leads to greater Aβ accumulation and worsened survival, whereas crossing with mice-lacking CD36 causes reduced brain cytokine production and Aβ accumulation and improved survival. CD33 is another receptor that is involved in uptake of Aβ peptides by microglia. CD33 is over-expressed in microglia of humans with AD and the CD33 mutations that were found to be protective vs AD caused decreased expression of CD33 [19, 26]. Crossing of mice-lacking CD33 with APP/PS1 mice leads to reduced Aβ peptide accumulation and plaque burden [19]. In vitro studies showed that CD33 actually reduces Aβ1-42 uptake by microglial cells.

Triggering receptor expressed on myeloid cells 2 (TREM2)—TREM2 has a more complex role in that it can mediate either phagocytic clearance or pro-inflammatory cytokine responses by myeloid cells [6]. Like CD33, it is highly expressed in microglia and monocytes in the brain. In particular, it is highly expressed in microglia surrounding amyloid plaques in APP/PS1 mice [16]. In one study using this mouse model, deletion of TREM2 reduced inflammatory pathology in the brain [27]. In contrast, in another study, over-expression of TREM2 in these mice improved pathology [28]. The GWAS studies suggest that polymorphisms associated with decreased TREM2 production increase risk of development of AD or other neuro-degenerative diseases [16]. Based on this, it has been postulated that loss of TREM2 impairs non-inflammatory phagocytic clearance of Aβ peptides or of damaged neurons. TREM2 is well described as a phagocytic receptor for bacteria. Further studies will be needed to understand the complex role of TREM2 in AD. Of interest, two recent studies provide potential links between the contributions of APOEε4 and TREM2 to inflammation in AD. APOE was shown to bind to wild-type (but not mutant) TREM2 [29] and the APOEε4 variant has distinctive effects (as compared to other APOE subtypes) in modulating microglial prostaglandin production and TREM2 expression [30].

Complement and complement receptors—The complement receptor CR-1 also appears to have a complex role in AD [20]. CR-1 is the receptor for complement factors C3b and C4b. Aβ can activate the complement cascade and bind to C3b. This in turn leads to binding of Aβ peptides to CR-1. CR-1 is expressed on myeloid cells and erythrocytes. In the case of erythro-cytes, it serves to mediate clearance of complement bound proteins or organisms from the circulation. There is some evidence that this may promote clearance of Aβ outside the brain [31]. CR-1 also mediates phagocytosis of complement bound proteins and pathogens by phagocytes. Aβ can activate the complement system via the alternative pathway. This could conceivably lead to increased inflammation in the brain. However, it has been found that C3 deficiency or inhibition of complement worsens Aβ accumulation and neurodegeneration in mice [32]. These finding suggest that the complement activation may overall be beneficial vs AD. A possible explanation for the role of CR-1 is that the polymorphism most tightly linked to increased risk for AD (CR1-S) has an increased C3b/C4b binding site and that CR-1 actually acts to inhibit further activation of the complement cascade after binding to C3b/C4b [20].

Toll like receptors—Toll-like receptors (TLRs) and the associated adaptor protein also have been found to mediate phagocyte activation by Aβ [24, 33–37]. Once again the exact role of TLRs in AD pathology is unclear. A simplistic hypothesis would assume that TLR activation should worsen AD pathology; however, there is also evidence that the reverse may be true [33, 38]. Of interest, IL-10 which is predominantly an anti-inflammatory cytokine has been found to have adverse effects in AD mouse models [39].

http://dx.doi.org/10.5772/63021

Inflammasomes—Another important line of evidence relates to the role of nucleotide-binding domain leucine-rich repeat containing 3 (NLRP3) inflammasomes in AD [4, 40, 41]. Inflammasomes are multi-molecular complexes in phagocytic cells which mediate production of the pro-inflammatory cytokines IL-1 and IL-18 through the action of caspase 1 and induction of an inflammatory form of cell death called pyroptosis [42, 43]. Inflammasomes are involved in phagocyte mediated host defense against various pathogens. In the case of bacteria, the inflammasomes are activated by pathogen-associated molecular patterns (or PAMPs), like LPS. Increasingly, however, inflammasomes have been implicated in various inflammatory states triggered by self molecules termed damage-associated molecular patterns or DAMPs. NLRP3 inflammasomes activation has been linked to inflammatory bowel diseases, celiac disease, gout, multiple sclerosis, and type II diabetes mellitus. It appears that NLRP3 inflammasomes also mediate chronic inflammatory responses to Aβ peptides. NLRP3 inflammasomes are one subtype among a variety of inflammasomes. **Figure 1** illustrates the potential mechanism of assembly and activation of NLRP3 inflammasomes by Aβ peptides. Aβ peptides appear to act as a DAMP. As noted, two signals are required for activation, both of which could be triggered by Aβ peptides. The NLRP3 inflammasome complex consists of oligomeric assemblies of the NLRP3 protein, the apoptosis-associated speck-like protein containing a caspase activation and recruitment domain (ASC) protein and caspase 1. Crossing of mice-lacking caspase 1 or NLRP3 with APP/PS1 mice results in increased clearance of Aβ peptides and plaques, reduced neurodegeneration and a skewing of microglia to the M2 phenotype. Pro-inflammatory signaling in response to Aβ peptides mediated through inflammasomes appears to lead to a vicious cycle in which microglia acquire and M1 phenotype and cause increasing injury and decreased Aβ clearance [21].

Chemokines—Chemokines and their receptors also appear to modulate Aβ-related pathology. The chemokine CXCL10 is expressed at high levels in AD brain. Deletion or inhibition of the receptor for this and other CXCL chemokines (CXCR3) increased microglial uptake of Aβ in vitro and in vivo [44]. Deletion of CXCR1 had a similar effect [45]. These findings imply that these chemokines worsen the inflammatory effects which lead to increased injury or impaired clearance of Aβ. An active area of investigation as well is the role of recruited monocyte macrophages to AD pathology or Aβ clearance. Deletion of the monocyte receptor CCR2 in mice reduces monocyte recruitment and increases amyloid pathology in APP/PS1 mice [46], indicating that these cells play a role in clearance. Similarly CCR5 deletion increased Aβ deposition and neurological loss [47]. Other cytokines, like IL-12, are linked to exacerbation of AD as is activation of oxidant production by microglia [48–50].

C. Epidemiological studies—Life-style or other factors which are known to increase AD incidence also may mediate their effects through chronic inflammation. Examples include obesity, lack of exercise, peri-odontitis, or diabetes [5]. Overall these studies lend strong support to the hypothesis that the innate immune system, and specifically, resident or recruited phagocytic cells play a pivotal role in determining the balance between protective Aβ clearance or damaging Aβ peptide-induced inflammation.

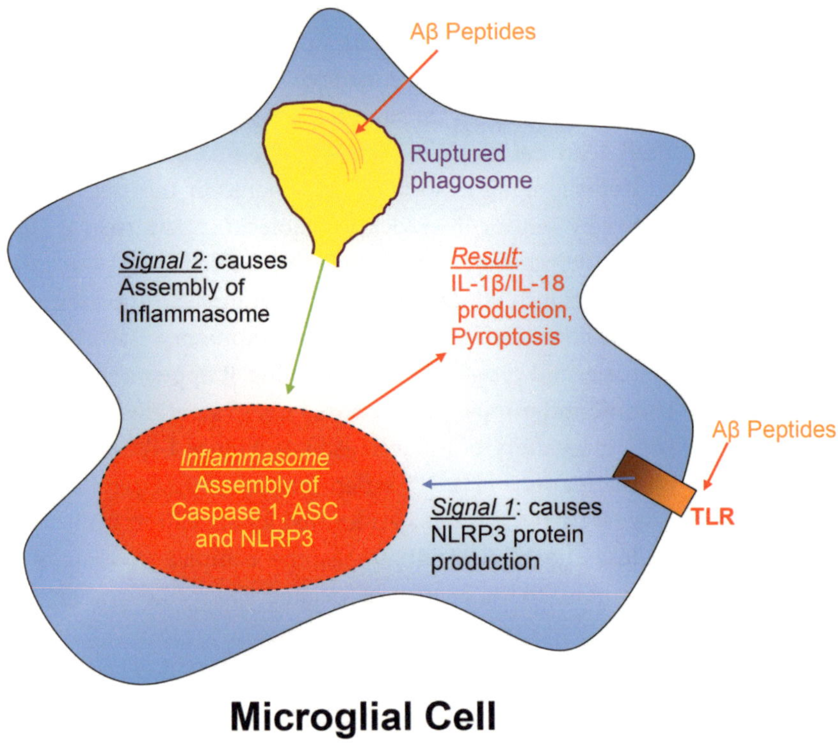

Figure 1. Microglial NLRP3 inflammasome activation by Aβ oligomers—the NLRP3 inflammasome can be activated by various PAMPs or DAMPS. Aβ oligomers can be considered as a DAMP which leads to NLRP3 activation in microglia. To induce NLRP3 activation, there needs to be at least two signals. The first signal causes increased production of the NLRP3 protein, and the second signal induces assembly of the multimolecular inflammasome complex. Other proteins involved in this complex include ASC and caspase 1. Activation of caspase 1 results in cleavage of pro-IL-1β and pro-IL-18 to form active IL-1β and IL-18. An additional effect of inflammasome activation is induction of a form of cell death caused pyroptosis. The result is a significant induction of local inflammation but also impairment of microglial phagocytosis, reducing further clearance of Aβ. The exact triggers of signal 1 and 2 are have not been fully elucidated. Since Aβ can trigger TLR activation, it is possible that this provides signal 1. In the case of some bacteria, rupture of phagosomes appears to provide signal 2, possibly by release of cathepsin B. We speculate that this could be involved in NLRP3 inflammasome activation by Aβ. Other possible mediators of the second signal include reactive oxygen species release or activation of plasma membrane ion channels.

III. What is the physiological stimulus for Aβ production?—Thus far most of the studies we, we have discussed consider the downstream effects of Aβ accumulation on inflammation or cellular dysfunction. For early onset AD, and for the APP/PS1 mice, increased Aβ accumulation is the result of alterations of the Aβ protein itself or of the enzymes involved in cleavage of the precursor protein. It is unclear, however, what triggers Aβ production under normal circumstances or in late onset AD. Attempts to directly reduce Aβ levels through the use of antibodies against Aβ peptides have not been highly successful, although it is possible that use in earlier stages of the disease (prior to major cognitive impairment) may be beneficial. There is also hope that intervention to reduce inflammatory response to Aβ may be beneficial, although here again it may be necessary to act early in the course of disease since the inflammatory phenotype seems to precede clinical AD.

If it was possible to determine the initial causes for Aβ accumulation in the brain, this might provide another approach to early intervention. One hypothesis is that infection initiates or sustains the process of Aβ accumulation. Excess accumulation of Aβ has been linked to Human Immunodeficiency Virus-related dementia [51, 52], and the virus can cause Aβ accumulation in vitro as well [53, 54]. Similarly Herpes Simplex Virus (HSV) induced encephalitis, and HSV infection in vitro is associated with Aβ accumulation [55–59], again implying that viruses may be a stimulus of Aβ production or impaired clearance. These findings suggest that viruses that infect the brain could be triggers for accumulation of Aβ, perhaps as part of an aberrant or sustained innate immune response. Antibodies to Cytomegalovirus, Epstein Barr Virus, or Human Herpes Virus 6 (HHV6) have also been associated with AD [60, 61] in some studies. In contrast, another study showed no link between AD and antibodies to HHV6 [62]. A variety of studies have also linked bacterial infection, including with chlamydia to development of AD [63, 64]. Of great interest, recent studies found fungal forms and sequences in brains of AD patients but not in controls [65–67]. Of course of a causal connection between these infections and AD is far from proven.

IV. Aβ peptides as antimicrobial agents—An alternative hypothesis to explain Aβ peptide and ultimately plaque production is that it is part of a host defense response to infectious or traumatic injury. Aβ peptides resemble some anti-microbial peptides or AMPs in their structure [68, 69]. Aβ peptides are similar to the porcine AMP, protegrin, in ability to form channels in membrane structures which is believed to be one of the anti-bacterial and anti-fungal mechanisms of AMPs. Recently, Soscia et al. demonstrated antibacterial and antifungal activity for Aβ peptides [70]. In addition, this study showed that Aβ isolated from the brain of AD patients had antimicrobial activity and that incubation of these brain-derived samples with antibodies to Aβ ablated the antimicrobial activity. More recently, we demonstrated that Aβ peptides also have antiviral activity using influenza A virus as a model [71]. In our study and that of Soscia et al., Aβ1-42 was found to have greater antimicrobial or antiviral activity than Aβ1-40. We demonstrated that Aβ1-42, but not Aβ1-40, caused viral aggregation which appears to contribute to its antiviral effects. This implies a possible connection between the ability of Aβ1-42 to assemble into oligomers and its antiviral activity, since this peptide has a greater propensity to form oligomers and fibrils than Aβ1-40.

The finding that Aβ peptides, especially, Aβ1-42 act like other cationic antimicrobial peptides may also explain its ability to activate phagocytic cells. AMPs have direct antimicrobial and antiviral activities but they also trigger recruitment and activation of immune cells [34, 36, 72]. We also recently showed that Aβ1-42 modulates responses of neutrophils and monocytes to the influenza virus [71]. Aβ1-42 increased neutrophil uptake of influenza A virus and potentiated neutrophil respiratory burst and neutrophil extracellular trap (NET) formation in response to the virus. Aβ1-42 also reduced inflammatory cytokine production triggered by influenza virus in monocytes. The opsonizing activity of Aβ1-42 was again not replicated with Aβ1-40. More recently, we found that Aβ peptides can increase neutrophil uptake of bacteria as well (unpublished data). Overall, these studies lend support to the hypothesis that Aβ peptides serve a host defense role and that chronic infectious or inflammatory stimuli may result in an aberrant prolongation of what normally would be a helpful response.

2. Conclusions

There is now abundant evidence from a variety of sources that AD is characterized by a chronic inflammatory response in the brain. The key elements in this process include the ability of Aβ peptides, especially Aβ1-42, to directly activate phagocytic cells, most notably microglia and, to a lesser extent, monocyte/macrophages. **Figure 2** summarizes the microglial receptors, cytokines, and signaling mechanisms known to be linked to responses to Aβ peptides. These phagocytic cells are at the cross-roads of innate immune responses in the brain, and they appear to play a pivotal role in determining whether the response to Aβ peptide accumulation is non-inflammatory phagocytosis or pro-inflammatory cytokine production. One conclusion from these studies is that inhibition of pro-inflammatory responses early in the evolution of Aβ related pathology could be protective. For example, inhibition of inflammasome activation has been proposed as an approach to treatment. One dilemma is that there is not a simple correlation between processes normally thought of as pro-inflammatory and reduction of neuronal injury in AD models. As prime examples, activation of the complement system or of toll-like receptor pathways appears to be protective in some studies. In addition, the role of TREM2, while clearly important, is not as simply as initially expected. The recent findings that Aβ peptides (especially Aβ1-42) function like other AMPs suggest that Aβ peptides may play a beneficial physiological role in vivo and may actually be part of an innate immune response to infection. If this is so then discovery of underlying infectious triggers of AD might provide a different modality of treatment.

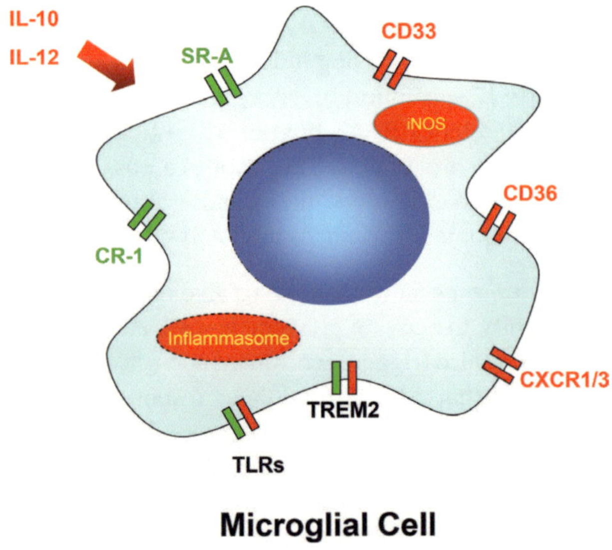

Figure 2. Microglial receptors and signaling pathways that are involved in response to Aβ—receptors, signaling pathways or extracellular cytokines shown to promote neuronal injury are shown in red, whereas those shown in green are protective vs neuronal injury or progression of AD like pathology. Receptors shown in as a mixture of green and red have been found to have both beneficial or adverse effects in various studies.

http://dx.doi.org/10.5772/63021

Author details

Ruth Kandel[1], Mitchell R White[2], I-Ni Hsieh[2] and Kevan L. Hartshorn[2*]

*Address all correspondence to: Khartsho@bu.edu

1 Hebrew Senior Life, Harvard Medical School, Boston, Massachusetts, USA

2 Department of Medicine, Boston University School of Medicine, Boston, Massachusetts, USA

References

[1] Dahlgren KN, Manelli AM, Stine WB, Jr., Baker LK, Krafft GA, LaDu MJ. Oligomeric and fibrillar species of amyloid-beta peptides differentially affect neuronal viability. J Biol Chem. 2002;277(35):32046–53. PubMed PMID: 12058030.

[2] Masters CL, Selkoe DJ. Biochemistry of amyloid beta-protein and amyloid deposits in Alzheimer disease. Cold Spring Harbor Perspect Med. 2012;2(6):a006262. doi:10.1101/cshperspect.a006262. PubMed PMID: 22675658; PubMed Central PMCID: PMC3367542.

[3] Selkoe DJ. Biochemistry and molecular biology of amyloid beta-protein and the mechanism of Alzheimer's disease. Handb Clin Neurol. 2008;89:245–60. doi:10.1016/S0072-9752(07)01223-7. PubMed PMID: 18631749.

[4] Heneka MT, Kummer MP, Stutz A, Delekate A, Schwartz S, Vieira-Saecker A, et al. NLRP3 is activated in Alzheimer's disease and contributes to pathology in APP/PS1 mice. Nature. 2013;493(7434):674–8. doi:10.1038/nature11729. PubMed PMID: 23254930; PubMed Central PMCID: PMC3812809.

[5] Heneka MT, Carson MJ, El Khoury J, Landreth GE, Brosseron F, Feinstein DL, et al. Neuroinflammation in Alzheimer's disease. Lancet Neurol. 2015;14(4):388–405. doi:10.1016/S1474-4422(15)70016-5. PubMed PMID: 25792098.

[6] Hickman SE, El Khoury J. TREM2 and the neuroimmunology of Alzheimer's disease. Biochem Pharmacol. 2014;88(4):495–8. doi:10.1016/j.bcp.2013.11.021. PubMed PMID: 24355566; PubMed Central PMCID: PMC3972304.

[7] Burton A. NSAIDS and Alzheimer's disease: it's only Rock and Rho. Lancet Neurol. 2004;3(1):6. PubMed PMID: 14700055.

[8] Weggen S, Eriksen JL, Das P, Sagi SA, Wang R, Pietrzik CU, et al. A subset of NSAIDs lower amyloidogenic Abeta42 independently of cyclooxygenase activity. Nature. 2001;414(6860):212–6. doi:10.1038/35102591. PubMed PMID: 11700559.

[9] Rogers J, Cooper NR, Webster S, Schultz J, McGeer PL, Styren SD, et al. Complement activation by beta-amyloid in Alzheimer disease. Proc Natl Acad Sci USA. 1992;89(21): 10016–20. PubMed PMID: 1438191; PubMed Central PMCID: PMC50268.

[10] Barrientos RM, Kitt MM, Watkins LR, Maier SF. Neuroinflammation in the normal aging hippocampus. Neuroscience. 2015;309:84–99. doi:10.1016/j.neuroscience.2015.03.007. PubMed PMID: 25772789; PubMed Central PMCID: PMC4567963.

[11] Jiang T, Yu JT, Zhu XC, Tan MS, Gu LZ, Zhang YD, et al. Triggering receptor expressed on myeloid cells 2 knockdown exacerbates aging-related neuroinflammation and cognitive deficiency in senescence-accelerated mouse prone 8 mice. Neurobiol Aging. 2014;35(6):1243–51. doi:10.1016/j.neurobiolaging.2013.11.026. PubMed PMID: 24368090.

[12] Liu CC, Kanekiyo T, Xu H, Bu G. Apolipoprotein E and Alzheimer disease: risk, mechanisms and therapy. Nat Rev Neurol. 2013;9(2):106–18. doi:10.1038/nrneurol.2012.263. PubMed PMID: 23296339; PubMed Central PMCID: PMC3726719.

[13] Holtzman DM, Herz J, Bu G. Apolipoprotein E and apolipoprotein E receptors: normal biology and roles in Alzheimer disease. Cold Spring Harbor Perspect Med. 2012;2(3):a006312. doi:10.1101/cshperspect.a006312. PubMed PMID: 22393530; PubMed Central PMCID: PMC3282491.

[14] Hartshorn KL. Role of surfactant protein A and D (SP-A and SP-D) in human antiviral host defense. Front Biosci (Schol Ed). 2010;2:527–46. PubMed PMID: 20036966.

[15] Nybo M, Andersen K, Sorensen GL, Lolk A, Kragh-Sorensen P, Holmskov U. Serum surfactant protein D is correlated to development of dementia and augmented mortality. Clin Immunol. 2007;123(3):333–7. PubMed PMID: 17449329.

[16] Neumann H, Daly MJ. Variant TREM2 as risk factor for Alzheimer's disease. N Engl J Med. 2013;368(2):182–4. doi:10.1056/NEJMe1213157. PubMed PMID: 23151315.

[17] Jonsson T, Stefansson H, Steinberg S, Jonsdottir I, Jonsson PV, Snaedal J, et al. Variant of TREM2 associated with the risk of Alzheimer's disease. N Engl J Med. 2013;368(2): 107–16. doi:10.1056/NEJMoa1211103. PubMed PMID: 23150908; PubMed Central PMCID: PMC3677583.

[18] Guerreiro R, Wojtas A, Bras J, Carrasquillo M, Rogaeva E, Majounie E, et al. TREM2 variants in Alzheimer's disease. N Engl J Med. 2013;368(2):117–27. doi:10.1056/NEJMoa1211851. PubMed PMID: 23150934; PubMed Central PMCID: PMC3631573.

[19] Griciuc A, Serrano-Pozo A, Parrado AR, Lesinski AN, Asselin CN, Mullin K, et al. Alzheimer's disease risk gene CD33 inhibits microglial uptake of amyloid beta. Neuron. 2013;78(4):631–43. doi:10.1016/j.neuron.2013.04.014. PubMed PMID: 23623698; PubMed Central PMCID: PMC3706457.

[20] Brouwers N, Van Cauwenberghe C, Engelborghs S, Lambert JC, Bettens K, Le Bastard N, et al. Alzheimer risk associated with a copy number variation in the complement

receptor 1 increasing C3b/C4b binding sites. Mol Psychiatry. 2012;17(2):223–33. doi: 10.1038/mp.2011.24. PubMed PMID: 21403675; PubMed Central PMCID: PMC3265835.

[21] Heneka MT, Golenbock DT, Latz E. Innate immunity in Alzheimer's disease. Nat Immunol. 2015;16(3):229–36. doi:10.1038/ni.3102. PubMed PMID: 25689443.

[22] Frenkel D, Wilkinson K, Zhao L, Hickman SE, Means TK, Puckett L, et al. Scara1 deficiency impairs clearance of soluble amyloid-beta by mononuclear phagocytes and accelerates Alzheimer's-like disease progression. Nat Commun. 2013;4:2030. doi: 10.1038/ncomms3030. PubMed PMID: 23799536; PubMed Central PMCID: PMC3702268.

[23] Wilkinson K, El Khoury J. Microglial scavenger receptors and their roles in the pathogenesis of Alzheimer's disease. Int J Alzheimer's Dis. 2012;2012:489456. doi: 10.1155/2012/489456. PubMed PMID: 22666621; PubMed Central PMCID: PMC3362056.

[24] Stewart CR, Stuart LM, Wilkinson K, van Gils JM, Deng J, Halle A, et al. CD36 ligands promote sterile inflammation through assembly of a Toll-like receptor 4 and 6 heterodimer. Nat Immunol. 2010;11(2):155–61. doi:10.1038/ni.1836. PubMed PMID: 20037584; PubMed Central PMCID: PMC2809046.

[25] Coraci IS, Husemann J, Berman JW, Hulette C, Dufour JH, Campanella GK, et al. CD36, a class B scavenger receptor, is expressed on microglia in Alzheimer's disease brains and can mediate production of reactive oxygen species in response to beta-amyloid fibrils. Am J Pathol. 2002;160(1):101–12. PubMed PMID: 11786404; PubMed Central PMCID: PMC1867121.

[26] Carlin AF, Chang YC, Areschoug T, Lindahl G, Hurtado-Ziola N, King CC, et al. Group B Streptococcus suppression of phagocyte functions by protein-mediated engagement of human Siglec-5. J Exp Med. 2009;206(8):1691–9. PubMed PMID: 19596804.

[27] Jay TR, Miller CM, Cheng PJ, Graham LC, Bemiller S, Broihier ML, et al. TREM2 deficiency eliminates TREM2+ inflammatory macrophages and ameliorates pathology in Alzheimer's disease mouse models. J Exp Med. 2015;212(3):287–95. doi:10.1084/jem.20142322. PubMed PMID: 25732305; PubMed Central PMCID: PMC4354365.

[28] Jiang T, Tan L, Zhu XC, Zhang QQ, Cao L, Tan MS, et al. Upregulation of TREM2 ameliorates neuropathology and rescues spatial cognitive impairment in a transgenic mouse model of Alzheimer's disease. Neuropsychopharmacology. 2014;39(13):2949–62. doi:10.1038/npp.2014.164. PubMed PMID: 25047746; PubMed Central PMCID: PMC4229581.

[29] Atagi Y, Liu CC, Painter MM, Chen XF, Verbeeck C, Zheng H, et al. Apolipoprotein E is a ligand for triggering receptor expressed on myeloid cells 2 (TREM2). J Biol Chem. 2015;290(43):26043–50. doi:10.1074/jbc.M115.679043. PubMed PMID: 26374899; PubMed Central PMCID: PMC4646257.

[30] Li X, Montine KS, Keene CD, Montine TJ. Different mechanisms of apolipoprotein E isoform-dependent modulation of prostaglandin E2 production and triggering receptor expressed on myeloid cells 2 (TREM2) expression after innate immune activation of microglia. FASEB J. 2015;29(5):1754–62. doi:10.1096/fj.14-262683. PubMed PMID: 25593125; PubMed Central PMCID: PMC4415020.

[31] Rogers J, Li R, Mastroeni D, Grover A, Leonard B, Ahern G, et al. Peripheral clearance of amyloid beta peptide by complement C3-dependent adherence to erythrocytes. Neurobiol Aging. 2006;27(12):1733–9. doi:10.1016/j.neurobiolaging.2005.09.043. PubMed PMID: 16290270.

[32] Wyss-Coray T, Yan F, Lin AH, Lambris JD, Alexander JJ, Quigg RJ, et al. Prominent neurodegeneration and increased plaque formation in complement-inhibited Alzheimer's mice. Proc Natl Acad Sci USA. 2002;99(16):10837–42. doi:10.1073/pnas.162350199. PubMed PMID: 12119423; PubMed Central PMCID: PMC125059.

[33] Michaud JP, Richard KL, Rivest S. MyD88-adaptor protein acts as a preventive mechanism for memory deficits in a mouse model of Alzheimer's disease. Mol Neurodegener. 2011;6(1):5. doi:10.1186/1750-1326-6-5. PubMed PMID: 21235801; PubMed Central PMCID: PMC3030527.

[34] Jana M, Palencia CA, Pahan K. Fibrillar amyloid-beta peptides activate microglia via TLR2: implications for Alzheimer's disease. J Immunol. 2008;181(10):7254–62. PubMed PMID: 18981147.

[35] Tang SC, Lathia JD, Selvaraj PK, Jo DG, Mughal MR, Cheng A, et al. Toll-like receptor-4 mediates neuronal apoptosis induced by amyloid beta-peptide and the membrane lipid peroxidation product 4-hydroxynonenal. Exp Neurol. 2008;213(1):114–21. PubMed PMID: 18586243.

[36] Richard KL, Filali M, Prefontaine P, Rivest S. Toll-like receptor 2 acts as a natural innate immune receptor to clear amyloid beta 1–42 and delay the cognitive decline in a mouse model of Alzheimer's disease. J Neurosci. 2008;28(22):5784–93. PubMed PMID: 18509040.

[37] Chen K, Iribarren P, Hu J, Chen J, Gong W, Cho EH, et al. Activation of Toll-like receptor 2 on microglia promotes cell uptake of Alzheimer disease-associated amyloid beta peptide. J Biol Chem. 2006;281(6):3651–9. PubMed PMID: 16339765.

[38] Michaud JP, Halle M, Lampron A, Theriault P, Prefontaine P, Filali M, et al. Toll-like receptor 4 stimulation with the detoxified ligand monophosphoryl lipid A improves Alzheimer's disease-related pathology. Proc Natl Acad Sci USA. 2013;110(5):1941–6. doi:10.1073/pnas.1215165110. PubMed PMID: 23322736; PubMed Central PMCID: PMC3562771.

[39] Michaud JP, Rivest S. Anti–inflammatory signaling in microglia exacerbates Alzheimer's disease-related pathology. Neuron. 2015;85(3):450–2. doi:10.1016/j.neuron.2015.01.021. PubMed PMID: 25654250.

[40] Sheedy FJ, Grebe A, Rayner KJ, Kalantari P, Ramkhelawon B, Carpenter SB, et al. CD36 coordinates NLRP3 inflammasome activation by facilitating intracellular nucleation of soluble ligands into particulate ligands in sterile inflammation. Nat Immunol. 2013;14(8):812–20. doi:10.1038/ni.2639. PubMed PMID: 23812099; PubMed Central PMCID: PMC3720827.

[41] Halle A, Hornung V, Petzold GC, Stewart CR, Monks BG, Reinheckel T, et al. The NALP3 inflammasome is involved in the innate immune response to amyloid-beta. Nat Immunol. 2008;9(8):857–65. doi:10.1038/ni.1636. PubMed PMID: 18604209; PubMed Central PMCID: PMC3101478.

[42] Gold M, El Khoury J. beta-amyloid, microglia, and the inflammasome in Alzheimer's disease. Semin Immunopathol. 2015;37(6):607–11. doi:10.1007/s00281-015-0518-0. PubMed PMID: 26251237; PubMed Central PMCID: PMC4618770.

[43] Lamkanfi M, Dixit VM. Inflammasomes and their roles in health and disease. Annu Rev Cell Dev Biol. 2012;28:137–61. PubMed PMID: 22974247.

[44] Krauthausen M, Kummer MP, Zimmermann J, Reyes-Irisarri E, Terwel D, Bulic B, et al. CXCR3 promotes plaque formation and behavioral deficits in an Alzheimer's disease model. J Clin Invest. 2015;125(1):365–78. doi:10.1172/JCI66771. PubMed PMID: 25500888; PubMed Central PMCID: PMC4382235.

[45] Fuhrmann M, Bittner T, Jung CK, Burgold S, Page RM, Mitteregger G, et al. Microglial Cx3cr1 knockout prevents neuron loss in a mouse model of Alzheimer's disease. Nat Neurosci. 2010;13(4):411–3. doi:10.1038/nn.2511. PubMed PMID: 20305648; PubMed Central PMCID: PMC4072212.

[46] Hickman SE, El Khoury J. Mechanisms of mononuclear phagocyte recruitment in Alzheimer's disease. CNS Neurol Disord Drug Targets. 2010;9(2):168–73. PubMed PMID: 20205643; PubMed Central PMCID: PMC3684802.

[47] Lee YK, Kwak DH, Oh KW, Nam SY, Lee BJ, Yun YW, et al. CCR5 deficiency induces astrocyte activation, Abeta deposit and impaired memory function. Neurobiol Learn Memory. 2009;92(3):356–63. doi:10.1016/j.nlm.2009.04.003. PubMed PMID: 19394434.

[48] Vom Berg J, Prokop S, Miller KR, Obst J, Kalin RE, Lopategui-Cabezas I, et al. Inhibition of IL-12/IL-23 signaling reduces Alzheimer's disease-like pathology and cognitive decline. Nat Med. 2012;18(12):1812–9. doi:10.1038/nm.2965. PubMed PMID: 23178247.

[49] Huang TC, Lu KT, Wo YY, Wu YJ, Yang YL. Resveratrol protects rats from Abeta-induced neurotoxicity by the reduction of iNOS expression and lipid peroxidation. PLoS One. 2011;6(12):e29102. doi:10.1371/journal.pone.0029102. PubMed PMID: 22220203; PubMed Central PMCID: PMC3248406.

[50] Medeiros R, Prediger RD, Passos GF, Pandolfo P, Duarte FS, Franco JL, et al. Connecting TNF-alpha signaling pathways to iNOS expression in a mouse model of Alzheimer's disease: relevance for the behavioral and synaptic deficits induced by amyloid beta

protein. J Neurosci. 2007;27(20):5394–404. doi:10.1523/JNEUROSCI.5047-06.2007. PubMed PMID: 17507561.

[51] Zhang J, Liu J, Katafiasz B, Fox H, Xiong H. HIV-1 gp120-induced axonal injury detected by accumulation of beta-amyloid precursor protein in adult rat corpus callosum. J Neuroimmune Pharmacol. 2011;6(4):650–7. PubMed PMID: 21286834.

[52] Andras IE, Eum SY, Toborek M. Lipid rafts and functional caveolae regulate HIV-induced amyloid beta accumulation in brain endothelial cells. Biochem Biophys Res Commun. 2012;421(2):177–83. PubMed PMID: 22490665.

[53] Lan X, Kiyota T, Hanamsagar R, Huang Y, Andrews S, Peng H, et al. The effect of HIV protease inhibitors on amyloid-beta peptide degradation and synthesis in human cells and Alzheimer's disease animal model. J Neuroimmune Pharmacol. 2012;7(2):412–23. doi:10.1007/s11481-011-9304-5. PubMed PMID: 21826404; PubMed Central PMCID: PMC3223330.

[54] Lan X, Xu J, Kiyota T, Peng H, Zheng JC, Ikezu T. HIV-1 reduces Abeta-degrading enzymatic activities in primary human mononuclear phagocytes. J Immunol. 186(12): 6925–32. PubMed PMID: 21551363.

[55] Wozniak MA, Itzhaki RF, Shipley SJ, Dobson CB. Herpes simplex virus infection causes cellular beta-amyloid accumulation and secretase upregulation. Neurosci Lett. 2007;429(2–3):95–100. PubMed PMID: 17980964.

[56] Wozniak MA, Frost AL, Preston CM, Itzhaki RF. Antivirals reduce the formation of key Alzheimer's disease molecules in cell cultures acutely infected with herpes simplex virus type 1. PLoS One. 2011;6(10):e25152. PubMed PMID: 22003387.

[57] De Chiara G, Marcocci ME, Civitelli L, Argnani R, Piacentini R, Ripoli C, et al. APP processing induced by herpes simplex virus type 1 (HSV-1) yields several APP fragments in human and rat neuronal cells. PLoS One. 2010;5(11):e13989. PubMed PMID: 21085580.

[58] Lukiw WJ, Cui JG, Yuan LY, Bhattacharjee PS, Corkern M, Clement C, et al. Acyclovir or Abeta42 peptides attenuate HSV-1-induced miRNA-146a levels in human primary brain cells. Neuroreport. 2010;21(14):922–7. PubMed PMID: 20683212.

[59] Piacentini R, Civitelli L, Ripoli C, Marcocci ME, De Chiara G, Garaci E, et al. HSV-1 promotes Ca2+ -mediated APP phosphorylation and Abeta accumulation in rat cortical neurons. Neurobiol Aging. 2010;32(12):2323 e13–26. PubMed PMID: 20674092.

[60] Lurain NS, Hanson BA, Martinson J, Leurgans SE, Landay AL, Bennett DA, et al. Virological and immunological characteristics of human cytomegalovirus infection associated with Alzheimer disease. J Infect Dis. 2013;208(4):564–72. PubMed PMID: 23661800.

[61] Carbone I, Lazzarotto T, Ianni M, Porcellini E, Forti P, Masliah E, et al. Herpes virus in Alzheimer's disease: relation to progression of the disease. Neurobiol Aging. 2013;35(1): 122–9. PubMed PMID: 23916950.

[62] Agostini S, Mancuso R, Baglio F, Cabinio M, Hernis A, Guerini FR, et al. Lack of evidence for a role of HHV-6 in the pathogenesis of Alzheimer's disease. J Alzheimers Dis. 2015;49(1):229–35. doi:10.3233/JAD-150464. PubMed PMID: 26444787.

[63] Hammond CJ, Hallock LR, Howanski RJ, Appelt DM, Little CS, Balin BJ. Immunohistological detection of Chlamydia pneumoniae in the Alzheimer's disease brain. BMC Neurosci. 2010;11:121. doi:10.1186/1471-2202-11-121. PubMed PMID: 20863379; PubMed Central PMCID: PMC2949767.

[64] Gerard HC, Dreses-Werringloer U, Wildt KS, Deka S, Oszust C, Balin BJ, et al. Chlamydophila (Chlamydia) pneumoniae in the Alzheimer's brain. FEMS Immunol Med Microbiol. 2006;48(3):355–66. doi:10.1111/j.1574-695X.2006.00154.x. PubMed PMID: 17052268.

[65] Pisa D, Alonso R, Rabano A, Rodal I, Carrasco L. Different brain regions are infected with Fungi in Alzheimer's disease. Sci Rep. 2015;5:15015. doi:10.1038/srep15015. PubMed PMID: 26468932; PubMed Central PMCID: PMC4606562.

[66] Alonso R, Pisa D, Rabano A, Rodal I, Carrasco L. Cerebrospinal fluid from Alzheimer's disease patients contains fungal proteins and DNA. J Alzheimers Dis. 2015;47(4): 873–6. doi:10.3233/JAD-150382. PubMed PMID: 26401766.

[67] Alonso R, Pisa D, Rabano A, Carrasco L. Alzheimer's disease and disseminated mycoses. Eur J Clin Microbiol Infect Dis. 2014;33(7):1125–32. doi:10.1007/s10096-013-2045-z. PubMed PMID: 24452965.

[68] Kagan BL, Jang H, Capone R, Teran Arce F, Ramachandran S, Lal R, et al. Antimicrobial properties of amyloid peptides. Mol Pharm. 2012;9(4):708–17. PubMed PMID: 22081976.

[69] Jang H, Ma B, Lal R, Nussinov R. Models of toxic beta-sheet channels of protegrin-1 suggest a common subunit organization motif shared with toxic alzheimer beta-amyloid ion channels. Biophys J. 2008;95(10):4631–42. PubMed PMID: 18708452.

[70] Soscia SJ, Kirby JE, Washicosky KJ, Tucker SM, Ingelsson M, Hyman B, et al. The Alzheimer's disease-associated amyloid beta-protein is an antimicrobial peptide. PLoS One. 2010;5(3):e9505. PubMed PMID: 20209079.

[71] White MR, Kandel R, Tripathi S, Condon D, Qi L, Taubenberger J, et al. Alzheimer's associated beta-amyloid protein inhibits influenza A virus and modulates viral interactions with phagocytes. PLoS One. 2014;9(7):e101364. doi:10.1371/journal.pone.0101364. PubMed PMID: 24988208; PubMed Central PMCID: PMC4079246.

[72] Oppenheim JJ, Yang D. Alarmins: chemotactic activators of immune responses. Curr Opin Immunol. 2005;17(4):359–65. PubMed PMID: 15955682.

Chapter 8

Amyloidogenesis and Responses to Stress

Magda de Eguileor, Rossana Girardello,
Annalisa Grimaldi, Laura Pulze and
Gianluca Tettamanti

Additional information is available at the end of the chapter

http://dx.doi.org/10.5772/64479

Abstract

Amyloidogenesis is a primitive, physiological response that seems to be an ancient process widely distributed in different cell types of evolutionary distant organisms. The amyloid fibril synthesis is part of a more general inflammatory response to stressful conditions all entailing overproduction of reactive oxygen species (ROS). Interestingly, this event has been integrated into additional physiological functions: (i) the formation of a scaffold promoting the activation and packaging of melanin; (ii) the formation of a scaffold to compartmentalize hormones in the cytoplasm; (iii) the ability to reversibly link different types of molecules to drive close to the nonself; (iv) the construction of a framework to close body lesions. Amyloid fibril formation is a cellular response harmonically integrated with the stress response but for a deregulation in assembling/dismantling, dangerous depots, as in a lot of pathologies, can occur.

Keywords: amyloidogenesis, ROS, melanin, invertebrates, vertebrates

1. Introduction

Bacteria, fungi, yeasts, unicellular algae, plants, invertebrates, and vertebrates can synthesize functional amyloids and physiological amyloidogenesis is a key process in response to stress. Even though the aggregation of proteins into amyloid fibrils is associated with human neurodegenerative diseases [1], including Alzheimer's, Parkinson's, and prion disease, it has been evidenced that amyloid is also a fundamental nonpathological protein folding process that spans from bacteria to humans [2–8]. There are many examples of functional and physiological amyloidogenesis: the bacterial biofilm, the insect silk to form the cocoon, the spider silk for constructing their webs, producing egg sacs, and wrapping in their prey, etc., the scaffold to package melanin in human melanocytes when activated by UV, etc.

The various proteins forming amyloids do not necessary display the same primary structure and/or the same biochemical function and/or similarities in biophysical properties: irrespective of the nature of the polypeptide, the proteins, under defined conditions, share the ability to change folding and adopt cross-β sheet conformation with high resistance to enzymatic cleavage, and denaturant. Amyloids can be easily recognized due to their ability to bind to specific dyes such as Thioflavin T/S and Congo Red (CR) and due to their ultrastructural features.

Once the aggregates, in form of amyloid fibrillar material, are formed and tailor-made for the intra- or extracellular space, they can contribute in numerous ways to cellular/tissue/organism activities.

In functional amyloidogenesis, the synthesis of fibrils, occurring in a controlled folding pathway, is balanced by mechanisms involved in their clearance through enzymatic cleavage. When there is a slow down or a total block in this complex balance between assembling and dismantling, a spatial or temporal accumulation of fibrillar material, responsible of deleterious/pathological state, occurs.

The exposure to any kind of chemical or physical nonlethal stress is responsible of an excessive production of cytoplasmic reactive oxygen species (ROS) that, if overpowering the endogenous antioxidant mechanisms, leads to a progressive cellular damage that, in turn, impairs the survival of the cell. In other words, transient or persistent increase of ROS, as a harmful bioproduct deriving from regular cellular metabolism, is coped in all cellular types with the same sequence of events. Constant basal ROS concentration is strictly maintained with the activation of enzymatic and nonenzymatic defences such as production of superoxide dismutase (SOD), catalase (CAT), glutathione peroxidase (GPX), methionine reductase, ascorbic acid (vitamin C), glutathione (GSH), and vitamin A. Uncontrolled, imbalanced production of ROS, and an inefficient free radical scavenging systems may result in inflammation, hypersensitivity, and in the pathogenesis of numerous human diseases such as neurodegenerative diseases, atherosclerosis, allergy, and cancer [9]. In healthy cells, ROS are produced in a small amount in mitochondria but the dysfunction of these organelles, resulting in increased ROS production, can be caused by rough endoplasmic reticulum (RER) stress. In stressed cells, RER cisternae release Ca^{2+} that in turn is taken up by mitochondria where determine the opening of membrane pores with the consequent enhancement of ROS production and release in cytoplasm. Resulted vicious cycle leads to impaired cellular homeostasis up to cellular death [10].

ROS overexpression, responsible of a change in cytoplasmic pH, can be considered the earliest event and an absolute prerequisite to induce proteins to adopt a β-sheet conformation, thus the amyloid fibril production is strictly linked to this event [2, 4, 5, 11].

1.1. Types of cells and subcellular districts involved in amyloid fibril synthesis

Even though the formation of amyloid or amyloid-like structure under physiological condition is a generic property of polypeptides across all kingdoms of life and can be considered as a response to different types of stimulations, it is of paramount importance to have an overview about which kinds of organisms, which types of cells, and for which purpose amyloid fibrils are synthesized.

Bacteria are able to produce and utilize amyloid material in adhesion to solid surfaces as a starting point to form the biofilm that is, for the most part of microorganisms, the guarantee to live in a consortium spatially and metabolically organized [12]. Amyloid proteins, contributing with exopolysaccharides to form the biofilm, provide a key component of this protective scaffold [13, 14].

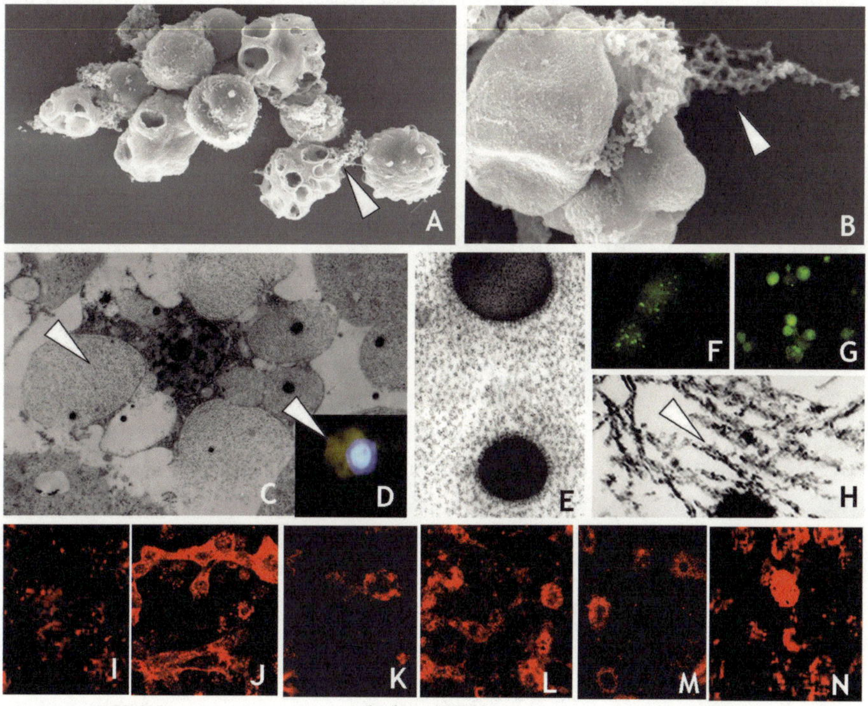

Figure 1. Unstimulated and stimulated H. virescens circulating cells. Optical and ultrastructural images (A–H). Scanning electron micrographs (SEMs) (A, B): the surface of several granulocytes shows bowl-shaped depression with exocytosed fibrillar material (white arrowheads). Transmission electron micrographs (TEMs) (C, E, H): the fibrillar material (white arrowhead) is spatially organized close to an electron dense core (E) in dilated RER cisternae surrounding the central nucleus (C). The Thioflavin positivity (green/yellow fluorescence), localized within RER cisternae (D, arrowhead), identify the amyloid fibrils. Melanin is ultrastructurally identified by using specific technique (the periodic acid-silver methenamine staining (PASM). Pigment deposition is localized on exocytosed amyloid fibrils (H, arrowhead). ROS generation is detected by monitoring the increase in fluorescence of the oxidized dye H_2DCFDA (F, G). The increase in ROS level is evident comparing control granulocytes (F) with those from activated hemocytes (G). Immunocytochemical characterizations for ACTH (I, J), α-MSH (K, L), and IL-18 (M, N) show higher positivity in activated granulocytes (J, L, N).

Moreover, many bacterial species, under stress condition, are able to induce not only the biofilm production but also melanin synthesis [15].

As in bacteria, many protozoa are able to secrete huge amounts of melanin and generally, the production of the pigment is strictly linked to the presence of an amyloid scaffold.

In 2006, Fowler et al. [4] demonstrated that, in mammals, nonpathogenic amyloids are involved in melanin synthesis in melanocytes where the glycoprotein Pmel17 polymerizes into amyloid fibrils forming a framework on which pigment assembled.

Our data (based on light microscopy (LM), transmission and scanning ultrastructural analysis paralleled by immunocytochemical ones) (see Section 3) about activated hemocytes in the lepidopteran-moth *Heliothis virescens* [7, 16], underline the relationship between melanin synthesis and the production of amyloid fibrils to template the pigment. Moreover, we have described and characterized the morpho-functional events sustaining the amyloid fibril assembly in relation to melanin production, in immune cells under stress condition, not only in insects such as *H. virescens* and *Spodoptera elicoverpa,* but also in different invertebrates (protostomes and deuterostomes) such as *Hirudo medicinalis* (Annelid), *Helix pomatia* (Mollusc), *Ciona intestinalis,* and *Botrillus schlosseri* (Ascidian). In all these animals, melanin synthesis/amyloid fibril assemblage always starts with ROS overproduction that, in turn, causes a cytoplasmic pH variation [8]. Amyloidogenesis takes place in RER where the large amount of fibrils, spatially organized, dilate them (**Figure 1**, panels **A** and **B**). RER is specialized in folding and maturation of a considerable number of secreted proteins and it is highly sensitive to external (chemical or physical) and internal stimuli (such as change in the redox state) [10].

This amyloid production due to RER deregulation/accumulation can be morphologically evidenced by Thioflavine S staining and by ultrastructural analysis. During this amyloid/pigment productive phase, a cross-talk between immune and endocrine systems, able to mutually influencing, occurs. These intercommunications are mediated by neuromodulators with the activation of stress-sensoring circuits to produce and release molecules such as adrenocorticotropic hormone (ACTH), melanocyte-stimulating hormone (α-MSH), and neutral endopeptidase (NEP) [7, 8, 16] (**Figure 1**, panels **I–N**). These molecules have a direct role in immune defences. ACTH is widely expressed in various tissues (as well demonstrated in immunocytochemical localizations) and it is synthesized not only by cells of nervous system but also by nonneural cells [17–19]. ACTH expression is induced in stress conditions (such as ROS increase, lipopolysaccharide (LPS) administration, presence of bacteria and proinflammatory cytokine administration) to regulate the immune cellular functions influencing proliferation, migration, production of immune mediators, and trafficking of immunocytes.

The temporal extend of ACTH action is restrained by the production of a neutral endopeptidase (NEP) that is concomitantly synthesized. This protease inactivates ACTH and the released cleaved product, α-MSH, is able to inhibit chemotaxis, production of proinflammatory cytokines (nuclear factor kappa-light-chain-enhancer of activated B cells) NFkB stimulation, as well as to stimulate melanin synthesis.

The pigment is accumulated in specific organelles where an amyloid scaffold sustains its packaging. Moreover, NEP can be also involved in the degradation of amyloid fibrils [20, 21].

Furthermore, the activation of amyloidogenesis is accompanied by the overexpression of a furin-like proprotein convertase, a specific enzyme that is activated in melanosomal biogenesis to liberate a fibrillogenic fragment [22] and by the overexpression of proinflammatory cytokines such as interleukin-18 (IL-18) [4, 8, 23, 24]. In particular, this is an important molecule that cooperates both in the activation of innate immune system and in amyloidogenic processes in Alzheimer disease (AD) [23, 24].

It is important to emphasize that in immune cells from phylogenetically distant metazoans (viz. molluscs, annelids, insects, ascidians, and vertebrates) [8, 16], the amyloid scaffold is produced to package melanin and to convey the pigment in close contact to the invader with a twofold advantage: to isolate the nonself from host tissues and to focus the toxic bio-product [7, 8, 16], thus minimizing the diffusion of highly reactive, toxic melanin precursors. This association may occur in intra- or extracell compartments. In several invertebrates, stimulated granulocytes (granular circulating cells) produce an amyloid lattice into the RER, that is exocytosed in the body cavity where it works as a template for melanin resulting from humoral prophenoloxidase (proPO) system reactions [25, 26]. proPOs synthesized primarily by hemocytes are present after their lysis in the hemolymph. The proPO activation cascade leads to the formation of quinones that undergo additional reactions leading to synthesis of melanin. This pigment is deposited on the parasite surface, on nodules made by hemocytes, and in wound sites.

In other invertebrates and in vertebrates, melanin and amyloid fibril synthesis are not disjoined and the molecules are produced and assembled in the same cell (melanocytes) [4]. In any case, amyloid fibrils, synthesized by circulating immunocytes (we use this generic term to identify the cells with the same morpho-functional characteristic that, in invertebrates, have been called, phagocytes, amebocytes, hemocytes), are a shuttle of melanin made to trap and isolate the nonself in capsules where the killing of pathogens is facilitated.

So far, we have described the formation of amyloid fibrils as an event absolutely necessary to activate, support, and store pigments, but this is also true, always as response to stress and due to its intrinsic adhesiveness [27], for the assembly and the compartmentalization of hormones such as ACTH in the cytoplasm [28].

The activation of vertebrates neutrophils, due to the presence of bacteria or fungi, culminates with the production of the neutrophil extracellular trap (NET). NETs, as we have immunocytochemically demonstrated, are characterized by a fibrillar backbone for addressing cytotoxic proteins and DNA against the nonself, that shows amyloid birefringence upon Congo red staining, Thioflavin S positivity, and harbors a basic mammalian protein, Pmel17 [4], as validated by the colocalization of signals [29] (**Figure 2**, panels **D–J**). In stimulated neutrophils, there is a correlation among amyloidogenesis and ROS generation, change in cytoplasmic pH, enhanced expression of the ACTH/α-MSH loop, synthesis of specific cytokine, and also autophagy and exosome release (**Figure 2**, panel **C**). These closely related partners appear to play a key role in the management of the amyloid fibrils that constitute the scaffold of NET [29].

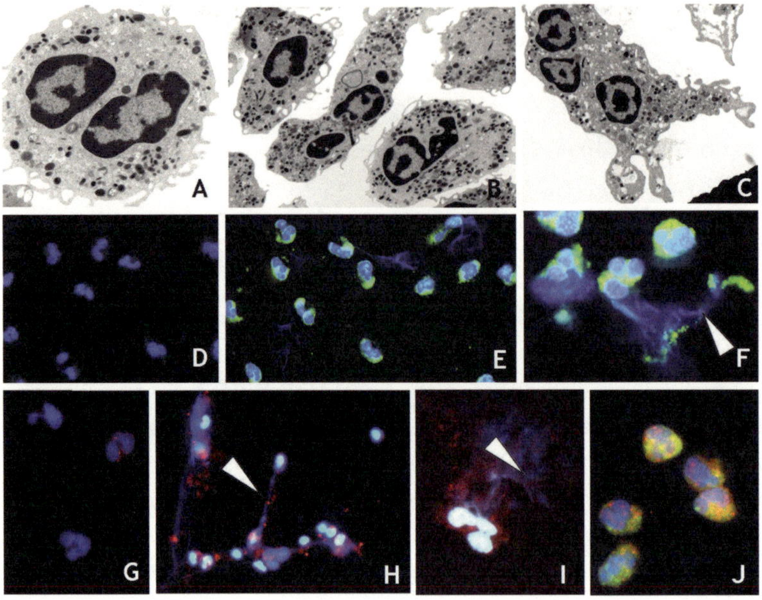

Figure 2. Unstimulated and stimulated human neutrophils. Thin and semithin sections of resting (A) and activated neutrophils (B, C). The unstimulated cells are roundish but after stimulation with LPS (B, C) they lose their globoid shape acquiring migratory phenotype (B, C). (D–F) Identification of amyloid fibrils with Thioflavin S (ThS): unstimulated neutrophils (D) in comparison with stimulated cells (E, F) from LPS administration. Within cells (E) and extracellularly (F), amyloid fibrils are localized by ThS brightly fluorescence. Nuclei and DNA material in NETs are marked in brilliant blue with DAPI staining. The blue (DAPI) and green (ThS) in NETs, released on stimulation, co-localize (white arrowhead). (G–J) Immunolocalization with a specific antibody directed against Pmel17 (a mammalian protein involved in amyloidogenesis): immunofluorescence staining show the increased Pmel17 expression that is present in the cytoplasm of stimulated neutrophils (H) and in the NETs (H, I) (arrowheads). DAPI (blue), staining for DNA, is localized in nuclei, as well as extracellularly in NETs. (J) Double labeling of neutrophils with ThS (green) and antibody against Pmel17 (red). Note the colocalization of two signals (merge in yellow). Nuclei (blue) are stained with DAPI.

Amyloid fibrils are also synthesized in inflammatory response induced by the presence of abiotic material such as nanotubes that, as waste, can be found in the air, in the soil, and into the water having a harmful effect to the health of many animals, including humans [30, 31]. Leeches, as animal model, exposed to multiwall carbon nanotubes (MWCNTs) powder dispersed in water, reflect the situation of aquatic animals subjected to uncontrolled carbon nanotube (CNT) exposition. MWCNTs, showing an average 9.5 nm external diameter and 1.5 μm mean length, are able to across the epithelial superficial barrier promoting inflammatory responses. MWCNTs in the leech body wall provoke nonspecific responses characterized by proliferation and migration of macrophages toward the stimulated area. Girardello et al. [32] show that these immune cells, recruited in the area of inflammation, produce amyloid material, as demonstrated by Thioflavin-T staining. In addition, the authors correlated this synthesis with a concomitant overexpression of IL-18, confirming the importance of this cytokine in the process. Extracellular amyloid fibrils entrap and isolate the nanotube aggregation but, forming a kind of spongy coating, can have an additional function in concentrating the cytokines produced by neighbor activated cells thus attracting and driving the macrophages engaged in immune responses [32] (**Figure 3**, panels **A–E**).

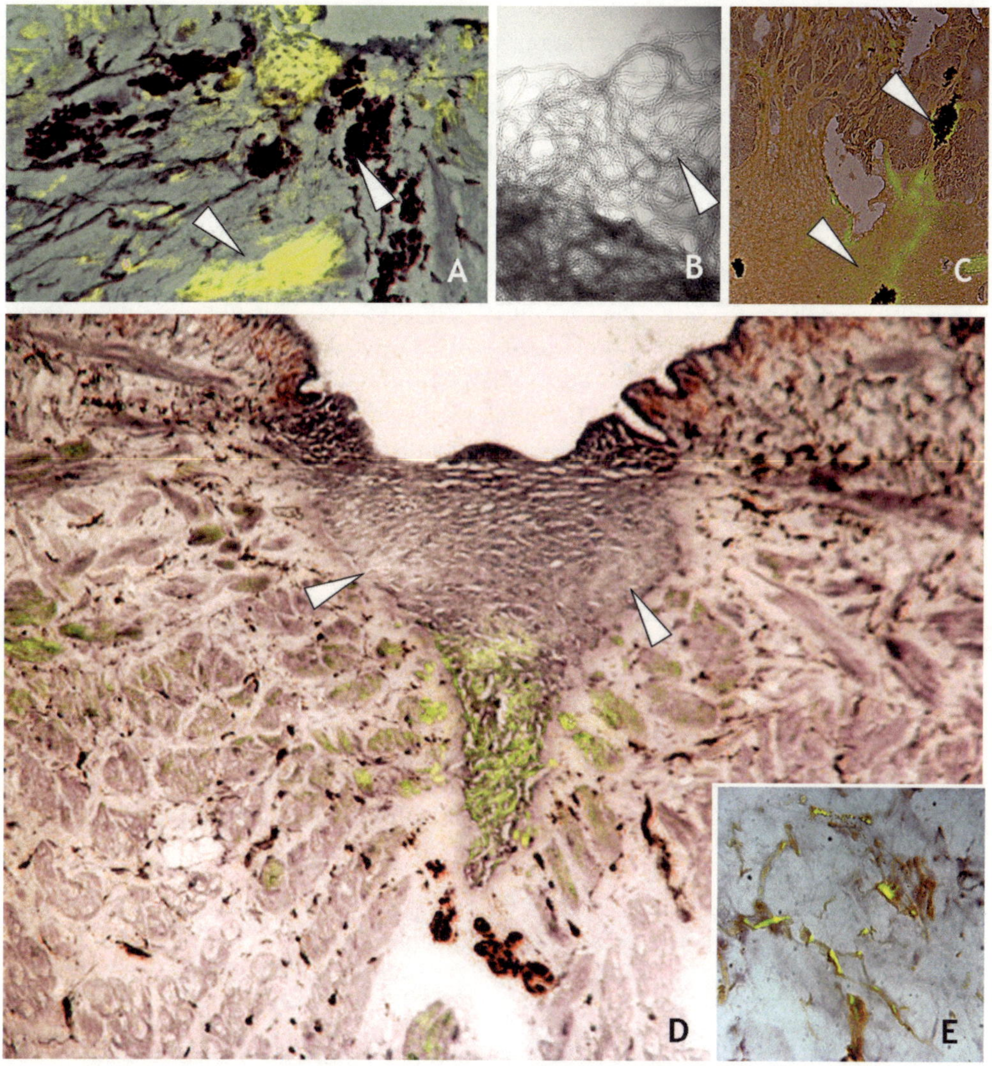

Figure 3. Effects of carbonanotube exposure and wound healing in leeches. Optical (A, C, D, E) and ultrastructural (B) images. Leech body wall sectioned in wound healing area (A, C, D, E). The specific Thioflavin-T colorimetric method evidences the presence of amyloid fibrils close to the aggregates of nanotubes (arrowheads). Ultrastructural (B) image of carbon nanotubes (CNTs) crude powder (used as control). The fibrillar material, Thioflavin-T positive, produced by migrating cells (E) contribute to form a plug (D) in the area of lesion (arrowheads).

Amyloids are also synthesized by the cells that are recruited in the lesioned body wall of diverse invertebrates to work as a "collision mat," the strategic solution patterned to close a boat leak, by forming a clot. The fibrillar material, Thioflavin-T positive, deposited in correspondence of damaged area, contributes to block the ingress of water/pathogens/external materials and prevent the loss of cells and hemolimph/blood from the body (unpublished data).

We have shown (combining light and electron microscopy, staining reactions, and immunocytochemical characterization—see paragraph about methodologies) that different types of cells characterized by different lineages (i.e., from mesoderm and ectoderm) and from diverse organisms, such as larval hemocytes, IPLB-LdFB and Drosophila Schneider's S2 cells from insects; NIH3T3 embryonic fibroblasts from mouse; human umbilical vein endothelial cells (HUVEC), and mesenchymal stem cells from human, under stress condition (for instance, LPS stimulation) are characterized by an increase of cytoplasmic ROS [33].

After stimulation, these cells are characterized by a morphological change and in the cytoplasm, empty vacuoles or RER cisternae filled with material showing staining properties typical of amyloid fibrils are visible (**Figure 4**, panels **A–L**). Moreover, the activation of amyloidogenesis is also linked with an extensive production of ACTH and α-MSH in all cultured cell types. These data suggest that amyloidogenesis could be a common, physiological cellular response to weak ROS, starting when other antistress cellular systems failed to restore homeostasis. Then the morphological evidence and/or functional characterization of synthesized amyloid fibrils could be an early indicator of oxidative stress that may lead to a general inflammatory process.

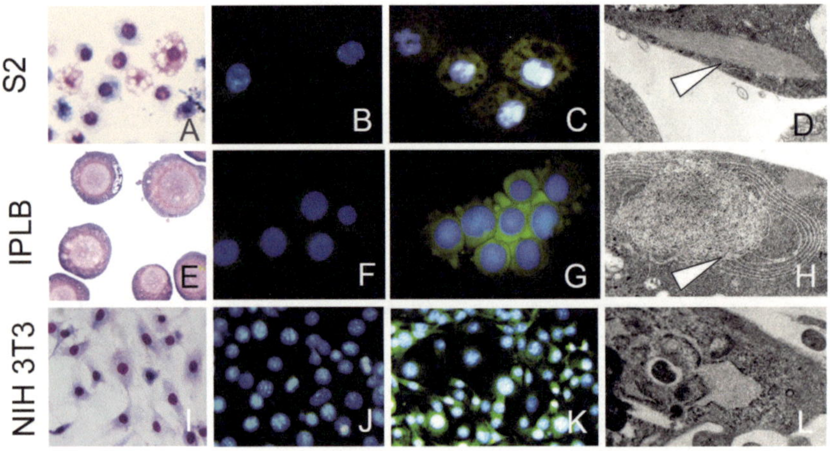

Figure 4. Effects of LPS stimulation on different cell types. Optical (A–C, E–G, I–K) and ultrastructural (D, H, I) images of S2 cells from *Drosophila melanogaster* (A–D), IPLB cells from insect (E–H) and NIH3T3 murine fibroblast (I–L). Amyloid fibril presence is detected with Thioflavin T. The yellow-green brightly fluorescence is more evident in stimulated cells (C, G, K) as compared to controls (B, F, J). Nuclei are stained with DAPI and marked in brilliant blue. TEM analysis: thin sections of LPS activated cells (D, H, L) show the presence of dilated reticulum cisternae filled with fibrillar material (arrowheads).

2. Conclusions

It is intriguing to underline that amyloid fibril synthesis is a cellular dynamic and versatile system evolutionary conserved. Recent evidence strengthen the idea that:

- Amyloidogenesis, shared by invertebrate and vertebrate cells, occurs as a protective response.
- Amyloid fibril synthesis that can be considered, in healthy cells, as a functional event, starts always, independently from their utilization, with an increase of ROS, real key player in defining this cellular response.
- The amyloid fibrillar material has unique features: it is versatile, extremely durable, can be assembled from any type of protein, it is able to paste, reversibly, different molecules due its residual charges, it can be disassembled only using specific enzymes such as NEP.
- The amyloid fibrils are utilized in different ways: they can be part of a more general response to stressful condition all entailing overproduction of ROS; they can form a scaffold to package pigment or hormones within the cell; can convey melanin or cytotoxic molecules; they can form a resistant structure to physically isolate the nonself, thus favoring the killing of pathogens, also conveying and concentrate toxic products; they can build a part of framework to close body lesions.

3. Methodologies

3.1. Light microscopy (LM) and transmission electron microscopy (TEM)

LM and TEM analysis give important information about morphology of cell and tissues.

Collected samples were fixed in 4% glutaraldehyde in 0.1 M Na-cacodylate buffer (pH 7.2) and washed in 0.1 M Na-cacodylate buffer at pH 7.2. The initial fixation is followed by a postfixation in 1% osmic acid in cacodylate buffer (pH 7.2) for 20 min. After standard dehydration in an ethanol series, samples were embedded in an Epon-Araldite 812 mixture and sectioned with a Reichert Ultracut S ultratome (Leica, Nussloch, Germany). Semithin sections were stained by conventional methods utilizing histological dyes such as crystal violet and basic fuchsine and then observed with a light microscope (Eclipse Nikon, Amsterdam, Netherlands). Thin sections were stained by uranyl acetate and lead citrate and observed with a Jeol 1010 electron microscope (Jeol, Tokyo, Japan).

3.2. Intracellular reactive oxygen species evaluation

Oxidative stress can induce proteins to adopt an insoluble β-pleated sheet conformation, and according to numerous authors, oxidative damage appears to be the earliest events preceding amyloid fibril formation. Thus, it is important to evaluate the overproduction of ROS in relation to LPS activation responsible for amyloid fibril production. ROS production and its derivation was validated by use of 2′,7′-dichlorodihydrofluorescein diacetate (H_2DCFDA, Molecular Probes, Eugene, OR, USA), a fluorigenic probe commonly used to detect the overall degree of intracellular level of ROS. H_2DCFDA is a nonfluorescent compound that readily crosses cell membranes. It is hydrolyzed to 2′,7′-dichlorofluorescein (DCF) within cells and becomes fluorescent when it is oxidized by ROS. Oxidation can be detected by monitoring the increase in fluorescence. Fluorescence was determined by excitation at 488 nm and emission at wavelength of 525 nm; fluorescent images visualized on a fluorescence Eclipse Nikon microscope, were acquired with a DS-5 M-L1 Nikon digital camera system.

3.3. Amyloid fibril characterization

Amyloid structures were identified by staining cells/tissues with Thioflavin S and visualizing the amyloid-specific green/yellow fluorescence with an Eclipse Nikon microscope. Images were acquired with a DS-5 M-L1 Nikon digital camera system. Amyloid fibrils were also characterized with Congo red staining, according to published methods and observed under cross-polarized light with an Axioskop 2 microscope (Carl Zeiss, Jena, Germany), equipped with a MC 80 DX camera (Carl Zeiss).

Amyloid fibrils (see the paragraph below) were also localized immunocytochemically using an antibody directed against Pmel17, protein that has amyloid characteristics and contributes to form fibrillar structures in mammals.

3.4. Immunocytochemistry for ACTH, α-MSH, NEP, interleukin 18, and Pmel17 localization

The presence of amyloid fibrils was confirmed by using the primary antibody antihuman Pmel17 (H-300) polyclonal antibody (1:100 dilution, Santa Cruz Biotechnology, Santa Cruz, CA, USA). The presence of ACTH and its cleavage product (due to degrading enzyme NEP), α-MSH, and of the proinflammatory interleukin 18 (IL-18) were assessed by using the following primary antibodies: antihuman ACTH polyclonal antibody (1:100 dilution, Abcam, Cambridge, UK); antihuman α-MSH polyclonal antibody (1:100 dilution, Abcam); antihuman IL-18 polyclonal antibody (1:100 dilution, Abnova, Taipei City, Taiwan); antihuman CD10/CALLA (NEP) monoclonal antibody (1:100 dilution, GeneTex, Hsinchu City, Taiwan). Incubations with suitable secondary antibodies conjugated with Cyanine5 (Cy5; 1:50 dilution, Abcam) were performed for 1 h in a dark humid chamber at room temperature. Nuclei were stained with 4′,6′-diamino-2-phenylindole (DAPI, Sigma-Aldrich). The PBS buffer used for washing steps and antibodies dilutions contained 2% bovine serum albumin (BSA, Sigma-Aldrich) and 0.1% Tween20.

In colocalization experiments, the cells were first stained with Thioflavin S (as described above) and then incubated with anti-Pmel17 antibody (as described above).

In control samples, primary antibodies were omitted, and samples were treated with BSA/Tween20-containing PBS. Coverslips were mounted in citifluor (citifluor Ltd., London, UK). Slides were observed under an Eclipse Nikon microscope.

Acknowledgements

R.G. is participants in the Biotechnology, Biosciences, and Surgical Technologies Doctoral programs of the University of Insubria. This work was supported by grant from FOCOVA (Fondazione Comunitaria del Varesotto, 2015).

Author details

Magda de Eguileor*, Rossana Girardello, Annalisa Grimaldi, Laura Pulze and Gianluca Tettamanti

*Address all correspondence to: magda.deeguileor@uninsubria.it

Department of Biotechnology and Life Sciences, University of Insubria, Varese, Italy

References

[1] Nogueira de Sousa Andrade L, Nathanson JL, Yeo GW, Mench CF, Muotri AR. Evidence for premature aging due to oxidative stress in iPSCs from Cockayne syndrome. Hum. Mol. Genet. 21: 3825–3834, 2012.

[2] Kelly JW, Balch WE. Amyloid as natural product. J. Cell Biol. 161: 461–466, 2003.

[3] Chiti F, Dobson CM. Protein misfolding, functional amyloid, and human disease. Annu. Rev. Biochem. 75: 333–366, 2006.

[4] Fowler DM, Koulov AV, Alory-Jost C, Marks M, Balch W, Kelly J. Functional amyloid formation within mammalian tissue. PLoS Biol. 4: 6–26, 2006.

[5] Maury CPI. The emerging concept of functional amyloid. J. Inter. Med. 265: 329–334, 2009.

[6] Eisenberg D, Jucker M. The amyloid state of proteins in human diseases. Cell 148: 1188–1198, 2012.

[7] Falabella P, Riviello L, Pascale M, Di Lelio I, Tettamanti G, Grimaldi A, et al. Functional amyloids in insect immune response. Insect. Biochem. Mol. Biol. 42: 203–211, 2012.

[8] Grimaldi A, Girardello R, Malagoli D, Falabella P, Tettamanti G, Valvassori R, et al. Amyloid/Melanin distinctive mark in invertebrate immunity. Inv. Surv. J. 9: 153–162, 2012.

[9] Bouayed J, Bohn T. Exogenous antioxidants-Double-edged swords in cellular redox state: Health beneficial effects at physiologic doses versus deleterious effects at high doses. Oxid. Med. Cell. Longev. 3: 228–237, 2010.

[10] Zeeshan HM, Lee GH, Kim HR, Chae HJ. Endoplasmic reticulum stress and associated ROS. Int. J. Mol. Sci. 17: E327, 2016.

[11] Hye A, Riddoch-Contreras J, Baird AL, Ashton NJ, Bazenet C, Leung R, et al. Plasma proteins predict conversion to dementia from prodromal disease. Alzheimers Dement. 10: 799–807, 2014.

[12] Nikolaev IuA and Plakunov VK. Biofilm—"City of microbes" or an analogue of multicellular organisms?. Mikrobiologiia. 76: 149–163, 2007.

[13] Hufnagel DA, Tükel C, Chapman MR. Disease to dirt: the biology of microbial amyloids. PLoS Pathog. 9: e1003740, 2013.

[14] Romero D, Sanabria-Valentin E, Vlamakis H, Kolter R. Biofilm inhibitors that target amyloid proteins. Chem. Biol. 20: 102–110, 2013.

[15] Plonka PM, Grabacka M. Melanin synthesis in microorganisms—biotechnological and medical aspects. Acta Biochim. Pol. 53: 429–443, 2006.

[16] Grimaldi A, Tettamanti G, Congiu T, Girardello R, Malagoli D, Falabella P, et al. The main actors involved in parasitization of *Heliotis virescens* larva. Cell Tissue Res. 350: 491–502, 2012.

[17] Slominski A, Zbytek B, Szczesniewski A, Semak I, Kaminski J, Sweatman T, et al. CRH stimulation of corticosteroids production in melanocytes is mediated by ACTH. Am. J. Physiol. Endocrinol. Metab. 288: E701–E706, 2005.

[18] Ottaviani E, Malagoli D, Franceschi C. Common evolutionary origin of the immune and neuroendocrine systems: from morphological and functional evidence to in silico approaches. Trends Immunol. 28: 497–502, 2007.

[19] Caruso C, Carniglia L, Durand D, Scimonelli TN, Lasaga M. Melanocortins: Anti-inflammatory and neuroprotective peptides. In: Martins LM et al., eds. Neurodegeneration, InTech, pp. 93–121, 2012.

[20] Marr RA, Rockenstein E, Mukherjee A, Kindy MS, Hersh LB, Gage FH, et al. Neprilysin gene transfer reduces human amyloid pathology in transgenic mice. J. Neurosci. 23: 1992–1996, 2003.

[21] Turner AJ, Nalivaeva NN New insights into the roles of metalloproteinases in neurodegeneration and neuroprotection. Int. Rev. Neurobiol. 82: 113–135, 2007.

[22] Berson JF, Theos AC, Harper DC, Tenza D, Raposo G, Marks MS. Proprotein convertase cleavage liberates a fibrillogenic fragment of a resident glycoprotein to initiate melanosome biogenesis. J. Cell Biol. 161: 521–533, 2003.

[23] Bossù P, Ciaramella A, Salani F, Vanni D, Palladino I, Caltagirone C, et al. Interleukin-18 from neuroinflammation to Alzheimer's disease. Curr. Pharm. Des. 16: 4213–4224, 2010.

[24] Alboni S, Montanari C, Benatti C, Blom JM, Simone ML, Brunello N, et al. Constitutive and LPS-regulated expression of interleukin-18 receptor beta variants in the mouse brain. Brain Behav. Immun. 25: 483–493, 2011.

[25] Duval C, Regnier M, Schmidt R. Distinct melanogenic response of human melanocytes in mono-culture, in co-culture with keratinocytes and in reconstructed epidermis, to UV exposure. Pigment Cell Res. 14: 348–355, 2001.

[26] Ferrarese R, Brivio M, Congiu T, Falabella P, Grimaldi A, Mastore M, et al. Early suppression of immune response in *Heliothis virescens* larvae by the endophagous. Invertebr. Surviv. J. 2: 60–68, 2005.

[27] Jarvis SP, Mostaert AS. Functional amyloid. Imaging Microsc. 9: 25–28, 2007.

[28] Rousseau K, Kauser S, Pritchard LE, Warhurst A, Oliver RL, Slominski A, et al. Proopiomelanocortin (POMC), the ACTH/melanocortin precursor, is secreted by human epidermal keratinocytes and melanocytes and stimulates melanogenesis. FASEB J. 21: 1844–1856, 2007.

[29] Pulze L, Bassani B, Gini E, D'Antona P, Grimaldi A, Luini A, et al. Net amyloidogenic backbone in human activated neutrophils. Clin. Exp. Immunol. 183: 469–479, 2015.

[30] Lam CW, James JT, McCluskey R, Arepalli S, Hunter RL. A review of carbon nanotube toxicity and assessment of potential occupational and environmental health risks. Crit. Rev. Toxicol. 36: 189–217, 2006.

[31] Simate GS, Iyuke SE, Ndlovu S, Heydenrych M, Walubita LF. Human health effects of residual carbon nanotubes and traditional water treatment chemicals in drinking water. Environ. Int. (Elsevier Ltd.) 39: 38–49, 2012.

[32] Girardello R, Tasselli S, Baranzini N, Valvassori R, de Eguileor M, Grimaldi A. Effects of carbon nanotube enviromental dispersion on an aquatic invertebrate, *Hirudo medicinalis*. PLoS One 10: e0144361, 2015.

[33] Grimaldi A, Tettamanti G, Girardello R, Pulze L, Valvassori R, Malagoli D, et al. Functional amyloid formation in LPS activated cells from invertebrates to vertebrates. ISJ. 11: 286–297, 2014.

Chapter 9

Developments in the Treatment of Amyloid A Amyloidosis Secondary to Rheumatoid Arthritis

Tadashi Nakamura

Additional information is available at the end of the chapter

http://dx.doi.org/10.5772/63132

Abstract

Amyloidosis refers to a heterogeneous group of diseases in which a soluble precursor, misfolded protein, and subsequently aggregates into highly structured protein fibrils with a cross-β-pleated structure. Of these diseases, amyloid A (AA) amyloidosis is a complication of long-standing inflammatory diseases such as rheumatoid arthritis (RA). Treatment of this amyloidosis with RA aims to stop serum AA protein production. Immunosuppressants have reportedly been useful for both RA inflammation and AA amyloidosis. Also, biologics are effective for these specific pathological processes by targeting key players in each inflammation. In addition to the above-mentioned medications, agents both inhibiting AA fibrillogenesis and destabilizing AA fibrils have recently been employed. Phagocytes play important roles in the regression of AA fibrils. Renal involvement is the most common complication in AA amyloidosis. Peritoneal dialysis, hemodialysis, and even renal transplantation are available for patients with end-stage renal disease and AA amyloidosis. This chapter thus discusses current developments in the treatment of AA amyloidosis secondary to RA.

Keywords: AA amyloidosis, rheumatoid arthritis, *SAA1.3* allele, biologics, fibrinolysis

1. Introduction

Amyloidosis is a rare disorder in which extracellular amyloid fibrils are deposited in various tissues. Those fibrils derive from the misfolding of precursor proteins, the result being multiple organs dysfunction. Systemic amyloidosis is thus characterized by failure of all sorts of organs and the presence of amyloid precursor protein in the serum. Reactive amyloid A (AA) amyloidosis is one of the most severe complications of a number of chronic disorders, especially rheumatoid arthritis (RA); most patients with this amyloidosis have an underlying rheumatic disease. AA amyloidosis, an extra-articular complication of RA, is a serious disorder, possibly life-threatening, that is caused by deposition in multiple organs of AA amyloid fibrils which originate from the circulatory acute-phase reactant, serum amyloid A protein (SAA) [1–4].

Both treatment and understanding of the roles of cytokines in RA have resulted in considerable progress. Remarkable advances, which not only provide insight into the pathophysiology of the disease but also aid discovery of new therapies to fight the deadly disease, have recently been made [5, 6]. For example, the introduction of biological therapies targeting specific inflammatory mediators revolutionized RA treatment. Focusing on essential components of the immune system allows effective suppression of the pathological inflammatory cascade that produces RA symptoms and the resulting joint destruction [7–10]. Several new biologics may permit AA amyloidosis secondary to RA to become a treatable, even manageable, disease. Furthermore, that the allele *SAA1.3* is not only a univariate predictor of survival but also a risk factor for the association of AA amyloidosis with RA in Japanese patients is very interesting [11].

Patients with RA, who have a less-than-optimal response to or cannot tolerate conventional synthetic disease-modifying antirheumatic drugs (csDMARDs) [12], such as methotrexate (MTX) [13, 14], are often prescribed biological DMARDs (bDMARDs). Treatment of AA amyloidosis caused by RA seeks to stop SAA production [15]. This approach to AA amyloidosis treatment is the most common and best-studied therapy; it interferes with synthesis of the precursor protein, with the goal of preventing continued amyloid fibril formation. Similarly, cytotoxic immunosuppressants, such as chlorambucil and cyclophosphamide (CYC), have reportedly been useful for both RA inflammation and AA amyloidosis [16–20].

An alternative approach to therapy involves developing drugs to inhibit amyloid fibrillogenesis. One technique targets AA amyloid deposits directly, by destabilizing AA amyloid fibrils so that they cannot maintain their structural configuration. Treatment with the drug (*R*)-1-[6-[(*R*)-2-carboxy-pyrrolidin-1-yl]-6-oxo-hexanoyl]pyrrolidine-2-carboxylic acid (CPHPC), a novel hexanoyl bis(D-proline), effectively removes the serum amyloid P component (SAP) from plasma but leaves some SAP in amyloid deposits that can then be specific targets of therapeutic IgG anti-SAP antibodies [21]. Also, eprodisate, which binds to glycosaminoglycan-binding sites on AA amyloid fibrils and in theory would destabilize them in tissues, may thereby cause regression of AA amyloidosis [22]. Although the mechanisms by which amyloid deposits are cleared are not well known, they supposedly involve breakdown of amyloid fibrils and associated molecules by macrophages and/or parenchymal cells [23, 24].

This chapter aims to review the advances in the treatment of AA amyloidosis secondary to RA and to describe the latest therapeutic developments based on our reports and literature reviews.

http://dx.doi.org/10.5772/63132

2. *SAA1.3* genotype and SAA concentration as predictive and prognostic factors of AA amyloidosis outcome

The frequency of *SAA1* gene polymorphism and that of *SAA1* alleles differ among races and regions worldwide. Three main *SAA1* alleles—*SAA1.1, SAA1.3,* and *SAA1.5*—are defined by two single-nucleotide polymorphisms (SNPs) in exon 3, which result in two amino acid differences at positions 52 and 57, respectively, [25]. In Japanese people, the three alleles occur approximately at the same frequency. The association between AA amyloidosis and the *SAA1* genotype was first observed in Japanese patients with RA, in whom *SAA1.3* allele homozygosity proved to be a risk factor [26]. The *SAA1.3/1.3* genotype in Japanese patients with RA was related to a shorter latency before the onset of AA amyloidosis and more severe AA amyloidosis-related symptoms [27, 28]. In addition, it was a univariate predictor of survival (**Figure 1**). Thus, the *SAA1.3* allele was a risk factor for AA amyloidosis, was associated with clinical severity of the disease, and poor prognosis [11]. In Caucasians, AA amyloidosis was often found in *SAA1.1* homozygous individuals, and the *SAA1.1* allele was believed to be a risk factor for AA amyloidosis [29]. As for SNPs of the *SAA1* gene promoter region, –13T was found to be a high-risk factor for AA amyloidosis in Japanese patients with RA, and –13T/T and –13T/C were more closely correlated with AA amyloidosis compared with –13C/C [30]. *SAA1* gene polymorphism affects both SAA transcriptional activity in hepatocytes and blood SAA levels, so differences in enzymatic SAA1 proteolysis have demonstrated a close association between *SAA1* gene polymorphism and the onset of AA amyloidosis [31]. However, the mechanism by which *SAA1* gene polymorphism is associated with of AA amyloidosis onset and the reason for ethnic differences in disease-susceptible SNPs are still unknown.

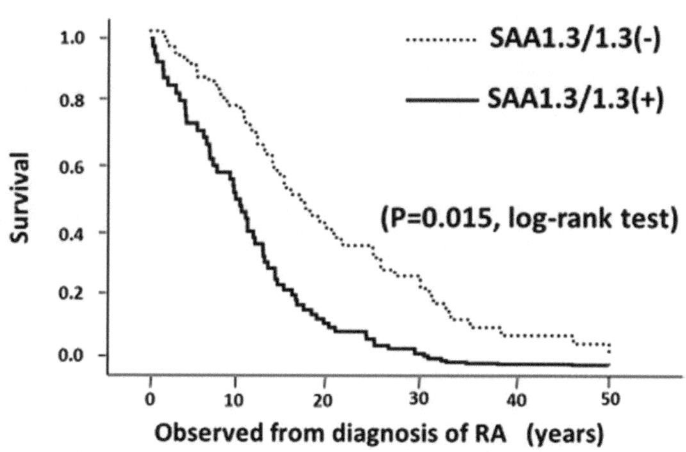

Figure 1. Kaplan-Meier survival curves for RA patients with and without *SAA1.3/1.3*. Statistical analysis of a large number of RA patients with AA amyloidosis who carried the *SAA1.3* allele revealed that the risk for association with AA amyloidosis was about eight times higher for *SAA1.3* homozygotes than for the control group and that homozygotes could develop AA amyloidosis very early after RA onset. Quoted from Nakamura et al. Rheumatology (Oxford) 2006; 45: 43–49.

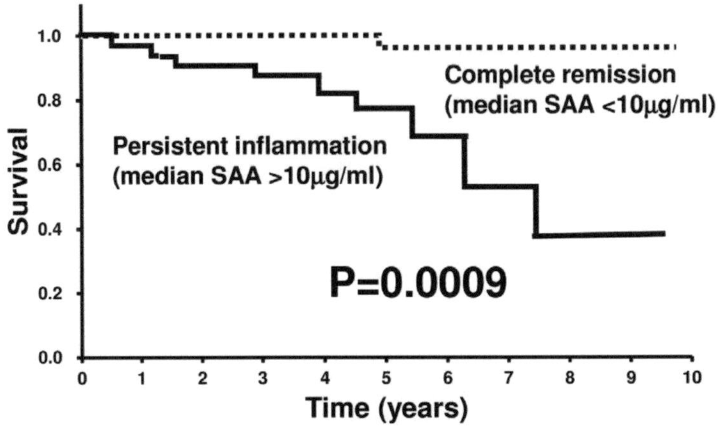

Figure 2. Kaplan-Meier survival curves for patients with systemic AA amyloidosis stratified according to whether the SAA concentration was above or below 10 μg/ml. During follow-up, the proportion of patients with AA amyloidosis who remained alive at 10 years was 90% in the group with median SAA values below 10 μg/ml and 40% in the group with SAA values above that value. Quoted and modified from Gillmore et al. Lancet 2011; 358: 24–29.

The current primary objective of therapy for all forms of amyloidosis was the reduction of the precursor protein supply [32]. In AA amyloidosis, long-term suppression of SAA levels is critical for patient and disease outcomes and for AA amyloidosis in patients with RA. The degree to which SAA concentration increased during follow-up was a strong predictor of outcome [33]. Sustained complete suppression of RA disease activity with the normalization of SAA levels should be the treatment aims in patients with AA amyloidosis, and monitoring the SAA levels is a vital part of patient management (**Figure 2**) [34].

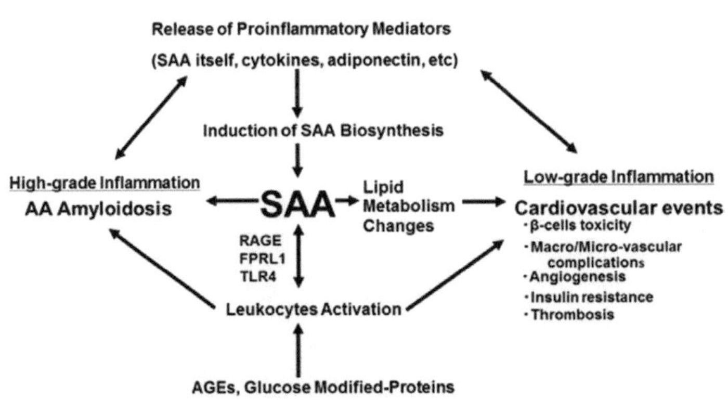

Figure 3. Biological versatility of SAA. SAA has important roles in high-grade and low-grade inflammation. Similar to cytokines, it utilizes autocrine, endocrine, and paracrine mechanisms. SAA, as a precursor protein of AA amyloidosis, induces this amyloidosis. Using different modes of action, SAA also affects metabolic syndrome. These humoral and cellular inflammatory events interact, with SAA as an essential factor. RAGE: receptor for advanced glycation end products; FPRL1: formyl peptide receptor-like 1; TLR2, 4: toll-like receptors 2 and 4; CLA-1: CD36, and LIMPII analogous-1, a human ortholog of the scavenger receptor class B type I (SR-BI); AGEs: advanced glycation end products. Quoted from Nakamura T. Clin Exp Rheumatol 2011; 29: 850–857.

SAA plays important roles in both high-grade and low-grade inflammation (**Figure 3**) [35]. Similar to cytokines, SAA operates by means of autocrine, endocrine, and paracrine mechanisms. SAA is a precursor protein of AA amyloid fibrils, and it induces AA amyloidosis. SAA also functions in metabolic syndrome by means of different modes of action. As a critical factor in the inflammatory interactions, SAA acts mutually among humoral and cellular events within inflammation.

3. Treatment with conventional synthetic DMARDs for AA amyloidosis secondary to RA

Treatment of patients with RA has focused on using immunosuppressants as conventional synthetic DMARDs (csDMARDs). Although case reports and studies of small series of patients showed that immunosuppressants can reverse nephrotic syndrome [36] and can even lead to complete resolution of proteinuria [37, 38], as **Table 1** shows, management of AA amyloidosis has focused on the RA process causing the inflammation as the underlying disease. We cannot, therefore, determine a clear difference in the effectiveness of therapies for RA and AA amyloidosis.

No. of cases	Diagnosis	Treatment	References
1	RA	CYC	Acta Med Scand 1979; 205: 651
11	RA	CYC/podophyllotoxin/ chlorambucil/ azathioprine	Clin Rheumatol 1987; 6: 27
9	RA	Chlorambucil/CYC	Ann Rheum Dis 1987; 46: 757
1	RA	Chlorambucil	S Afr Med J 1988; 73: 55
4	JIA	Chlorambucil	Pediatr Nephrol 1990; 4: 463
3	RA/JIA	CYC/methotrexate	Medicine (Baltimore) 1991; 70: 246
12	RA/JIA	Chlorambucil/CYC	J Rheumatol 1993; 20: 2051
1	RA	CYC	Clin Nephrol 1994; 42: 30
1	RA	Azathioprine	Arthritis Rheum 1995; 38: 1851
1	RA	CYC	Mod Rheumatol 2000; 10: 160
4	RA	CYC	Arthritis Rheum 2001; 44: 66
15	RA	CYC	Rheumatology (Oxford) 2001; 40: 821
15	RA	CYC	Clin Rheumatol 2003; 22: 371

AA: amyloid A; RA: rheumatoid arthritis; JIA: juvenile idiopathic arthritis; CYC: cyclophosphamide.

Table 1. Reported cases in the treatment for AA amyloidosis secondary to RA/JIA with immunosuppressants.

The efficacy of corticosteroid treatment with regard to AA amyloidosis secondary to RA is still controversial [39]. Corticosteroids can reduce the magnitude of acute phase reactions including synthesis of C-reactive protein (CRP) and SAA. In cultures of human hepatocyte, corticosteroids stimulated SAA production but not CRP production. Although corticosteroids reduced SAA and CRP levels in longitudinal studies of patients with RA, the effect was somewhat greater for CRP than for SAA [40]. Growing evidence suggests that SAA is sensitive to change, achieves much higher levels than CRP, declines rapidly, and may therefore accurately reflect disease activity. The advantages of SAA as a biomarker of disease activity include the rapid production and exceptionally wide dynamic range of the inflammatory response. During acute inflammation, serum SAA levels may rise up to 1000-fold and the biologic half-life of SAA levels are significantly shorter than that of CRP [41]. Monitoring SAA instead of CRP levels would thus be advisable, especially if corticosteroids are used. Treating patients with AA amyloidosis secondary to RA using cytotoxic drugs either alone or together with prednisolone, which is a synthetic glucocorticoid and a cortisol derivative, seems reasonable [42]. Because the effect of immunosuppressants may require weeks or months to be obvious, giving steroids in addition to immunosuppressants is recommended to ensure an immediate reduction in the acute phase response and, in particular, SAA synthesis [43].

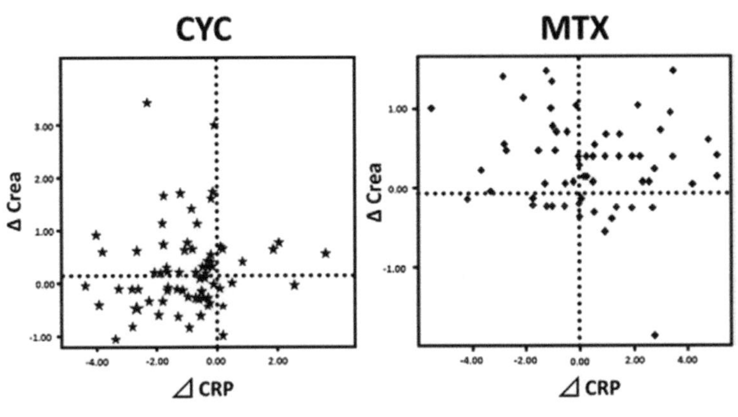

Figure 4. Differences between CYC and methotrexate (MTX) treatments in RA patients with AA amyloidosis. The deducted value (in the figure) was determined by subtracting the starting CRP and serum creatinine values from the corresponding ending values in each treatment. Quoted from Nakamura et al. Rheumatology (Oxford) 2006; 45: 43–49.

Although no evidence is available that csDMARDs have a particular effect on amyloidogenesis and AA amyloidosis in RA, reports provided encouraging description of the beneficial results of alkylating agents in clinical trials in RA patients with AA amyloidosis [44–46]. Using immunosuppressive agents may improve prognosis, and CYC has proved to be superior compared with methotrexate (MTX) for the treatment of RA patients with AA amyloidosis (**Figure 4**) [11]. Because between before and during CYC treatment, the values of Lansbury index, which implies a statistical approach to indices of disease activity, have lowered more; CYC may be more effective mainly in patients with *SAA1.3* homozygosity than in patients with *SAA1.3* heterozygosity, which suggests that *SAA1.3* homozygosity is a CYC treatment-susceptible factor (**Figure 5**) [20].

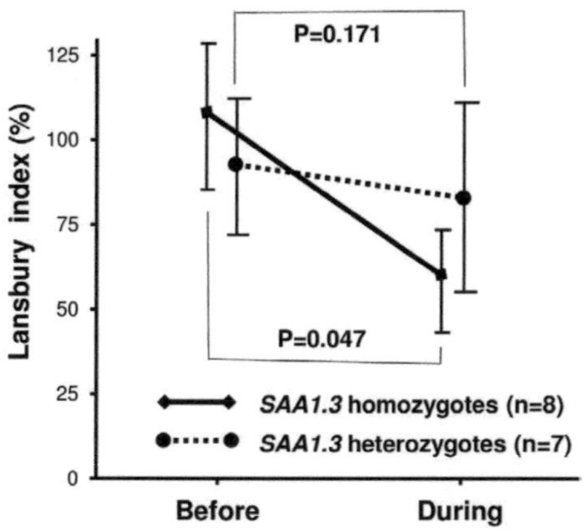

Figure 5. Changes in Lansbury index after CYC or prednisolone treatment in RA patients with AA amyloidosis with *SAA1.3* heterozygosity or homozygosity. In *SAA1.3* homozygous patients, a statistically significant difference occurred between before and during, whereas *SAA1.3* heterozygous patients showed no such significant difference. Quoted from Nakamura et al. Clin Rheumatol 2003; 22: 371–375.

During signal transduction, interleukin-6 (IL-6) binds to the membrane-bound IL-6 receptor gp80 [47], and after which the IL-6-gp80 dimer interacts with gp130. Formation of gp130-containing complexes activates Janus kinases, which stimulates signal transducers and activators of transcription (STATs) [48–50]. Some evidence suggests that STAT3 is the critical transcription factor that is responsible for IL-6 activation of SAA gene transcription [51]. The function of Janus kinase inhibition in the IL-6-signaling pathway will thus be one target of RA treatment. Suppressing IL-6-mediated pro-inflammatory signaling pathways using Janus kinase inhibitors may be a novel anti-inflammatory therapeutic strategy for RA and AA amyloidosis.

Another agent, tacrolimus, may inhibit T-cell function in the pathogenesis of AA amyloidosis. In experimental murine models of AA amyloidosis, blocking the function of T lymphocytes with the calcineurin inhibitor tacrolimus showed that it inhibited deposition of AA amyloid fibril in a dose-dependent manner. Also, the location of $CD4^+$ T lymphocytes in the spleen was identical to that of AA amyloid fibril deposits, which suggests that T lymphocytes have a role in the pathogenesis of AA amyloidosis [52].

4. Treatment with biological DMARDs for AA amyloidosis secondary to RA

Tight control of RA during treatment is important for obtaining clinical remission or for low disease activity [53]. This control is achieved via periodic assessments of RA disease activity and aggressive investigation of additional more effective treatments [54]. Biological DMARDs (bDMARDs) therapy is expected to be effective against systemic inflammation and local inflammation such as those occurring in RA.

Type of agent	Biologic	References
TNFα antagonist		
	IFX	Arthritis Rheum 2002; 46: 2571
	ETN/IFX	Arthritis Rheum 2003; 48: 2019
	ETN/IFX	Rheumatology (Oxford) 2003; 42:1425
	ETN	Intern Med J 2004; 34: 570
	ETN/IFX	Rheumatology (Oxford) 2004; 43: 669
	ETN/IFX	Am J Med 2005; 118: 552
	ETN	Clin Exp Rheumatol 2007; 25: 518
	IFX	Rheumatol Int 2008; 28: 1155
	ETN/IFX	J Rheumatol 2009; 36: 2409
	ETN	Clin Rheumatol 2010; 29: 1395
	ETN	Rev Bras Reumatol 2010; 50: 205
	ETN	Rheumatol Int 2011; 31: 247
	ETN/ADA	Joint Bone Spine 2013; 80: 223
IL-6 receptor antagonist		
	TCZ	Arthritis Rheum 2006; 54: 2997
	TCZ	Clin Rheumatol 2009; 28: 1113
	TCZ	Clin Rheumatol 2010; 29: 1195
	TCZ	Mod Rheumatol 2014; 24: 405
	TCZ	Amyloid 2015; 22:84
	TCZ	Clin Exp Rheumatol 2015; 33 (Suppl. 94): S46
Selective costimulation modulator of T-cell function		
	ABT	Clin Exp Rheumatol 2014; 32: 501
Anti-CD20 antibody		
	RTX	Joint Bone Spine 2011; 78: 98

DMARDs: disease-modifying antirheumatic drugs; AA: amyloid A; RA: rheumatoid arthritis; TNFα: tumor necrosis factor α; IFX: infliximab; ETN: etanercept; ADA: adalimumab; IL-6: interleukin6; TCZ: tocilizumab; ABT: abatacept; CD: cluster of differentiation; RTX: rituximab.

Table 2. Biological DMARDs for patients with AA amyloidosis secondary to RA.

Etanercept (ETN) and infliximab (IFX), both tumor necrosis factor α (TNFα) antagonists, can lower SAA levels in RA patients with AA amyloidosis [55, 56]. This effect ameliorates both RA inflammation and AA amyloidosis, reduces the number of swollen and tender joints, lowers or normalizes proteinuria, and improves renal function [57, 58]. Although a small number of patients with AA amyloidosis secondary to RA received ETN, this drug had benefits for both RA inflammation and AA amyloidosis, even in *SAA1.3/1.3* allele-carrying RA patients (**Table 2**) [59–62]. Such benefits were determined by evaluating the surrogate markers disease activity score 28-erythrocyte sedimentation rate, CRP, SAA, and proteinuria (**Table 3**). Also, patients with mild RA disease and renal dysfunction demonstrated significantly improved serum creatinine levels. This result suggests that an earlier intervention with bDMARDs produces a better outcome for RA patients with AA amyloidosis (**Table 4**) [63, 64].

Parameter	Initial visit	Last visit	P-value
DAS28-ESR	5.99 ± 0.69	2.99 ± 0.15	<0.01
CRP (mg/dl)	4.68 ± 0.87	0.48 ± 0.29	<0.01
SAA (μg/ml)	250 ± 129	26 ± 15	<0.01
Proteinuria (g/day)	2.24 ± 0.81	0.57 ± 0.41	<0.01
Creatinine (mg/dl)*	2.54 ± 1.38	2.50 ± 2.21	0.896

ETN: etanercept; AA: amyloid A; RA: rheumatoid arthritis; DAS: disease activity score; ESR: erythrocyte sedimentation rate; CRP: C-reactive protein; SAA: serum amyloid A protein.
*Serum levels.
ETN was significantly effective for RA patients with AA amyloidosis. DAS28-ESR and CRP indicated RA inflammation, and SAA and proteinuria-indicated AA amyloidosis. Quoted and modified from Nakamura et al. Clin Rheumatol 2010; 29: 1395–1401.

Table 3. Effect of ETN on AA amyloidosis secondary to RA.

Creatinine value less than 2.0 (mg/dl) (n = 6)		Creatinine value more than 2.0 (mg/dl) (n = 8)	
Initial visit (mg/dl)	Last visit (mg/dl)	Initial visit (mg/dl)	Last visit (mg/dl)
1.37 ± 0.49[a]	1.07 ± 0.59[a]	3.43 ± 1.14[b]	3.56 ± 2.39[b]

ETN: etanercept; AA: amyloid A; RA: rheumatoid arthritis.
Although a statistical significance of serum levels of creatinine was not observed as shown in **Table 3**, when cutting levels of serum creatinine by 2.0 mg/dl, the group with values lower than 2.0 mg/dl revealed to be significant. Regarding with renal dysfunction because of AA amyloidosis secondary to RA, the earlier the intervention, the better the outcome was suggested. Quoted and modified from Nakamura et al. Clin Rheumatol 2010; 29: 1395–1401.
[a] P = 0.021, [b] not significant.

Table 4. Effect of ETN on renal dysfunction in AA amyloidosis secondary to RA.

Tocilizumab, an IL-6 receptor antagonist, also produced excellent SAA suppression and may show promise as a therapeutic agent for AA amyloidosis [65–67]. Circulating SAA levels usually indicate changes in CRP, and levels of these acute phase reactants usually increase at the same time, but certain differences can occur. SAA and CRP seem to be somewhat affected by different cytokines [68, 69]. As mentioned earlier, therapy in which IL-6 is blocked, rather than therapy utilizing TNF-α blockade, should influence multiple signal transduction systems and may normalize SAA levels in RA patients (**Figure 6**) [70].

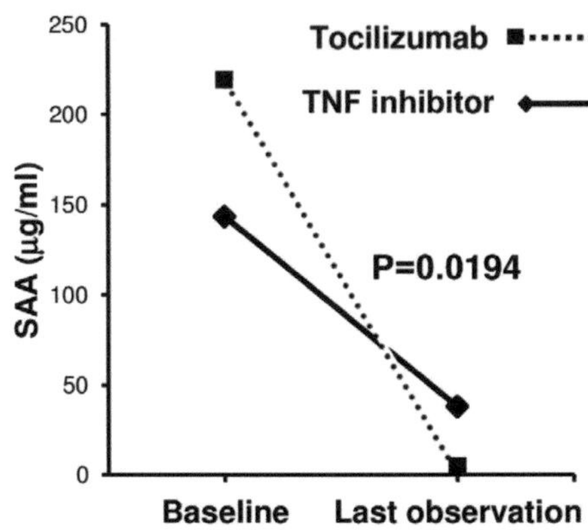

Figure 6. Changes in serum values of SAA between the first and last observations for each biologic. SAA values showed more significant suppression in the tocilizumab group than in the TNF inhibitor group (P = 0.0194, Wilcoxon rank sum test). Quoted and modified from Okuda et al. Mod Rheumatol 2014; 24: 137–143.

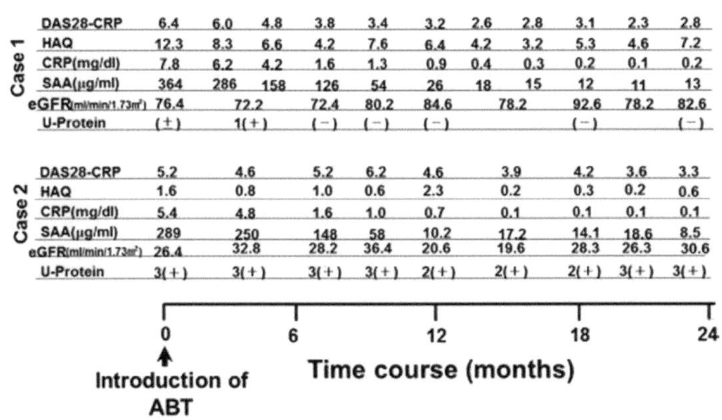

Figure 7. Clinical course of two RA patients with AA amyloidosis who received abatacept treatment. Clinical parameters were related to RA inflammation and AA amyloidosis after treatment. DAS28-CRP: disease activity score in 28 joints based on the CRP level; HAQ: Health Assessment Questionnaire; eGFR: estimated glomerular filtration rate; U-protein: qualitative protein analysis of spot urine. Quoted and modified from Nakamura et al. Clin Exp Rheumatol 2014; 32: 501–508.

Abatacept (ABT) is a soluble fusion protein consisting of the extracellular domain of recombinant human cytotoxic T lymphocyte-associated antigen 4 plus a fragment of the Fc domain human immunoglobulin IgG1 (CTLA-4Ig) [71]. CTLA-4Ig may reduce T lymphocyte responses by competing with CD80/CD86 to access CD28 and thus limit the CD28 signaling that T lymphocyte activation requires [72]. ABT may also affect more than just T lymphocytes [73]. Whether intracellular signaling or other CTLA-4Ig-mediated effects contribute to a favorable outcome or a poor outcome, especially during the treatment of RA patients, is not entirely clear, and the exact role of CTLA-4Ig in biological systems, including patients with AA amyloidosis secondary to RA, is also unresolved. Although accumulating clinical data on ABT treatment suggest an advantage for ABT in RA management [74, 75], the safety and efficacy of ABT in patients with AA amyloidosis secondary to RA have not yet been studied. **Figure 7** illustrates that in two patients, who had more than 20 years of RA history and who carried the *SAA1.3* allele, which is a risk factor for AA amyloidosis in Japanese RA patients, ABT gradually improved RA disease activities, proteinuria, and various gastrointestinal symptoms and was clinically effective to some degree in one case and completely in the other for both RA inflammation and AA amyloidosis. Study results also suggest that ABT targeting of costimulatory molecules may be useful for treating patients with AA amyloidosis secondary to RA and that ABT may be an alternative to anti-cytokine therapies for AA amyloidosis complicating RA [76].

Rituximab, an anti-CD20 monoclonal antibody, was effective for treating patients with severe active RA who had an inadequate response to TNFα inhibitor (or inhibitors) [77]. The efficacy and safety of rituximab for patients with AA amyloidosis secondary to RA together with substantial clinical improvement in articular symptoms, marked reduction in acute phase reactants, and stabilization of renal function and proteinuria were demonstrated [78].

5. Inhibiting AA amyloid fibrillogenesis in AA amyloidosis secondary to RA

Highly sulfated glycosaminoglycans, especially heparan sulfate and dermatan sulfate proteoglycans, are universal constituents of amyloid deposits and promote fibril assembly and help maintain conformational changes related to amyloidogenesis [79, 80]. Eprodisate is a negatively charged, sulfonated low molecular weight molecule that has a structure which is similar to that of heparan sulfate [81]. It binds to the SAA binding site to prevent interaction of SAA with glycosaminoglycans and thereby inhibits a conformational change required to cause SAA to become amyloidogenic. In in vivo studies with murine models, eprodisate inhibited the development of amyloid deposits [82, 83].

Eprodisate is still the only drug that was tested in a phase II/III multicenter, placebo-controlled, double-blinded study of amyloidosis [84]. Patients were stratified according to the presence of nephrotic syndrome and the treatment center, after of which they were randomized to receive eprodisate or placebo twice daily for up to 2 years. Outcome measures were a composite endpoint of serum creatinine, creatinine clearance, and progression to end-stage renal disease (ESRD) or death. Secondary outcome measures included the creatinine clearance slope, change in proteinuria, improvement in diarrhea, and alteration in amyloid content of abdominal fat. The study demonstrated that eprodisate may have contributed to the failure to achieve the study's primary endpoints, although the eprodisate-treated group did show renal benefits (**Figure 8**). The study, however, did not demonstrate a significant benefit from active therapy on progression to ESRD or risk of death, although a trend to benefit was seen. A phase III clinical study is currently under way in Japan.

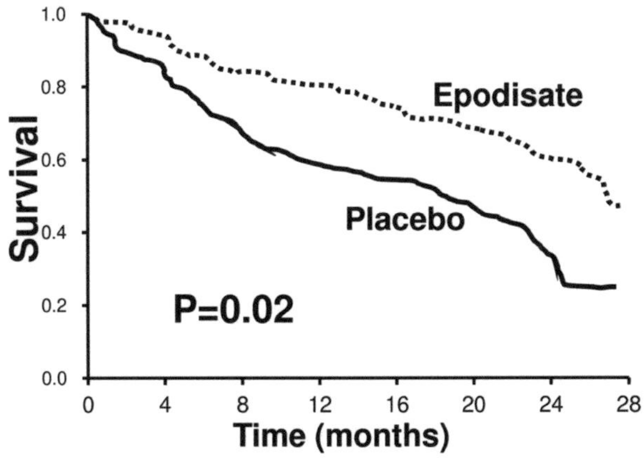

Figure 8. Kaplan-Meier survival curves for patients with AA amyloidosis who were given eprodisate or placebo. In terms of event-free survival, eprodisate demonstrated superior effectiveness compared with placebo, but this effect was not statistically significant. An event was defined as any component of the composite endpoint of worsened disease. Quoted and modified from Dember et al. N Engl J Med 2007; 356: 2349–2360.

6. Immunotherapy for AA amyloidosis secondary to RA

An alternative therapeutic approach was to target other components of amyloid deposits to destabilize amyloid fibrils. SAP is a normal plasma component and is a universal constituent of amyloid deposits. Its presence may therefore mask the presence of amyloid deposits and inhibit effective clearance of amyloid [85]. In fact, SAP knockout mice showed inhibited amyloid formation [86]. SAP was identified as a therapeutic target, which then led to development of CPHPC, a drug that inhibits the binding of SAP to amyloid deposits [87]. The activity of this agent relates to its ability to cross-link SAP molecule pairs face to face, which results in rapid hepatic clearance and completely blocks the binding face of the SAP molecule [88]. A preliminary study demonstrated that regular administration resulted in sustained and profound SAP depletion. Several patients received the drug for many years with no obvious adverse effects, although the degree of potential clinical benefit was not great enough to be determined in this open, non-controlled study (**Table 5**) [89].

Antibodies recognizing a common fibril epitope were raised and given to mice [90] with systemic AA amyloidosis, which resulted in reduced amyloid levels. CPHPC effectively removed SAP from the blood, but only very slowly from amyloid deposits, which allowed the development of an antibody directed at SAP. CPHPC was used to remove the SAP from plasma followed by use of an anti-SAP antibody, which led to rapid clearance by macrophages of experimentally induced amyloid deposits; this method begin developed for use in patients [91].

http://dx.doi.org/10.5772/63132

Patient no.	Amyloid type	Anti-SAP dose (mg)	SAP scan	Change in amyloid load
1	AA	5	Not improved	None detected
2	AApoA1	637	Improved	Liver reduction
3	AA	650	Improved	Kidney reduction

AA: amyloid A; SAP: serum amyloid P component; CPHPC: (*R*)-1-[6-[(*R*)-2-carboxy-pyrrolidin-1-yl]-6-oxo-hexanoyl]pyrrolidine-2-carboxylic acid; AApoA1: apolipoprotein A1.
Improved SAP scan: an improved scan was defined as a ^{123}I-SAP scintigram revealing a reduction in organ amyloid load at day 42 after SAP-antibody administration.
Combination treatment with CPHPC and anti-SAP antibody was effective to some extent for AA amyloidosis. Quoted and modified from Richards et al. N Engl J Med 2015; 373: 1106–1114.

Table 5. Response of patients with AA amyloidosis to anti-SAP antibody after depletion of plasma SAP with CPHPC.

7. Biomarkers predicting effectiveness of treatment for AA amyloidosis secondary to RA

Because renal dysfunction is the most common symptom in AA amyloidosis secondary to RA, surrogate markers representing the effectiveness of each treatment were investigated, with a focus on kidney function, in RA patients with AA amyloidosis who carried the *SAA 1.3* allele and who were treated with CYC or ETN focusing [92]. Identifying patients with a poor prognosis when it may be possible to modify the disease process and in whom any therapy may be justified is important. The presence of *SAA1.3* allele in Japanese RA patients may be a critical indicator for maintaining tight control of RA inflammation via vigorous treatment during the early phase of the RA disease course [11]. The rationale for using biologics in AA amyloidosis relates to their ability to lower levels of serum pro-inflammatory cytokines, which regulate SAA synthesis [93, 94]. A retrospective study reported the efficacy and safety of ETN for patients with AA amyloidosis secondary to RA who carried *SAA1.3* allele [64]. Using ETN for RA patients with AA amyloidosis may be possible, even for those undergoing dialysis [95, 96]. The efficacy of ETN was compared with that of CYC for treating AA amyloidosis secondary to RA as related to the *SAA1.3* allele, which was not a factor affecting therapeutic susceptibility (**Figure 9**). Demonstrable endpoints included recovery of serum albumin biosynthesis, improvement in the acute phase response, and amelioration of estimated glomerular filtration rate (eGFR). *SAA1.3* allele polymorphism was not affected on these parameters (**Table 6**). Albumin in fact reflects the severity of AA amyloidosis [97]. The changes in CRP and albumin were influenced by the difference between therapies rather than *SAA1.3* allele polymorphism (**Figure 10**). In contrast, the eGFR in patients with end-stage renal damage may reflect diminished urinary flow and may indicate improvement in renal function. Only ETN aided the amelioration of the eGFR, which indicated the greater efficacy of ETN compared with CYC for treating AA amyloidosis secondary to RA.

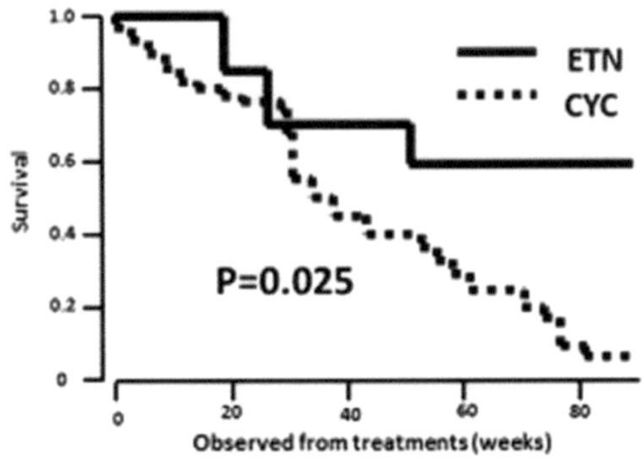

Figure 9. Kaplan-Meier survival curves after the treatment with ETN or CYC. ETN clearly demonstrated more effectiveness for RA patients with AA amyloidosis than did CYC. Quoted and modified from Nakamura et al. Rheumatology (Oxford) 2012; 51: 2064–2069.

Category	CRP	Alb	eGFR	Crea
Within-subject	<0.01	<0.01	0.035	0.085
Interaction with				
SAA1.3 allele polymorphism	0.777	0.715	0.465	0.228
Treatment (ETN/CYC)	<0.01	<0.01	0.032	0.148

ETN: etanercept; CYC: cyclophosphamide; CRP: C-reactive protein; Alb: albumin; eGFR: estimated glomerular filtration rate; Crea: creatinine.
Except creatinine, recovery of serum albumin biosynthesis, improvement in the acute phase response, and amelioration of estimated glomerular filtration rate (eGFR) were valuable parameters to show effectiveness in the treatment with etanercept. *SAA1.3* allele polymorphism was not affected on these parameters. Quoted from Nakamura et al. Rheumatology (Oxford) 2012; 51: 2064–2069.

Table 6. Parameters showing effectiveness of treatment with ETN or CYC.

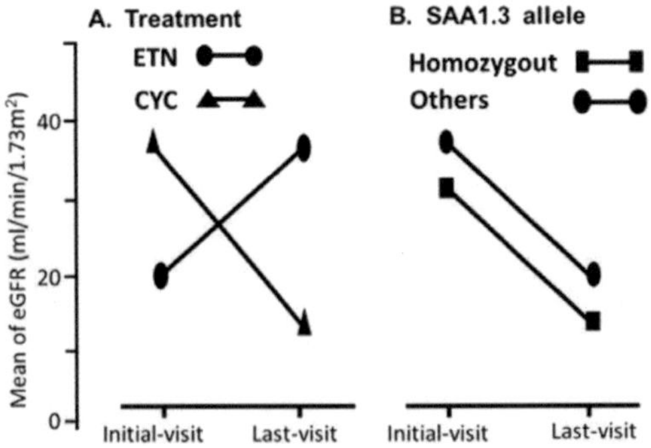

Figure 10. Changes in the eGFR between initial and last visits according to the effectiveness of treatment with ETN or CYC (A) and as a function of the *SAA1.3* allele homozygosity or other polymorphisms (B). ETN increased the eGFR, which improved the reduced renal function caused by AA amyloidosis, more than did CYC, and *SAA1.3* did not affect treatment in both groups of patients. Quoted from Nakamura et al. Rheumatology (Oxford) 2012; 51: 2064–2069.

http://dx.doi.org/10.5772/63132

8. End-stage renal disease treatment in AA amyloidosis secondary to RA

Kidneys that have extensive AA amyloid deposits are extremely susceptible to intercurrent insults such as hypoperfusion, hypertension, nephrotoxic drug effects, and surgical injuries, which should all be avoided in AA amyloidosis [98, 99]. Renal involvement is the most common problem in AA amyloidosis, and patients with AA amyloidosis frequently progress to end-stage renal disease (ESRD) and poor prognosis (**Figure 11**). When evaluating therapies for renal dysfunction related to AA amyloidosis, renal transplantation has been thought to be a suitable method [100]. However, existing data on patient survival and graft prognosis do not provide conclusive results about whether renal plantation is suitable for patients with AA amyloidosis [101]. An alternative to transplantation is chronic dialysis, but experience with dialysis in patients with AA amyloidosis has not yet as been encouraging [102, 103]. Peritoneal dialysis increases the susceptibility to infection and protein loss [104]. Hypoalbuminemia is well known to predict overall mortality in hemodialysis patients [105]. An elevated CRP value is associated with an increased risk of death in dialysis patients [106], and CRP has been found to be an independent predictor of major adverse cardiac events [107]. Because patients with AA amyloidosis who have progressed to ESRD have already been exposed to significant levels of inflammation, which may be ongoing, they may have an additional cardiovascular risk [108]. Patients with marked proteinuria have an increased risk of thrombosis, and the decision to use anticoagulants must be made on an individual basis [109]. General management principles apply to patients with AA amyloidosis secondary to RA for lowering high lipid levels and modifying diet as other causes of renal dysfunction.

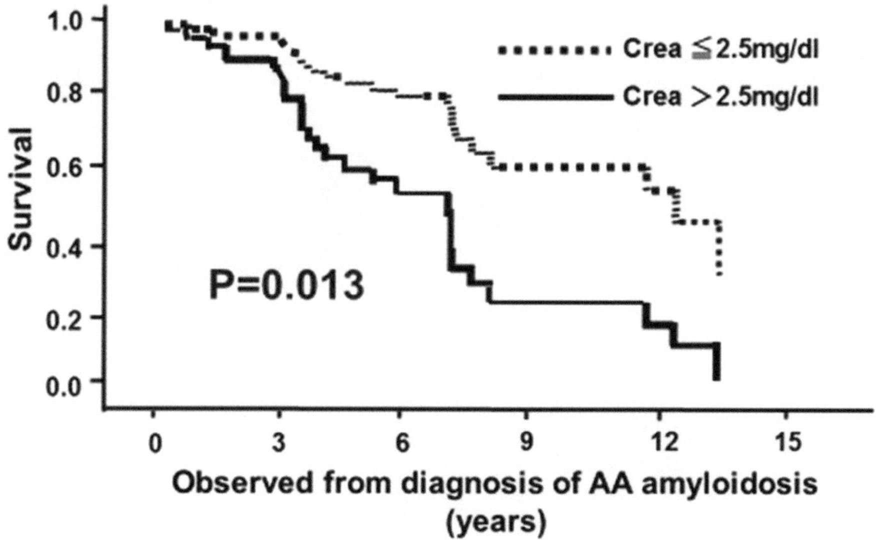

Figure 11. Kaplan-Meier survival curves after diagnosis of AA amyloidosis for patients with serum creatinine values of >2.5 or ≤2.5 mg/dl. Renal dysfunction, the most common symptom in AA amyloidosis secondary to RA, is a factor indicating a poor prognosis for survival. Quoted from Nakamura et al. Rheumatology (Oxford) 2006; 45: 43–49.

9. Possible involvement of phagocytes in degeneration of AA amyloid fibrils

Macrophages participate in SAA processing and deposition [110, 111], and cell surface-expressed heparan sulfate proteoglycans have an essential function in amyloidogenesis through the binding of high-density lipoprotein-associated SAA [112]. In addition, Fc-receptor-positive macrophages have been implicated in the reduction of the amyloid load after inflammation has resolved [113]. Phagocytes such as neutrophils and macrophages will serve an important function for reducing AA amyloid deposits during ABT treatment (**Figure 12**).

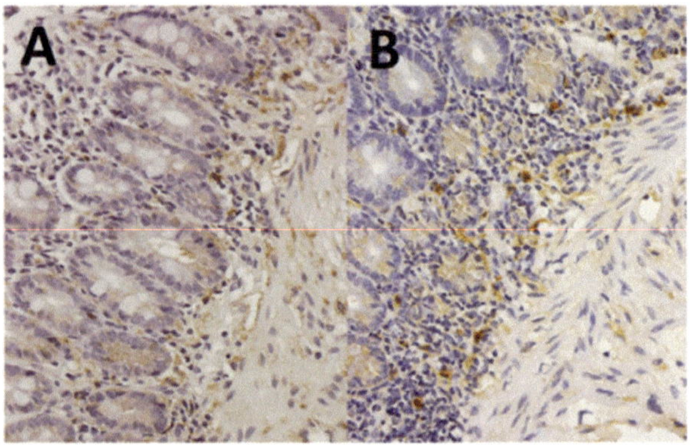

Figure 12. Immunohistochemical analysis of a biopsy specimen from a patient with RA and AA amyloidosis who received abatacept (ABT). (A) Stained with the antibody anti-formyl peptide receptor-like 1 (fPRL-1, the receptor involved in production of reactive oxygen species, degradation, and phagocyte migration) and (B) anti-human CD68 antibody staining. Phagocytes, polymorphonuclear leukocytes, and macrophages stained positively in the upper gastrointestinal mucosa specimen. Quoted and modified from Nakamura et al. Clin Exp Rheumatol 2014; 32: 501–508.

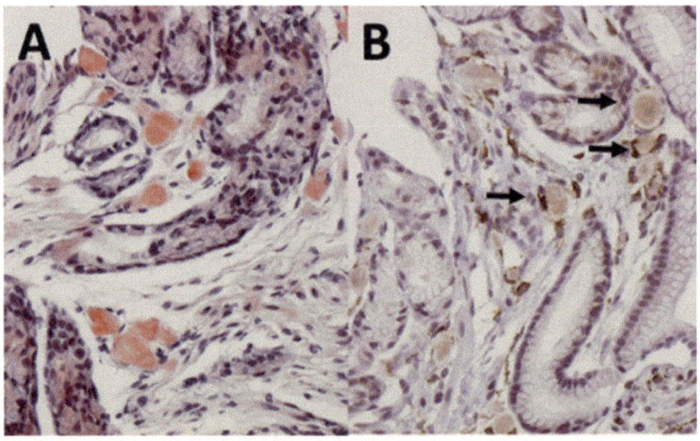

Figure 13. Relation between macrophages and AA amyloid deposits. AA amyloid deposits showed positive Congo-red staining (A), and anti-CD68 antibody-positive macrophages (arrows) surrounded AA amyloid deposits (B). These findings suggest an interaction between macrophages and amyloid deposits for the reduction in AA amyloid deposits. Quoted and modified from Nakamura et al. Clin Exp Rheumatol 2014; 32: 501–508.

T lymphocytes may influence the formation or metabolism of these amyloid fibrils. These cells colocalized within AA amyloid deposits, which indicates that phagocytes may participate in the metabolism or turnover of these amyloid deposits (**Figure 13**). Involvement of macrophages in AA amyloid reduction was proposed [114], and this hypothesis was supported by observations that macrophage-derived proteases completely degraded AA amyloid [115]. Resolution of AA amyloid deposits appears to start when inflammation subsides and SAA levels normalize. Additional data on the natural clearance of AA amyloid are vital [116], for both a better understanding of the dynamics of amyloidogenesis and the development of effective treatments for patients with AA amyloidosis secondary to RA.

10. Conclusion

AA amyloidosis is an uncommon yet important complication of chronic inflammatory conditions. Significant progress has been made in understanding of pathology, pathogenesis, and clinical treatment of AA amyloidosis secondary to RA, but AA amyloidosis is still a serious problem that deserves continued investigation. The *SAA1.3* allele is both a risk factor for AA amyloidosis and a factor related to poor prognosis and shortened survival in Japanese patients with RA. The incidence of AA amyloidosis secondary to RA will likely decrease because of remarkable advances in RA treatments such as bDMARDs and intracellular signal transduction inhibitors. However, when rheumatologists first meet patients with AA amyloidosis secondary to RA, the patients may be facing a serious, life-threatening disorder such as ESRD and/or cardiac complications, even given the present medical milieu in developed countries. The pathological process in RA patients with AA amyloidosis is likely to be more complicated and subtle than previously realized. Clarification of the formation and degeneration of AA amyloid fibrils induced by not only drugs but also cellular mechanisms and elucidation of the biological significance of SAA in health and disease is indispensable prerequisites to the management of AA amyloidosis secondary to RA. Novel therapies that target AA fibril formation and immunotherapy are currently under investigation and will lead to improved prognosis in the near future.

Acknowledgements

The author would like to thank his colleagues Hirokazu Takaoka, MD, and Tetsuhiro Maesaki, MD, at Kumamoto Shinto General Hospital; Masahiro Shono, MD, Ph.D., at Kumamoto Yuge Hospital; Michishi Tsukano, MD, Ph.D., Kunihiro Tomoda, MD, Ph.D., at Kumamoto Orthopaedic Hospital; Takeshi Kambara, MD, Ph.D., Tetsuro Yamamoto, MD, Ph.D., Yukio Ando, MD, Ph.D., and Mitsuharu Ueda, MD, Ph.D., at Kumamoto University; Takami Matsuyama, MD, Ph.D., at Kagoshima University, in Japan; and Laurence A. Boxer, MD, Ph.D., at University of Michigan Medical Center, Ann Arbor, MI, USA. This work was supported in part by a Grant-in-Aid for scientific research from the Japanese Ministry of Health, Labor, and

Welfare and the Amyloidosis Research Committee for Intractable Diseases, Epochal Diagnosis, and Treatment in Japan.

Conflict of interest

The author has declared no conflicts of interest.

Author details

Tadashi Nakamura

Address all correspondence to: nakamura@k-shinto.or.jp

Director, Section of Clinical Rheumatology, Kumamoto Shinto General Hospital, and Clinical Professor, Graduate School of Medical Sciences, Kumamoto University, Kumamoto, Japan

References

[1] Pinney JH, Hawkins PN. Amyloidosis. Ann Clin Biochem 2012; 49: 229–241.

[2] Hazenberg BPC. Amyloidosis: a clinical overview. Rheum Dis Clin N Am 2013; 39: 323–345.

[3] de Asua DR, Costa R, Galvan JM, Filigheddu MT, Trujillo D, Cadinanos J. Systemic AA amyloidosis: epidemiology, diagnosis, and management. Clin Epidemiol 2014; 6: 369–377.

[4] Westermark GT, Fändrich M, Westermark P. AA amyloidosis: pathogenesis and targeted therapy. Annu Rev Pathol 2015; 10: 321–344.

[5] Mijinheer G, Prakken BJ, van Wijk F. The effect of autoimmune arthritis treatment strategies on regulatory T-cell dynamics. Curr Opin Rheumatol 2013; 25: 260–267.

[6] Hunt L, Emery P. Defining populations at risk of rheumatoid arthritis: the first steps to prevention. Nat Rev Rheumatol 2014; 10: 521–530.

[7] Plant MJ, Jones PW, Saklavala J, Ollier WE, Dawes PT. Patterns of radiographic progression in early rheumatoid arthritis: results of an 8 year prospective study. J Rheumatol 1998; 25: 417–426.

[8] Chiche L, Jorde-Chiche N, Pascual V, Chaussabel D. Current perspectives on systemic immunology approaches to rheumatic diseases. Arthritis Rheum 2013; 65: 1407–1417.

[9] Sattar N, McInnes IB. Vascular comorbidity in rheumatoid arthritis: potential mechanisms and solutions. Curr Opin Rheumatol 2005; 17: 286–292.

[10] Saleem B, Keen H, Goeb V, Parmar R, Nizam S, Hensor EMA, Churchman SM, Quinn M, Wakefield R, Conaghan PG, Ponchel F, Emery P. Patients with RA in remission on TNF blockers: when and in whom can TNF blocker therapy be stopped? Ann Rheum Dis 2010; 69: 1636–1642.

[11] Nakamura T, Higashi S, Tomoda K, Tsukano M, Baba S, Shono M. Significance of SAA1.3 allele genotype in Japanese patients with amyloidosis secondary to rheumatoid arthritis. Rheumatology (Oxford) 2006; 45: 43–49.

[12] Smolen JS, van der Heijde D, Machold KS, Aletaha D, Landewe R. Proposal for a new nomenclature of disease-modifying antirheumatic drugs. Ann Rheum Dis 2014; 73: 3–5.

[13] Smolen JS, Aletaha D, Bijlsma JW, Breedvelt FC, Boumpas G, Burmester G, Combe B, Cutolo M, de Wit M, Dougados M, Emery P, Gibofsky A, Gomez-Reino JJ, Haraoui B, Kalden J, Keystone EC, Kvien TK, McInnes I, Martin-Mola E, Montecucco C, Schoels M, van der Heijde D; T2T Expert Committee. Treatingrheumatoid arthritis to target: recommendations of an international task force. Ann Rheum Dis 2010; 69: 631–637.

[14] Scott DL, Wolfe F, Huizinga TW. Rheumatoid arthritis. Lancet 2010; 376: 1094–1108.

[15] Nakamura T. Clinical strategies for amyloid A amyloidosis secondary to rheumatoid arthritis. Mod Rheumatol 2008; 18: 109–118.

[16] Berglund K, Thysell H, Keller C. Results, principles and pitfalls in the management of renal AA-amyloidosis; a 10–21 year followup of patients with rheumatic disease treated with alkylating cytostatics. J Rheumatol 1993; 20: 2015–2017.

[17] Chevrel G, Jenvrin C, McGregor B, Miossec P. Renal type AA amyloidosis associated with rheumatoid arthritis: a cohort study showing improved survival on treatment with pulse cyclophosphamide. Rheumatology (Oxford) 2001; 40: 821–825.

[18] Maezawa A, Hiromura K, Mitsuhashi H, Tsukada Y, Kanai H, Yano S, Naruse T. Combined treatment with cyclophosphamide and prednisolone can induce remission of nephrotic syndrome in a patient with renal amyloidosis, associated with rheumatoid arthritis. Clin Nephrol 1994; 42: 30–32.

[19] Shapiro DL, Spiera H. Regression of the nephrotic syndrome in rheumatoid arthritis and amyloidosis treated with azathioprine. A case report. Arthritis Rheum 1995; 38: 1851–1854.

[20] Nakamura T, Yamanura Y, Tomoda K, Tsukano M, Shono M, Baba S. Efficacy of cyclophosphamide combined with prednisolone in patients with AA amyloidosis secondary to rheumatoid arthritis. Clin Rheumatol 2003; 22: 371–375.

[21] Gillmore JD, Tennent GA, Hutchinson WL, Gallimore JR, Lachmann HJ, Goodman HJB, Offer M, Millar DJ, Petrie A, Hawkins PN, Pepys MB. Sustained pharmacological depletion of serum amyloid P component in patients with systemic amyloidosis. Br J Haematol 2010; 148: 760–767.

[22] Rumjon A, Coats T, Javaid MM. Review of eprodisate for the treatment of renal disease in AA amyloidosis. Int J Nephrol Renovasc Dis 2012; 5: 37–43.

[23] Nystrom SN, Westermark GT. AA-amyloid is cleared by endogenous immunological mechanisms. Amyloid 2012; 19: 138–145.

[24] Wynn TA, Chawla A, Pollard JW. Macrophage biology in development, homeostasis and disease. Nature 2013; 496: 445–455.

[25] Nakamura T. Amyloid A amyloidosis secondary to rheumatoid arthritis: an uncommon yet important complication. Curr Rheumatol Rev 2007; 3: 231–241.

[26] Baba S, Masago SA, Takahashi T, Kasama T, Sugimura H, Tsugane S, Tsutsui Y, Shirasawa H. A novel allelic variant of serum amyloid A, SAA1γ: genomic evidence, evolution, frequency, and implication as a risk factor for reactive systemic AA-amyloidosis. Hum Mol Genet 1995; 4: 1083–1087.

[27] Nakamura T, Yamamura Y, Tomoda K, Tsukano M, Baba S. Massive hematuria due to bladder amyloidosis in patients with rheumatoid arthritis: three case reports. Clin Exp Rheumatol 2003; 21: 673–674.

[28] Nakamura T, Tomoda K, Tsukano M, Yamamura Y, Baba S. Gustatory sweating due to autonomic neuropathy in a patient with amyloidosis secondary to rheumatoid arthritis. Mod Rheumatol 2004; 14: 498–501.

[29] Utku U, Dilek M, Akpolat I, Bedir A, Akpolat T. *SAA1* α/α alleles in Behçet's disease related amyloidosis. Clin Rheumatol 2007; 26: 927–929.

[30] Moriguchi M, Kaneko H, Terai C, Koseki Y, Kajiyama H, Inada S, Kitamura Y, Kamatani N. Relative transcriptional activities of *SAA1* promoters polymorphic at position -13(T/C): potential association between increased transcription and amyloidosis. Amyloid 2005; 12: 26–32.

[31] Turesson C, Weyand CM, Matteson EL. Genetics of rheumatoid arthritis: is there a pattern predicting extraarticular manifestations? Arthritis Rheum 2004; 51: 853–863.

[32] Ebert EC, Nagar MN. Gastrointestinal manifestations of amyloidosis. Am J Gastroenterol 2008; 103: 776–787.

[33] Herrera GA, Teng J, Turbat-Herrera EA. Renal amyloidosis: current views on pathogenesis and impact on diagnosis. In: Herrera GA, editor. Experimental Models for Renal Diseases: Pathogenesis and Diagnosis. Contrib Nephrol. Basel: Karger; 2011, vol. 169, pp 232–246.

[34] Gillmore JD, Lovat LB, Persey MR, Pepys MB, Hawkins PN. Amyloid load and clinical outcome in AA amyloidosis in relation to circulating concentration of serum amyloid A protein. Lancet 2001; 358: 24–29.

[35] Nakamura T. Amyloid A amyloidosis secondary to rheumatoid arthritis: pathophysiology and treatment. Clin Exp Rheumatol 2011; 29: 850–857.

[36] Pamuk ON, Donmez S, Pamuk GE, Puyan FO, Keystone EC. Turkish experience in rheumatoid arthritis patients with clinical apparent amyloid deposition. Amyloid 2013; 20: 245–250.

[37] Berglund K, Keller C, Thysell H. Alkylating cytostatic treatment in renal amyloidosis secondary to rheumatic disease. Ann Rheum Dis 1987; 46: 757–762.

[38] Nakamura T, Baba S, Yamamura Y, Tsuruta T, Matsubara S, Tomoda K, Tsukano M. Combined treatment with cyclophosphamide and prednisolone is effective for secondary amyloidosis with SAA1γ/γ genotype in a patient with rheumatoid arthritis. Mod Rheumatol 2000; 10: 160–164.

[39] Bakker MF, Jacobs JWG, Welsing PMJ, Verstappen SMM, Tekstra J, Ton E, Geurts MA, van der Werf JH, van Albada-Kuipers GA, Jahangier-de Veen ZN, van der Veen MJ, Verhoef CM, Lafeber FP, Bijlsma JW; Utrecht Rheumatoid Arthritis Cohort Study Group. Low-dose prednisone inclusion in a methotrexate-based, tight control strategy for early rheumatoid arthritis: a randomized trial. Ann Intern Med 2012; 156: 329–339.

[40] Migita K, Yamasaki K, Shibatomi H, Ida H, Kita M, Kawakami A, Eguchi K. Impaired degradation of serum amyloid A (SAA) protein by cytokine-stimulated monocytes. Clin Exp Immunol 2001; 123: 408–411.

[41] Eklund KK, Niemi K, Kovanen PT. Immune functions of serum amyloid A. Crit Rev Immunol 2012; 32: 355–348.

[42] Matsuda M, Morita H, Ikeda S. Long-term follow-up of systemic reactive AA amyloidosis secondary to rheumatoid arthritis: successful treatment with intermediate-dose corticosteroid. Intern Med 2002; 41: 403–407.

[43] Fushimi T, Takahashi Y, Kashima Y, Fukushima K, Ishii W, Kaneko K, Yazaki M, Nakamura A, Tokuda T, Matsuda M, Furuya R, Ikeda S. Severe protein losing enteropathy with intractable diarrhea due to systemic AA amyloidosis, successfully treated with corticosteroid and octreotide. Amyloid 2005; 12: 48–53.

[44] Getz MA, Kyle RA. Secondary amyloidosis: response and survival in 64 patients. Medicine (Baltimore) 1991; 70: 246–256.

[45] Shapiro DL, Spiera H. Regression of the nephrotic syndrome in rheumatoid arthritis and amyloidosis treated with azathioprine. A case report. Arthritis Rheum 1995; 38: 1851–1854.

[46] Gómez-Casanovas E, Sanmartí R, Solé M, Cañete JD, Muñoz-Gómez J. The clinical significance of amyloid fat deposits in rheumatoid arthritis: a systemic long-term followup study using abdominal fat aspiration. Arthritis Rheum 2001; 44: 46–72.

[47] Nishimoto N, Yoshizaki K, Miyasaka N, Yamamoto K, Kawai S, Takeuchi T, Hashimoto J, Azuma J, Kishimoto T. Treatment of rheumatoid arthritis with humanized anti-

interleukin-6 receptor antibody: a multicenter, double-blind, placebo-controlled trial. Arthritis Rheum 2004; 50: 1761–1769.

[48] Hagiwara K, Nishikawa T, Isobe T, Song J, Sugamata Y, Yoshizaki K. IL-6 plays a critical role in the synergistic induction of human serum amyloid A (SAA) gene when stimulated with proinflammatory cytokines as analyzed with an SAA isoform real-time quantitative RT-PCR assay system. Biochem Biophys Res Commun 2004; 314: 363–369.

[49] Kishimoto T, Akira S, Taga T. IL-6 receptor and mechanism of signal transduction. Int J Immunopharmacol 1992; 14: 431–438.

[50] Hirano T, Ishihara K, Hibi M. Roles of STAT3 in mediating the cell growth, differentiation and survival signals relayed through the IL-6 family of cytokine receptors. Oncogene 2000; 19: 2548–2556.

[51] Cutolo M, Soldona S, Contini P, Sulli A, Seriolo B, Montagna P, Brizzolara R. Intracellular NF-κB-decrease and IκBα increase in human macrophages following CTLA4-Ig treatment. Clin Exp Rheumatol 2013; 31: 943–946.

[52] Ueda M, Ando Y, Nakamura M, Yamashita T, Himeno S, Kim J, Sun X, Saito S, Tateishi T, Bergström J, Uchino M. FK506 inhibits murine AA amyloidosis: possible involvement of T cells in amyloidogenesis. J Rheumatol 2006; 33: 2260–2270.

[53] Aletaha D, Neogi T, Silman AJ, Funovits J, Felson DT, Bingham CO, III, Birnbaum NS, Burmester GR, Bykerk VP, Cohen MD, Combe B, Costenbader KH, Dougados M, Emery P, Ferraccioli G, Hazes JM, Hobbs K, Huizinga TW, Kavanaugh A, Kay J, Kvien TK, Laing T, Mease P, Ménard HA, Moreland LW, Naden RL, Pincus T, Smolen JS, Stanislawska-Biernat E, Symmons D, Tak PP, Upchurch KS, Vencovský J, Wolfe F, Hawker G. 2010 Rheumatoid arthritis classification criteria. An American College of Rheumatology/European League Against Rheumatism Collaborative Initiative. Arthritis Rheum 2010; 62: 2569–2581.

[54] Smolen JS, Landewé R, Breedveld FC, Buch M, Bumester G, Dougados M, Emery P, Gaujoux-Viala C, Gossec L, Nam J, Ramiro S, Winthrop K, de Wit M, Aletaha D, Betteridge N, Bijlsma JW, Boers M, Buttgereit F, Combe B, Cutolo M, Damjanov N, Hazes JM, Kouloumas M, Kvien TK, Mariette X, Pavelka K, van Riel PL, Rubbert-Roth A, Scholte-Voshaar M, Scott DL, Sokka-Isler T, Wong JB, van der Heijde D. EULAR recommendations for the management of rheumatoid arthritis with synthetic and biological disease-modifying antirheumatic drugs: 2013 update. Ann Rheum Dis 2014; 73: 492–509.

[55] Pettersson T, Konttinen YT, Maury CPJ. Treatment strategies for amyloid A amyloidosis. Expert Opin Pharmacother 2008; 9: 2117–2128.

[56] Dember LM. Modern treatment of amyloidosis: unsolved questions. J Am Soc Nephrol 2009; 20: 469–472.

[57] Roque R, Ramiro S, Corderio A, Goncalves P, da Canas S, Santos MJ. Development of amyloidosis in patients with rheumatoid arthritis under TNF-blocking agents. Clin Rheumatol 2011; 30: 869–870.

[58] Kuroda T, Tanabe N, Kobayashi D, Sato H, Wada Y, Murakami S, Saeki T, Nakano M, Narita I. Treatment with biologic agents improves the prognosis of patients with rheumatoid arthritis and amyloidosis. J Rheumatol 2012; 39: 1348–1354.

[59] Gottenberg J-E, Merle-Vincent F, Bentaberry F, Allanore Y, Berenbaum FY, Berenbaum F, Fautrel B, Combe B, Durbach A, Sibilia J, Dougados M, Mariette X. Anti-tumor necrosis factor α therapy in fifteen patients with AA amyloidosis secondary to inflammatory arthritides. A followup report of tolerability and efficacy. Arthritis Rheum 2003; 48: 2019–2024.

[60] Perry ME, Stirling A, Hunter JA. Effect of etanercept on serum amyloid A protein (SAA) levels in patients with AA amyloidosis complicating inflammatory arthritis. Clin Rheumatol 2008; 27: 923–925.

[61] Nobre CA, Callado MRM, Rodriges CEM, de Menezes DB, Viera WP. Anti-TNF therapy in renal amyloidosis in refractory rheumatoid arthritis: a new therapeutic perspective. Bras J Rheumatol 2010; 50: 205–210.

[62] Kuroda T, Wada Y, Kobayashi D, Murakami S, Sakai T, Hirose S, Tanabe N, Saeki T, Nakano M, Narita I. Effective anti-TNF-α therapy can induce rapid resolution and sustained decrease of gastrointestinal mucosal amyloid deposits in reactive amyloidosis associated with rheumatoid arthritis. J Rheumatol 2009; 36: 2409–2415.

[63] Ravindan J, Shenker N, Bhalla AK, Lachmann H, Hawkins P. Case report: response in proteinuria due to AA amyloidosis but not Felty's syndrome in a patient with rheumatoid arthritis treated with TNF-α blockade. Rheumatology (Oxford) 2004; 43: 669–672.

[64] Nakamura T, Higashi S, Tomoda K, Tsukano M, Shono M. Etanercept can induce resolution of renal deterioration in patients with amyloid A amyloidosis secondary to rheumatoid arthritis. Clin Rheumatol 2010; 29: 1395–1401.

[65] Okuda Y, Takasugi K. Successful use of a humanized anti-interleukin-6 receptor antibody, tocilizumab, to treat amyloid A amyloidosis complicating juvenile idiopathic arthritis. Arthritis Rheum 2006; 54: 2997–3000.

[66] Lane T, Gillmore JD, Wechalekar AD, Hawkins PN, Lachmann HJ. Therapeutic blockade of interleukin-6 by tocilizumab in the management of AA amyloidosis and chronic inflammatory disorders: a case series and review of the literature. Clin Exp Rheumatol 2015; 33 (Suppl. 94): S46–S53.

[67] Courties A, Grateau G, Philippe P, Flipo R-M, Astudillo L, Aubry-Rozier B. AA amyloidosis treated with tocilizumab: case series and updated literature review. Amyloid 2015; 22: 84-92.

[68] Fernández-Nebro A, Olivé A, Castro MC, Varela AH, Riera E, Irigoyen MV, García de Yébenes MJ, García-Vicuña R. Long-term TNF-α blockade in patients with amyloid A amyloidosis complicating rheumatic diseases. Am J Med 2010; 123: 454–461.

[69] Miyagawa I, Nakayamada S, Saito K, Hanami K, Nawata M, Sawamukai N, Nakano K, Yamaoka K, Tanaka Y. Study on the safety and efficacy of tocilizumab, an anti-IL-6 receptor antibody, in patients with rheumatoid arthritis complicated with AA amyloidosis. Mod Rheumatol 2014; 24: 405–409.

[70] Okuda Y, Ohnishi M, Matoba K, Jouyama K, Yamada A, Sawada N, Mokuda S, Murata Y, Takasugi K. Comparison of the clinical utility of tocilizumab and anti-TNF therapy in AA amyloidosis complicating rheumatic diseases. Mod Rheumatol 2014; 24: 137–143.

[71] Haggerty HG, Abbott MA, Reilly TP, DeVona DA, Gleason CR, Tay L, Dodge R, Aranda R. Evaluation of immunogenicity of T cell costimulation modulator abatacept in patients treated for rheumatoid arthritis. J Rheumatol 2007; 34: 2365–2373.

[72] Fiocco U, Sfriso P, Oliviero F, Pagnin E, Scaglioni E, Campana C, Dainese S, Cozzi L, Punzi L. Co-stimulatory modulation in rheumatoid arthritis: the role of (CTLA4-Ig) abatacept. Autoimmun Rev 2008; 8: 76–82.

[73] Cope AP, Schulze-Koops H, Aringger M. The central role of T cells in rheumatoid arthritis. Clin Exp Rheumatol 2007; 25 (Suppl. 46): S4–S11.

[74] Benucci M, Stam WB, Gilloteau I, Sennfält K, Leclerc A, Maetzel A, Lucioni C. Abatacept or infliximab for patients with rheumatoid arthritis and inadequate response to methotrexate: an Italian trial-based and real-life cost-consequence analysis. Clin Exp Rheumatol 2013; 31: 575–583.

[75] Innone F, Lapadula G. The inhibition of costimulation of T cells: abatacept. J Rheumatol 2012; 89: 100–102.

[76] Nakamura T, Kumon Y, Hirata S, Takaoka H. Abatacept may be effective and safe in patients with amyloid A amyloidosis secondary to rheumatoid arthritis. Clin Exp Rheumatol 2014; 32: 501–508.

[77] Rubber-Roth A, Finckh A. Treatment options in patients with rheumatoid arthritis failing TNF inhibitor therapy: a critical review. Arthritis Res Ther 2009; 11 (Suppl. 1): S1.

[78] Narváez J, Hernández MV, Ruiz JM, Vaquero CG, Juanola X, Nollaa JM. Rituximab therapy for AA-amyloidosis secondary to rheumatoid arthritis. Joint Bone Spine 2011; 48: 101–103.

[79] Kisilevsky R, Lemieux LJ, Fraser PE, Kong X, Hultin PG, Szarek WA. Arresting amyloidosis in vivo using small molecule anionic sulphonates or sulphate: implications for Alzheimer's disease. Nat Med 1995; 1: 143–148.

[80] Snow AD, Kisilevsky R, Sobh MA, Mohamed NA, Sheashaa HA, Ghoneim MA. Long-term outcome of live donor kidney transplantation for renal amyloidosis. Am J Kidney Dis 2003; 42: 370–375.

[81] Khalighi MA, Wallace WD, Palma-Diaz MF. Amyloid nephropathy. Clin Kidney J 2014; 7: 97–106.

[82] Gervais F, Chalifour R, Garceau D, Kong X, Laurin J, McLaughlin R, Morissette C, Paquette J. Glycosamoinoglycan mimetics: a therapeutic approach to cerebral amyloid angiopathy. Amyloid 2001; 8 (Suppl. 1): S28–S35.

[83] Gervais F, Morissette C, Kong X. Proteoglycans and amyloidogenic proteins in peripheral amyloidosis. Curr Med Chem Immunol Endocr Metab Agents 2003; 3: 361–370.

[84] Dember LM, Hawkins PN, Hazenberg PBC, Gorevic P, Merlini G, Butrimiene I, Livneh A, Lesnyak O, Puéchal X, Lachmann HJ, Obici L, Balshaw R, Garceau D, Hauck W, Skinner M; Eprodisate for AA Amyloidosis Trial Group. Eprodisate for the treatment of renal disease in AA amyloidosis. N Engl J Med 2007; 356: 2349–2360.

[85] Tennent GA, Brennan SO, Stangou AJ, O'Grady J, Hawkins PN, Pepys MB. Human plasma fibrinogen is synthesized in the liver. Blood 2007; 109: 1971–1974.

[86] Botto M, Hawkins PN, Bickerstaff MCM, Herbert J, Bygrave AE, McBride A, Hutchinson WL, Tennent GA, Walport MJ, Pepys MB. Amyloid deposition is delayed in mice with targeted deletion of the serum amyloid P component gene. Nat Med 1997; 3: 855–859.

[87] Kolstoe SE, Jenvey MC, Purvis A, Light ME, Thompson D, Hughes P, Pepys MB, Wood SP. Interaction of serum amyloid P component with hexanoyl bis(D-proline) (CPHCP). Acta Crystallogr D Biol Crystallogr 2014; 70: 2232–2240.

[88] Pepys MB, Herbert J, Hutchinson WL, Tennent GA, Lachmann HJ, Gallimore JR, Lovat LB, Bartfai T, Alanine A, Hertel C, Hoffmann T, Jakob-Roetne R, Norcross RD, Kemp JA, Yamamura K, Suzuki M, Taylor GW, Murray S, Thompson D, Purvis A, Kolstoe S, Wood SP, Hawkins PN. Targeted pharmacological depletion of serum amyloid P component for treatment of human amyloidosis. Nature 2002; 417: 254–259.

[89] Richards DB, Cookson LM, Berges AC, Barton SV, Lane T, Ritter JM, Fontana M, Moon JC, Pinzani M, Gillmore JD, Hawkins PN, Pepys MB. Therapeutic clearance of amyloid by antibodies to serum amyloid P component. N Engl J Med 2015; 373: 1106–1114.

[90] O'Nuallain B, Wetzel R. Conformational Abs recognizing a genetic amyloid fibril epitope. Proc Natl Acad Sci USA 2002; 99: 1485–1490.

[91] Bodin K, Ellmerich S, Kahan MC, Tennent GA, Loesch A, Gilbertson JA, Hutchinson WL, Mangione PP, Gallimore JR, Millar DJ, Minogue S, Dhillon AP, Taylor GW, Bradwell AR, Petrie A, Gillmore JD, Bellotti V, Botto M, Hawkins PN, Pepys MB.

Antibodies to human serum amyloid P component eliminate visceral amyloid deposits. Nature 2010; 468: 93–97.

[92] Nakamura T, Higashi S, Tomoda K, Tsukano M, Shono M. Effectiveness of etanercept *vs* cyclophosphamide as treatment of patients with amyloid A amyloidosis secondary to rheumatoid arthritis. Rheumatology (Oxford) 2012; 51: 2064–2069.

[93] Chiche L, Jorde-Chiche N, Pascual V, Chaussabel D. Current perspectives on systems immunology approaches to rheumatic diseases. Arthritis Rheum 2013; 65: 1407–1417.

[94] Obici L, Raimondi S, Lavetelli F, Bellotti V, Merlini G. Susceptibility to AA amyloidosis in rheumatic diseases: a critical overview. Arthritis Care Res 2009; 61: 1435–1440.

[95] Don BR, Spin G, Nestorov I, Hutmacher M, Rose A, Kaysen GA. The pharmacokinetics of etanercept in patients with end-stage renal disease on haemodialysis. J Pharm Pharmacol 2005; 57: 1407–1413.

[96] Nakamura T, Higashi S, Tomda K, Tsukano M, Arizono K, Nakamura T. Etanercept treatment in patients with rheumatoid arthritis on dialysis. Rheumatol Int 2010; 30: 1527–1528.

[97] Maury CPJ, Teppo A-M. Mechanism of reduced amyloid-A-degrading activity in serum of patients with secondary amyloidosis. Lancet 1982; 2: 234–237.

[98] Kuroda K, Tanabe N, Sato H, Ajiro J, Wada Y, Murakami S, Hasegawa H, Sakatsume M, Nakano M, Gejyo F. Outcome of patients with reactive amyloidosis associated with rheumatoid arthritis in dialysis treatment. Rheumatol Int 2006; 26: 1147–1153.

[99] Sahin S, Sahin GM, Ergin H, Kantarci G. The effect of dialytic modalities on clinical outcomes in ESRD patients with familial Mediterranean fever. Ren Fail 2007; 29: 315–319.

[100] Heering P, Hetzel R, Grabensee B, Opelz G. Renal transplantation in secondary systemic amyloidosis. Clin Transpl 1998; 12: 159–164.

[101] Kofman T, Grimbert P, Canouï-Poitrine F, Zuber J, Garrigue V, Mousson C, Frimat L, Kamar N, Couvrat G, Bouvier N, Albano L, Le Thuaut A, Pillebout E, Choukroun G, Couzi L, Peltier J, Mariat C, Delahousse M, Buchler M, Le Pogamp P, Bridoux F, Pouteil-Noble C, Lang P, Audard V. Renal transplantation in patients with AA amyloidosis nephropathy: results from a French multicenter study. Am J Transpl 2011; 11: 2423–2431.

[102] Iwamoto M, Honma S, Asano Y, Minota S. Effective and safe administration of tocilizumab to a patient with rheumatoid arthritis on haemodialysis. Rheumatol Int 2011; 31: 559–560.

[103] Kuroda T, Tanabe N, Kobayashi D, Sato H, Wada Y, Murakami S, Sakatsume M, Nakano M, Narita I. Programmed initiation of hemodialysis for systemic amyloidosis patients associated with rheumatoid arthritis. Rheumatol Int 2011; 31: 1177–1182.

[104] John B, Tan BK, Dainty S, Spanel D, Smith D, Davies SJ. Plasma volume, albumin, and fluid status in peritoneal dialysis patients. Clin J Am Soc Nephrol 2010; 5: 1463–1470.

[105] Lowrie EG, Lew NL. Death risk in hemodialysis patients: the predictive value of commonly measured variables and an elevation of death differences between facilities. Am J Kidney Dis 1990; 15: 458–482.

[106] Bollée G, Guery B, Joly D, Snanoudj R, Terrier B, Allouache M, Mercadal L, Peraldi MN, Viron B, Fumeron C, Elie C, Fakhouri F. Presentation and outcome of patients with systemic amyloidosis undergoing dialysis. Clin J Am Soc Nephrol 2008; 3: 375–381.

[107] Falk RH. Cardiac amyloidosis. Circulation 2011; 124: 1079–1085.

[108] Muhammad N, Murakami T, Inoshita Y, Ishiguro N. Long-term kinetics of AA amyloidosis and effects of inflammatory restimulation after disappearance of amyloid depositions in mice. Clin Exp Immunol 2015; 181: 133–141.

[109] Hallén J, Madsen L, Ladefoged S, Fagerland MW, Serebruany VL, Agewall S, Atar D. Incremental value of a combination of cardiac troponin T, N-terminal pro-brain natriuretic peptide and C-reactive protein for prediction of mortality in end-stage renal disease. Scand J Urol Nephrol 2011; 45: 151–158.

[110] Elimova E, Kisilevsky R, Ancin JB. Heparin sulfate promotes the aggregation of HDL-associated serum amyloid A: evidence for a proamyloidogenic histidine molecule switch. FASEB J 2009; 23: 3436–3448.

[111] Kennel SJ, Macy S, Wooliver C, Huang Y, Richey T, Heidel E, Wall JS. Phagocyte depletion inhibits AA amyloid accumulation in AEF-induced huIL-6 transgenic mice. Amyloid 2014; 21: 45–53.

[112] Simons JP, Al-Shawi R, Ellmerich S, Speck I, Aslam S, Hutchinson WL, Mangione PP, Disterer P, Gilbertson JA, Hunt T, Millar DJ, Minogue S, Bodin K, Pepys MB, Hawkins PN. Pathogenetic mechanisms of amyloid A amyloidosis. Proc Natl Acad Sci USA 2013; 110: 16115–16120.

[113] Nystrom SN, Westermark GT. AA-amyloid is cleared by endogenous immunological mechanisms. Amyloid 2012; 19: 138–145.

[114] Lu J, Yu Y, Zhu I, Cheng Y, Sun PD. Structural mechanism of serum amyloid A-mediated inflammatory amyloidosis. Proc Natl Acad Sci USA 2014 111: 5189–5194.

[115] van der Hilst JC, Kluve-Beckerman B, van der Meer JW, Simon A. Cathepsin D activity protects against development of type AA amyloid fibrils. Eur J Clin Investig 2009; 39: 412–416.

[116] Westermark GT, Westermark P. Serum amyloid A and protein AA: molecular mechanisms of a transmissible amyloidosis. FEBS Lett 2009; 583: 2685–2690.

Chapter 10

The Role of Human IAPP in Stress and Inflammatory Processes in Type 2 Diabetes

Joel Montane and Anna Novials

Additional information is available at the end of the chapter

http://dx.doi.org/10.5772/102425

Abstract

Understanding the mechanisms regulating whole-body glucose homeostasis is important in order to understand what happens in a disease such as type 2 diabetes (T2D). Insulin resistance, inflammation, dysfunction of islet β-cells, and the presence of amyloid deposits in the pancreas are some of the major causes involved in the process of β-cell deterioration. The unique peptide constituent of amyloid deposits, human islet amyloid polypeptide (hIAPP), is capable of inducing endoplasmic reticulum (ER) stress and the resulting unfolded-protein response activation. Additionally, hIAPP has been shown to induce interleukin-1β expression, the main cytokine involved in inflammation and T2D causing inflammation and eventually, inducing apoptosis. Nevertheless, the mechanisms behind the process of hIAPP aggregation and amyloid formation are still unknown. In this chapter, we describe the different mechanisms by which hIAPP induces ER stress and inflammation. This should open the door for designing therapeutic interventions aimed at modulating the immune system and the ER stress response.

Keywords: Diabetes, pancreatic amyloid, inflammation, ER stress, IAPP, chaperones, diabetes

1. Introduction

Type 2 diabetes (T2D) is a chronic metabolic disease characterized by hyperglycemia resulting from defects in insulin secretion, insulin action, or both. The chronic hyperglycemia is associated with long-term damage, dysfunction and failure of different organs, especially the eyes, kidneys, nerves, heart and blood vessels. The genetic and molecular basis of the pathogenesis of T2D is not completely elucidated; however, a growing body of evidence has reported that the progression from normal to impaired blood glucose level regulation in individuals with T2D is mostly influenced by insulin resistance and β-cell dysfunction. During the last decade, the reduction in β-cell function has been attributed mostly to a decrease in β-cell mass; however, its precise role for the etiology of T2D remains controversial due to the lack of longitudinal studies. In spite of this, several studies in patients with T2D have shown a significant β-cell mass reduction ranging from 20 to 65% [1, 2]. Although, the reasons underlying this deficit are not clearly understood, some factors responsible for this decline have been suggested, for example, metabolic abnormalities (gluco- and lipotoxicity), hormonal changes (inadequate incretin secretion and action), aging, genetic abnormalities, etc. [3]. Additionally, a growing body of evidence has demonstrated the contribution of the hypersecretion of islet amyloid polypeptide (IAPP), together with amyloid deposition for the establishment of T2D.

The process of amyloid deposition is a remarkable physiopathological finding in individuals with T2D (**Figure 1**). The term amyloid emerged from the Latin word *amylum*, which means starch. For a long time, it was thought that these deposits were starch-like, but later it was discovered that they were actually a mass of proteins with a particular β-sheet structure. From that, pathologies with conformational changes in normally soluble proteins or peptides that result in the formation of intermolecular hydrogen bonds, β-sheet conformation, and fibril formation are namely conformational diseases [4]. Besides T2D, these conditions have been also implicated in different human disorders, including Alzheimer's disease (AD), Parkinson's disease, and Huntington's disease.

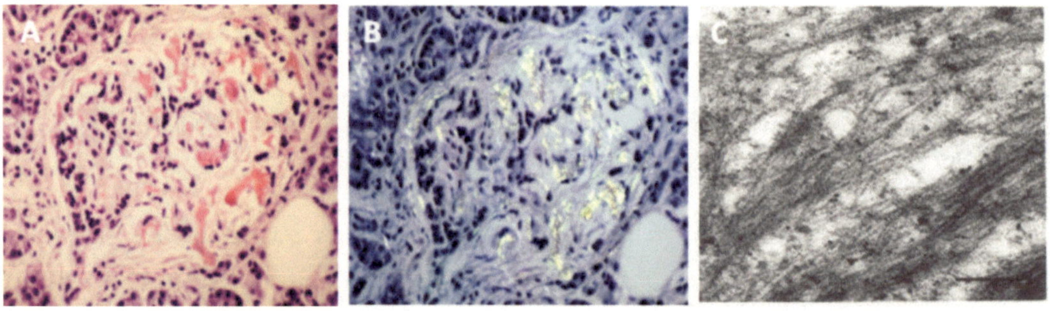

Figure 1. Amyloid deposits from cadaveric human pancreata. Amyloid deposits are observed in human pancreas by (A) hematoxylin/eosin staining, (B) Congo Red staining, or (C) electron microscopy, kindly provided by Anne Clark (unpublished data).

The contribution of IAPP in T2D is still controversial; several studies question whether amyloid deposition is a cause or a consequence of islet decline and whether it occurs intra- or extracellularly [5, 6]. However, numerous evidences correlate the role of IAPP with the severity of the disease. The facts indicate that amyloid deposits are seen in 90% of patients with T2D at autopsy and can possibly correspond to stages of the pathology [7, 8].

While IAPP and amyloid formation seem to have a substantial relation in T2D, it is unknown whether aggregation of IAPP plays any role in the development of type 1 diabetes (T1D). One can assume that during β-cell destruction, as in T2D, cells are exposed to high levels of IAPP. Indeed, children with new onset of T1D presented with high levels of IAPP [9]. Nevertheless, further studies need to be done in order to determine the importance of IAPP in the development of T1D.

2. IAPP and T2D

2.1. Islet amyloid polypeptide

Islet amyloid polypeptide or IAPP, also known as amylin, is a normal product of pancreatic β-cells. It is stored along with insulin in secretory granules and co-secreted in response to nutrient stimuli. This 37-amino acid peptide was identified in 1987, although the gene was isolated and characterized in 1989 [7]. Nishi et al. located it in chromosome 12, containing three exons and two introns that codified for an 89-amino acid precursor termed preproIAPP with an amino-terminal signal sequence. This signal peptide is then cleaved from the precursor to generate a 67-amino acid propeptide termed proIAPP. This peptide undergoes further translational modifications by the prohormone convertases, which include the formation of disulfide bridges between cysteine residues and an amidation of a C-terminal tyrosine. These prohormone convertases are as well responsible for proteolytic conversion of proinsulin to insulin, supporting the idea that the processing of proIAPP might also be impaired in T2D [10].

The function of IAPP has been suggested to be involved with glucose homeostasis. In general, this hormone inhibits gastric emptying and is important in controlling and delaying the rate of meal-derived glucose. It has also been shown to inhibit secretion of other pancreatic hormones, such as glucagon and somatostatin. Indeed, physiological concentrations of IAPP are responsible for the regulation of food intake and body weight. Several other effects have been described, including the regulation of renal filtration [11], calcium homeostasis [12], and vasodilatation [13]. Nevertheless, a critical role positions IAPP as the main responsible for the pathogenesis of T2D through formation of amyloid deposits and destruction of pancreatic β-cells.

Non-toxic bioactive variants of IAPP have been shown to be clinically important for the treatment of T1D, T2D, and obesity. For example, co-administration of modified non-toxic variants of IAPP and insulin helped normalization of oscillating glucose levels to a greater extent than insulin alone [14, 15]. Furthermore, combinations of IAPP and leptin have also been used for the treatment of obesity [16]. Nevertheless, aggregation, engineering, and solubility problems at physiological pHs have been affecting the different approaches.

2.2. Molecular mechanisms of IAPP aggregation and amyloid formation

Although there has been considerable progress, the exact mechanism of abnormal aggregation of IAPP is still largely unknown; however, several studies pointed the overproduction or mutations in IAPP as the main causes of amyloid formation. The role of overproduction of IAPP is associated with the increased secretory demand for insulin due to insulin resistance and increasing hyperglycemia [17]. Because IAPP and insulin are co-secreted in β-secretory granules, this increased production and secretion could result in accumulation and aggregation of IAPP. Many studies have reported that transgenic mice overexpressing hIAPP develop islet amyloid deposits [18, 19]. However, other studies contradicted this hypothesis, claiming that IAPP levels are several times higher than normally. To confirm these findings, Kahn et al. demonstrated that non-diabetic obese and/or insulin-resistant individuals with elevated IAPP levels do not develop amyloid deposits per se. However, in both cases, the presence of some factors, such as genetic predisposition, high fat diet, and obesity, might be critical for the development of extensive islet amyloid [18, 19].

Another possible mechanism for amyloid formation concerns the mutations in the IAPP gene or promoter regions, by producing more fibrillogenic forms [20]. For example, based on several studies, the S20G mutation in the IAPP gene appears to be associated with an early onset and more severe form of T2D [21].

In addition, the existence of hydrophobic amino acids in the mid-portion of IAPP could also be responsible for its propensity to aggregate into β-pleated sheets. Several algorithms, such as discrete molecular dynamics simulations [22] or specifically designed software such as TANGO [23–25], have been developed to identify the amyloidogenic regions of hIAPP. In this line, the residues at positions 20–29 of the polypeptide chain have been determined to be the amyloidogenic region of the peptide. Accordingly, the proline substitutions in the 24–29 regions of rodent IAPP are thought to prevent amyloid fibril formation completely [26]. Proline is known to be a β-sheet breaker, and a total inhibition of amyloid formation was seen when substitutions in the 20–29 wild-type area were performed [27]. Proteoglycans, the major components of the extracellular matrix, have been implicated with several pathologies, including AD and T2D, and have been associated with amyloid deposits in the human body [28]. In particular, together with IAPP, heparan sulfate proteoglycan perlecan is the main component of amyloid deposits in pancreatic islets. Several hypotheses indicate that the impaired processing of proIAPP may result in an elevated secretion of the IAPP precursor with a strong affinity for heparan sulfate proteoglycans, which could eventually result in a generation of a nucleus from amyloid formation [17, 18].

2.3. IAPP toxicity

Aggregated hIAPP has cytotoxic properties and is believed to be of critical importance for the progression in patients with T2D. Early studies have shown that the formation of islet amyloid is strongly associated with reduction of insulin secretion and with loss of approximately 50% of the β-cell mass [29, 30]. Human IAPP aggregation has been suggested to occur in a stepwise manner, with soluble monomeric hIAPP forming oligomeric structures, protofibrils, and eventually amyloid fibrils (**Figure 2**).

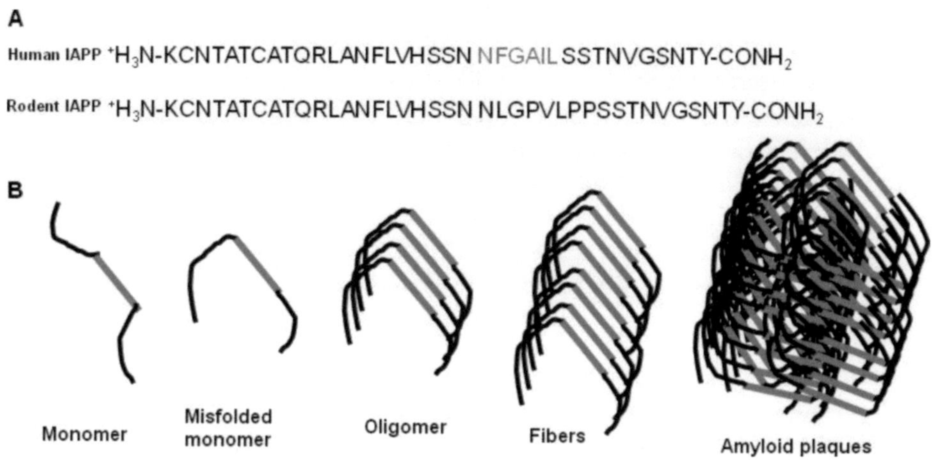

Figure 2. Proposed model of amyloid formation. (A) Primary sequences of human and murine islet amyloid polypeptide. Amyloidogenic region predicted by intrinsic propensities for aggregation is indicated in gray. Note the presence of proline residues in rodent IAPP sequence. (B) Folding or trafficking alterations can induce hIAPP misfolding leading to aggregation. Misfolded monomers aggregate to oligomers that eventually form the characteristic amyloid plaques from T2D.

Initially, there was general acceptance about the concept that the fibrillar forms of hIAPP are the toxic species [31]. Moreover, amyloid fibrils are less toxic than small oligomers formed by aggregates of IAPP. Studies have shown a strong correlation between islet amyloidosis and hIAPP cytotoxicity and eventually β-cell death. Yanker et al. have demonstrated that toxicity is mediated by IAPP fibrils by direct contact of fibrils with the cell surface causing DNA fragmentation, chromatin condensation, and protuberances in the plasma membrane leading to islet cell apoptosis [32]. The common feature for hIAPP fibrils lies on the classical cross β-structure, polymorphic, and typically unbranched [33]. Additionally, in vitro studies have provided evidences that synthetic hIAPP readily forms fibrils and amyloid deposits, which allowed studying the overall morphology and formation process [33, 34].

According to the structural information available for hIAPP fibrils and oligomers, it is clear that hIAPP as an amyloid protein has shown to be toxic through similar mechanisms as other amyloid proteins. One of the most widely accepted mechanisms refers to membrane interaction which leads to cell membrane permeabilization or disruptions [35]. Concerning hIAPP oligomers, the membrane leakage occurs via direct interaction and/or formation of ionic pores and depends on the lipid composition, peptide ratio, pH, and ionic strength. In the case of fibril formation, the damage in the membrane may happen through interaction of fibrils with specific channels located on the cell surface, such as potassium channels [36]. Moreover, oligomers of hIAPP have been shown to increase inflammation in β-cells via the inflammasome, a large group of intracellular multiprotein complexes that induce inflammation and play a central role in immunity [37].

Comparably, hIAPP can form oligomers and fibrils that contribute to islet inflammation. In this line, hIAPP oligomers and fibrils (but not rodent IAPP) have been shown to induce synthesis of interleukins and other inflammatory mediators by pancreatic islets that recruit and activate macrophages in vivo [38]. Further, endoplasmic reticulum (ER) stress has been proposed to be an important contributor to hIAPP-induced-β-cell death since exogenously added hIAPP has been confirmed to induce ER stress. Some reports showed that ER stress-mediated apoptosis is exacerbated in rodent β-cells expressing amyloidogenic isoforms of hIAPP, leading to a reduction of β-cell mass in hIAPP transgenic mice and rats [6, 39]. In addition, Casas et al. [40] demonstrated that extracellular hIAPP aggregation is associated with ER stress responses in mouse β-cells. Although the mechanism responsible for β-cell cytotoxicity during the process of hIAPP aggregation is still not well defined, a growing body of evidence firmly indicates that IAPP fibrils or oligomers have a crucial role in the progressive β-cell dysfunction in T2D.

Prevention of IAPP amyloid formation may represent a potential treatment for T2D. Thus, the use of several small-molecule inhibitors is being exploited. Several small inhibitory peptides [26, 41], natural polyphenols (such as resveratrol and epigallocatechin gallate; EGCG) [42, 43] or specific antibodies [44, 45] have been successfully used to validate the application of anti-amyloid compounds. For example, the peptide D-ANFLVH inhibited the formation of islet amyloid deposits and contributed to the preservation of β-cell area and improved glucose tolerance in mice [46]. These results validate the application of anti-amyloid compounds as therapeutic strategies to maintain β-cell function in patients with T2D.

3. The endoplasmic reticulum

3.1. Physiological role

Protein folding begins as the nascent polypeptide chain is co-translationally translocated through the ER membrane into the ER lumen. The unique environment of the ER lumen allows for both oxidative protein folding and post-translational modification such as glycosylation and disulfide bond formation, and accounts for approximately one-third of all proteins in eukaryotic cells. Since ER is mainly associated with protein synthesis, if the protein is not properly folded/maturated, it will remain in the ER and will eventually be degraded without reaching its normal cellular site of action [47]. This sophisticated supervision carried by the ER is regulated by sensitive quality control systems that can discriminate between the proper folded proteins from the misfolded ones. For example, folding chaperones consist of a considerable number of proteins that have the capacity to recognize properties common to non-native proteins, such as exposed hydrophobic areas and in most cases through the expenditure of ATP [48]. Thus, chaperones have the role of correctly folding and assembling secreted proteins, aiding oligomerization, and performing post-translational modifications [49]. The other quality control system is the ubiquitin-proteasome system (UPS) in which irreparably damaged proteins are identified and sorted for degradation. This system is responsible for the clearance of intracellular misfolded and aggregated proteins [50]. Many stimuli can disrupt this process, and its failure can give rise to the malfunctioning of living systems leading to the development of an increasing number of disorders, including Parkinson, AD, Huntington, and T2D [51].

3.2. ER stress and the unfolded protein response

Some situations (oxidative stress, energy deprivation, metabolic challenge, or inflammatory stimuli) can represent a major problem for the cell due to a probable production of unfolded or misfolded proteins. These physiological and pathological conditions may interfere with protein maturation and trafficking processes, leading to the accumulation of unfolded and/or misfolded proteins.

A complex homeostatic mechanism known as the unfolded protein response (UPR) has evolved linking the load of newly synthesized proteins with the capacity of the ER to mature them. The UPR works as a multifaceted strategy to protect the integrity of the ER and the associated functionality of the secretory pathway. In mammalians, the first response consists in attenuating the translation of most peptides, followed by an induction of ER chaperone translation that promotes the correct folding [52] and finally, the activation of the ER-associated degradation (ERAD), in which misfolded proteins are retrotranslocated from the ER lumen to the cytosol and degraded by the ubiquitin-proteasome [52, 53]. Conversely, if this mechanism of adaptation and survival fails to relieve ER stress, a continued accumulation of misfolded proteins takes place within the ER, and consequently UPR will generate pro-apoptotic signals to eliminate the diseased cell [52].

In mammals, the UPR consists of three main classes of proteins that act as sensors of ER stress: inositol-requiring enzyme 1 (IRE1), double-stranded RNA-activated 9 protein kinase RNA (PKR)-like ER kinase (PERK), and activating transcription factor 6 (ATF6) (**Figure 3**). Despite the difference, each of these proteins activates different signaling pathways and activates transcription factors that mediate the induction of several ER stress genes. IRE1 is considered a central regulator of the ER stress signaling and plays an important role in protein biosynthesis. Under non-stressed conditions, IRE1 remains in an inactive monomeric form. Upon accumulation of unfolded proteins, IRE1 is activated and released by the binding immunoglobulin protein or BiP, an endogenous chaperone located in the lumen of the ER that binds newly synthesized proteins and helps them through the process of folding and maturation. Subsequently, IRE1 activates a transcription factor named X-box-binding protein (XPB1), which once translocated into the nucleus initiates several transcriptional programs that upregulate UPR-associated genes. In a similar way, once chaperone BiP releases from its interaction with PERK, PERK is able to dimerize, promoting autophosphorylation and activation [54]. Once activated, PERK phosphorylates eukaryotic initiation factor 2a (elF2α), its only recognized target. Once activated, elF2α leads to a rapid reduction in the number of proteins entering the already overwhelmed ER [55]. However, in some circumstances, other transcription factors such as activating transcription factor 4 (ATF4) are translated and modulate the expression of C/EBP homologous protein (CHOP). CHOP acts by inducing apoptosis [56]. A major mediator of transcriptional induction by ER stress is the basic leucine zipper domain transcription factor ATF6. This protein is also regulated not only by BiP but also by intra- and inter-molecular disulfide bridges which are thought to keep ATF6 inactive [57, 58]. In response to ER stress, BiP is released from ATF6 and disulfide bonds are reduced, which eventually target the expression of transcription chaperones, upregulation of XBP1, and transcription of elements of the ERAD (**Figure 3**).

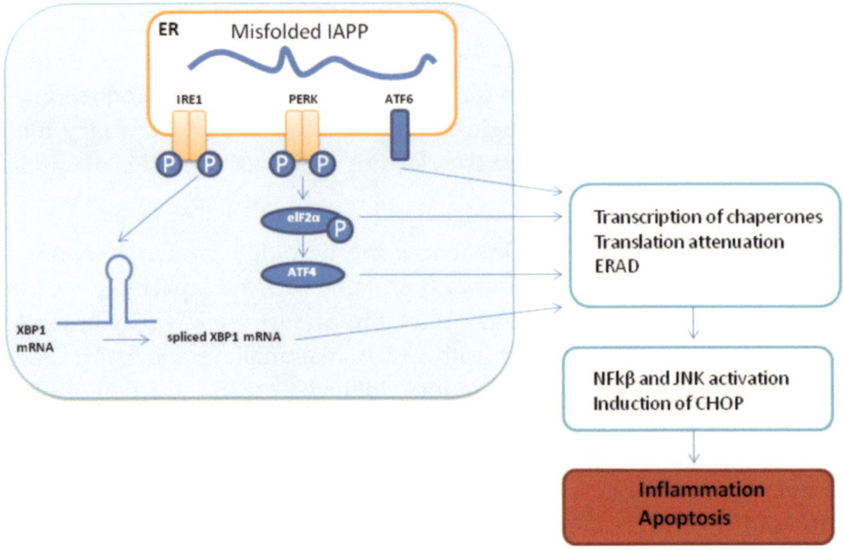

Figure 3. Branches of the UPR and inflammation signaling pathways. The three sensor-transducers of the UPR are inositol-requiring protein-1 (IRE-1), PERK, and ATF6. These three sensor-transducers determine the state of unfolded proteins in the ER lumen. If persistent, NF-κβ and JNK become activated, leading to inflammation and apoptosis.

3.3. Link between ER stress and apoptosis

A growing number of studies implicate ER stress with β-cell death during the evolution of T2D [59, 60]. Several physiological, environmental, and genetic factors can provoke alterations in ER homeostasis leading to a state of stress. Evidences suggest that a continuous increase in insulin biosynthesis might overwhelm the folding capacity of the ER, leading to a chronic state. As a consequence, the UPR signaling pathways are triggered with the objective of maintaining β-cell function and promoting β-cell survival. In general, cells have the capacity to adapt to substantial ER stress, but if the ER stress is too severe and long-standing, the UPR-mediated efforts ultimately fail and the apoptotic pathway is activated in order to protect the organism by eliminating damaged cells (**Figure 3**). At least, three parallel pathways are involved in the stress-mediated apoptosis: activation of CHOP (recognized as a key mediator of apoptosis in ER stress), activation of IRE1–JNK pathway, and activation of caspase 12 [61, 62]. β-Cell apoptosis is also observed in human pancreatic sections and post-mortem islet grafts in correlation with amyloid deposition levels [6, 63, 64].

As previously discussed, ER stress-mediated apoptosis is exacerbated in rodent β-cells expressing hIAPP in β-cells, leading to a reduction of β-cell mass [39]. In addition, extracellular hIAPP aggregation is associated with ER stress, contributing to β-cell apoptosis [40, 65]. Nevertheless, in a rat pancreatic β-cell line overexpressing hIAPP, the detection of toxic intracellular oligomers, which lead to defective insulin and IAPP secretion levels in response to glucose, did not change the expression of genes involved in ER stress and apoptosis was not induced [36]. These results agree with other findings with hIAPP transgenic mice, in which the authors demonstrated that amyloid formation was not associated with significant increases in the expression of ER stress markers [66]. As discussed elsewhere, the discrepancy in these results may be explained by differences in the ratio of IAPP and insulin produced by the different models used in vitro and in vivo, ranging from low to significantly high levels of hIAPP [67].

4. ER stress and inflammation

The three branches of UPR response can trigger inflammatory signals through different branches that converge in signaling pathways involving c-Jun N-terminal kinases (JNKs) and the nuclear factor κ-light-chain-enhancer of activated B cells (NF-κβ). JNK is considered to play an important role in ER stress in mouse models of diabetes. For instance, an increase in JNK activity promotes insulin resistance in peripheral tissues and in pancreatic β-cells without affecting cell viability [68]. The importance of the JNK pathway in stress has also been observed in knock-out (KO) mice where suppression of the JNK pathway protects β-cells against oxidative stress induction [69].

The pathway of the UPR involving IRE1 can, by different mechanisms, trigger an inflammatory signaling pathway through the activation of JNK (**Figure 3**) [70]. In addition, through multiple mechanisms, both the IRE1 and PERK pathways can also lead to the activation of the NF-κβ pathway, which also plays a critical role in the induction of multiple inflammatory mediators and has been implicated in insulin resistance [60, 71]. ATF6 has also been linked to inflammatory signaling. Genetic and pharmacological inhibition of ATF6 significantly suppresses NF-κβ activation, which can transcriptionally regulate many other inflammatory genes [72]. Activation of either JNK or NF-κB pathways in pancreatic β-cells has been reported to cause increased expression of proinflammatory molecules that can act as mediators, such as inflammatory interleukins 8 (IL8) and 6 (IL6), monocyte chemotactic protein-1 (MCP-1 or CCL2), and the cytotoxin tumor necrosis factor-α (TNF-α), which may have a detrimental effect on cell survival and function [73, 74]. Local chemokine and cytokine release can also contribute to the inflammatory milieu, attracting host macrophages to the pancreatic β-cells, which further propagate local inflammation [38, 75]. In addition, the NF-κβ pathway has been shown to activate the NLRP3 inflammasome, a multiprotein, cytosolic molecular platform that controls the activation of caspase 1, and the secretion of other proinflammatory cytokines such as interleukin-1β (IL-1β) and interleukin 18 (IL-18) in metabolic stress [76]. Inflammation induced by inflammasome-dependent proinflammatory cytokines may produce insulin resistance or cause the death of pancreatic β-cells, leading to the development of diabetes [37, 77].

NLRP3 inflammasome formation is reported to be induced by a variety of compounds, including hIAPP [37]. Oligomeric hIAPP has been shown to induce inflammasome activation and subsequent production of IL-1β. This is supported by observations with a transplantation model, in which hIAPP-expressing islets were transplanted into immunodeficient NOD-SCID mice treated with and without the IL-1β receptor agonist (IL1Ra) [38]. In this study, IL-1Ra was able to protect transplanted hIAPP-expressing islets from impaired glucose tolerance. Islet grafts expressing hIAPP contained amyloid deposits in close association with macrophages. Moreover, early aggregates of hIAPP induced production of inflammatory cytokines and chemokines, such as CCL2, TNF-α, IL-1α, IL-1β, chemokine (C–C motif) ligand 3 (CCL3), and the chemokine (C–X–C motif) ligand 1, 2, and 10 (CXCL1, CXCL2, and CXCL10, respectively) [38].

5. The role of hIAPP in ER stress, inflammation, and apoptosis

Multiple physiological and pathological conditions, including the accumulation of misfolded proteins, such as insulin or hIAPP, are responsible for the loss of ER homeostasis in β-cells [6, 60].

5.1. Exogenous hIAPP induces ER stress and apoptosis in vitro

Several approaches have been applied to study amyloid toxicity in vitro; synthetic peptides, corresponding to either fragments or the whole protein, have been useful attempt in defining the amyloidogenic pathology. Several studies have reported that amyloid peptide is proficient to induce cytotoxic cell death by external addition of synthetic hIAPP [32, 40, 78–80]. Although the precise mechanism by which IAPP aggregates lead to β-cell death is still unknown, it has been recognized that this aggregation is a concentration dependent on synthetic hIAPP in vitro. Bailey et al. suggested a progressive increase in cell toxicity according to the initial peptide concentration, as well as the time exposed for the process of IAPP fibrillation [34]. In addition, Casas et al. demonstrated that extracellular hIAPP aggregation is associated with ER stress responses in mouse β-cells, by an intracellular signaling that involves downstream inhibition of the ubiquitin-proteasome pathway, contributing to β-cell apoptosis [40]. In line with these studies, evidences have demonstrated that in aqueous solution, synthetic hIAPP spontaneously forms β-sheets and aggregates, whereas synthetic rat IAPP does not [81, 82], and the aggregation process seems to be extremely sensitive to amyloid concentrations [83].

5.2. Intracellular hIAPP

The mechanism by which amyloid oligomers and/or fibrils are formed within the β-cell is not completely understood. For that reason, many attempts to express this protein in various vectors and hosts have been designed. O'Brien et al. [84] were able to transfect fibroblast-like cell line (COS-1) cells with vectors expressing amyloidogenic IAPP; however, those cells containing amyloid fibrils were degenerated or dead when compared to rat IAPP overexpression. Years later, the same group, with the effort to understand the mechanism by which intracellular hIAPP causes cell death, demonstrated that in transfected COS-1 cells, the accumulation of hIAPP initiates a cascade of intracellular signaling events that trigger the apoptotic pathway [85]. However, this cell line was not expected to prevent such event due to the lack of the cellular machinery needed for the processing and trafficking of immature IAPP, such as secretory granules or the presence of prohormone convertases.

Recent studies have also reported successful cloning and expression of recombinant hIAPP in cultured mammalian cells. Several in vitro approaches allowed the successful expression, purification, and characterization of the amyloidogenicity and cytotoxicity of the human mature IAPP in sufficient amounts using, for example, the Lacl-T7 RNA polymerase-based heterologous expression system for *Escherichia coli*. This *E. coli* expression system has been shown to remove potential toxic proteins and, at the same time, generate high levels of recombinant proteins [86]. Likewise, other studies were capable to clone the hIAPP full-length peptide into not only COS-1 cells but also in rat insulinoma (RIN) and Chinese hamster ovary (CHO) cells [87]. Nevertheless, when studies were performed in INS1E cells, a β-cell line with all the equipment for the processing and regulation of IAPP, the expression of hIAPP by adenovirus has not resulted in cell death unless hIAPP was high enough to cause impaired proIAPP processing [88].

Furthermore, Soty et al. established an in vitro model in which INS1E cells were stably transfected with hIAPP cDNA under the cytomegalovirus promoter (CMV). Under hIAPP overexpression, these cells showed intracellular oligomers and a strong alteration of glucose-stimulated insulin and IAPP secretion. Moreover, inhibition of insulin and secretion of IAPP affected the activity of K_{ATP} channels, leading to an increased mitochondrial metabolism in order to counteract the secretory defects of the β-cells [36]. Nevertheless, hIAPP-expressing INS1E cells were able to completely restore insulin secretion and prevent ER stress upon treatment with molecular (BiP and protein disulfide isomerase; PDI) and chemical (taurour-sodeoxycholic acid; TUDCA and 4-phenylbutyrate; PBA) chaperones [89]. Amelioration of insulin secretion upon high glucose stimulation and prevention of β-cell death was further confirmed by the same group using hIAPP transgenic mouse islets and molecular chaperone PDI [90].

5.3. In vivo models of hIAPP overexpression

One of the most active research areas that have contributed substantially to our current understanding of the molecular basis in a multifactorial disease such as T2D is the creation and development of diverse animal models. Nowadays, in vivo studies of human pancreas morphology are not possible by obvious ethical considerations, and the collective human material comes from either autopsy or surgical resection from pancreatic cancer. It is interesting that apart from humans, the only species capable of spontaneously developing T2D are non-human primates and cats; nevertheless, besides the cost of working with such big species, these models not always progress toward T2D, making the use of these models not optimal for research [91]. Studies performed with rodent models of diabetes are then greatly useful and advantageous, especially regarding islet amyloidosis studies. As previously mentioned, unlike the human IAPP, the rodent IAPP is not amyloidogenic due to the proline substitutions in the 20–29 amino acid region. This lack of amyloid development in these models makes impossible to assess the role of IAPP aggregation in islet physiology. Since only a limited number of species spontaneously form islet amyloid, several groups have developed transgenic mice strains choosing hIAPP as a model for islet amyloidogenesis [91].

Nonetheless, some reports showed that the mere hIAPP overproduction did not lead to amyloid formation or deposition despite elevated plasma concentration of hIAPP. Thus, other factors beyond overexpression had to be involved in the mechanism of islet amyloid formation since these mice were normoglycemic and normoinsulinemic (94–96). Islet amyloid was reported in transgenic mice fed a diet high in fat. Verchere et al. [18] have shown that approximately 80% of male transgenic mice (<13 months old) presented amyloid deposits and were always associated with severe hyperglycemia. In the case of hemizygous transgenic mice for hIAPP, the treatment with growth hormone or dexamethasone induced small intra- and extracellular amyloid deposits [92].

Another strategy used to overexpress hIAPP was to cross-bread hIAPP mice onto a mouse with obese background (ob/ob) [19] or obese Agouti viable yellow (Avy/Agouti) [93]. These mice developed amyloid formation and loss of β-cells, which was associated with progression of diabetes (**Figure 4**).

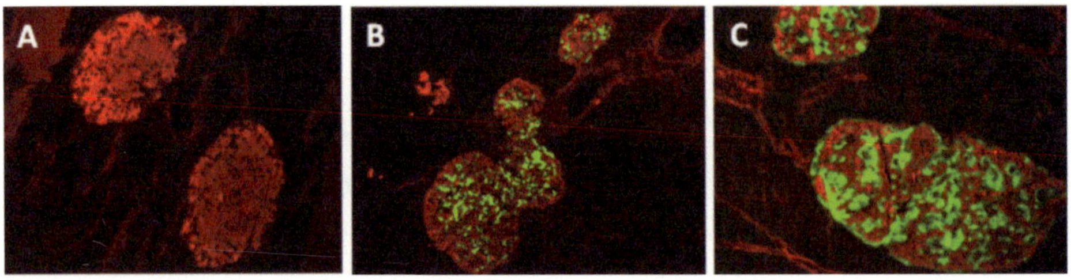

Figure 4. Amyloid formation in hIAPP transgenic mouse islets in obese Agouti yellow mice. Amyloid staining of hIAPP Tg mice in (A) FVB background, Avy/Agouti background at (B) 16 weeks of age and (C) 22 weeks of age. Note the presence of amyloid deposits in Avy/Agouti background as shown by Thioflavin S staining (unpublished data).

Moreover, it was found that female transgenic mice do not increase the occurrence of amyloid when oophorectomized, suggesting a protective role of ovarian hormones in islet amyloidosis. In recent years, Butler et al. showed that transgenic β-cell expression of human proIAPP in rats (HIP rats) that are homozygous for hIAPP develop diabetes within 5-10 months, together with the presence of extracellular amyloid, decreased β-cell mass, and increased β-cell apoptosis [94]. In addition, the loss of approximately 60% of β-cell mass at diabetes onset is comparable to the loss observed in humans with T2D [1].

In conclusion, with a variety of transgenic hIAPP models, it has been possible to clearly highlight that the process of islet amyloid formation is a complex event associated with a great number of factors considered important in the pathogenesis of T2D.

Acknowledgements

This work was supported by grants PI11/00679 and PI14/00447, integrated in the Plan Estatal I+D+I 2013-2016, and co-financed by the ISCIII-Subdirección General de Evaluación y Fomento de la investigación el Fondo Europeo de Desarrollo Regional (FEDER), by Centro de Investigación Biomédica en Red de Diabetes y Enfermedades Metabólicas Asociadas (CIBERDEM) and with the support of project number 2014_SGR_520 of the Department of Universities, Research and Information Society of the Government of Catalonia.

Author details

Joel Montane[1,2] and Anna Novials[1,2*]

*Address all correspondence to: anovials@clinic.ub.es

1 The August Pi i Sunyer Biomedical Research Institute (IDIBAPS), Barcelona, Spain

2 Biomedical Research Centre in Diabetes and Associated Metabolic Disorders (CIBER-DEM), Barcelona, Spain

References

[1] Butler AE, Janson J, Bonner-Weir S, Ritzel R, Rizza RA, Butler PC. Beta-cell deficit and increased beta-cell apoptosis in humans with type 2 diabetes. Diabetes. 2003;52: 102–110. doi:10.2337/diabetes.52.1.102

[2] Henquin JC, Rahier J. Pancreatic alpha cell mass in European subjects with type 2 diabetes. Diabetologia. 2011;54: 1720–1725. doi:10.1007/s00125-011-2118-4

[3] Vaag a, Henriksen JE, Madsbad S, Holm N, Beck-Nielsen H. Insulin secretion, insulin action, and hepatic glucose production in identical twins discordant for non-insulin-dependent diabetes mellitus. J Clin Invest. 1995;95: 690–698. doi:10.1172/JCI117715

[4] Carrell RW, Lomas DA. Conformational disease. Lancet. 1997;Jul 12;350(9071):134–138. doi:10.1016/S0140-6736(97)02073-4

[5] Zraika S, Hull RL, Verchere CB, Clark A, Potter KJ, Fraser PE, et al. Toxic oligomers and islet beta cell death: guilty by association or convicted by circumstantial evidence? Diabetologia. 2010 Jun;53(6):1046–1056. doi:10.1007/s00125-010-1671-6

[6] Montane J, Klimek-Abercrombie A, Potter KJ, Westwell-Roper C, Bruce Verchere C. Metabolic stress, IAPP and islet amyloid. Diabetes Obes Metab. 2012;Oct;14 Suppl 3:68–77. doi:10.1111/j.1463-1326.2012.01657.x

[7] Westermark P, Wernstedt C, Wilander E, Sletten K. A novel peptide in the calcitonin gene related peptide family as an amyloid fibril protein in the endocrine pancreas. Biochem Biophys Res Commun. Diabetes Metab Syndr Obes. 2014 Feb 1986;140: 827–831.

[8] Marzban L, Trigo-Gonzalez G, Verchere CB. Processing of pro-islet amyloid polypeptide in the constitutive and regulated secretory pathways of beta cells. Mol Endocrinol. 2005;19: 2154–2163. doi:10.1210/me.2004-0407

[9] Paulsson JF, Ludvigsson J, Carlsson A, Casas R, Forsander G, Ivarsson SA, et al. High plasma levels of islet amyloid polypeptide in young with new-onset of type 1 diabetes mellitus. PLoS One. 2014 Mar 26;9(3):e93053. doi:10.1371/journal.pone.0093053

[10] Higham CE, Hull RL, Lawrie L, Shennan KIJ, Morris JF, Birch NP, et al. Processing of synthetic pro-islet amyloid polypeptide (proIAPP) "amylin" by recombinant prohormone convertase enzymes, PC2 and PC3, in vitro. Eur J Biochem. 2000;267: 4998–5004. doi:10.1046/j.1432-1327.2000.01548.x

[11] Harris PJ, Cooper ME, Hiranyachattada S, Berka JL, Kelly DJ, Nobes M, et al. Amylin stimulates proximal tubular sodium transport and cell proliferation in the rat kidney. Am J Physiol Ren Physiol. 1997;272: F13–F21.

[12] Dacquin R, Davey RA, Laplace C, Levasseur R, Morris HA, Goldring SR, et al. Amylin inhibits bone resorption while the calcitonin receptor controls bone formation in vivo. J Cell Biol. 2004;164: 509–514. doi:10.1083/jcb.200312135

[13] Chin SY, Hall JM, Brain SD, Morton IK. Vasodilator responses to calcitonin gene-related peptide (CGRP) and amylin in the rat isolated perfused kidney are mediated via CGRP1 receptors. J Pharmacol Exp Ther. 1994;269: 989–992.

[14] Ratner RE, Dickey R, Fineman M, Maggs DG, Shen L, Strobel S a, et al. Amylin replacement with pramlintide as an adjunct to insulin therapy improves long-term glycaemic and weight control in type 1 diabetes mellitus: a 1-year, randomized controlled trial. Diabet Med. 2004;21: 1204–1212. doi:10.1111/j.1464-5491.2004.01319.x

[15] Lebovitz HE. Adjunct therapy for type 1 diabetes mellitus. Nat Rev Endocrinol. 2010;6: 326–34. doi:10.1038/nrendo.2010.49

[16] Roth JD, Roland BL, Cole RL, Trevaskis JL, Weyer C, Koda JE, et al. Leptin responsiveness restored by amylin agonism in diet-induced obesity: evidence from nonclinical and clinical studies. Proc Natl Acad Sci USA. 2008;105: 7257–7262. doi:10.1073/pnas.0706473105

[17] Marzban L, Park K, Verchere CB. Islet amyloid polypeptide and type 2 diabetes. Exp Gerontol. 2003;Apr;38(4):347–351. doi:10.1016/S0531-5565(03)00004-4

[18] Verchere CB, D'Alessio D a, Palmiter RD, Weir GC, Bonner-Weir S, Baskin DG, et al. Islet amyloid formation associated with hyperglycemia in transgenic mice with pancreatic beta cell expression of human islet amyloid polypeptide. Proc Natl Acad Sci USA. 1996;93: 3492–3496. doi:10.1073/pnas.93.8.3492

[19] Höppener JWM, Jacobs HM, Wierup N, Sotthewes G, Sprong M, de Vos P, et al. Human islet amyloid polypeptide transgenic mice: in vivo and ex vivo models for the role of

hIAPP in type 2 diabetes mellitus. Exp Diabetes Res. 2008;2008: 697035. doi: 10.1155/2008/697035

[20] Novials a, Mato E, Lucas M, Franco C, Rivas M, Santisteban P, et al. Mutation at position-132 in the islet amyloid polypeptide (IAPP) gene promoter enhances basal transcriptional activity through a new CRE-like binding site. Diabetologia. 2004;47: 1167–1174. doi:10.1007/s00125-004-1439-y

[21] Sakagashira S, Hiddinga HJ, Tateishi K, Sanke T, Hanabusa T, Nanjo K, et al. S20G mutant amylin exhibits increased in vitro amyloidogenicity and increased intracellular cytotoxicity compared to wild-type amylin. Am J Pathol. 2000;157: 2101–2109. doi: 10.1016/S0002-9440(10)64848-1

[22] Nedumpully-Govindan P, Ding F. Inhibition of IAPP aggregation by insulin depends on the insulin oligomeric state regulated by zinc ion concentration. Sci Rep. 2015;5: 8240. doi:10.1038/srep08240

[23] Fernandez-Escamilla A-M, Rousseau F, Schymkowitz J, Serrano L. Prediction of sequence-dependent and mutational effects on the aggregation of peptides and proteins. Nat Biotechnol. 2004;22: 1302–1306. doi:10.1038/nbt1012

[24] Linding R, Schymkowitz JWH, Rousseau F, Diella F, Serrano L. A comparative study of the relationship between protein structure and beta-aggregation in globular and intrinsically disordered proteins. J Mol Biol. 2004;342: 345–353. doi:10.1016/j.jmb.2004.06.088

[25] Fox A, Snollaerts T, Errecart Casanova C, Calciano A, Nogaj LA, Moffet DA. Selection for nonamyloidogenic mutants of islet amyloid polypeptide (IAPP) identifies an extended region for amyloidogenicity. Biochemistry. 2010;49: 7783–7789. doi:10.1021/bi100337p

[26] Hull RL, Westermark GT, Westermark P, Kahn SE. Islet amyloid: a critical entity in the pathogenesis of type 2 diabetes. J Clin Endocrinol Metab. 2004;89: 3629–3643. doi: 10.1210/jc.2004-0405

[27] Moriarty DF, Raleigh DP. Effects of sequential proline substitutions on amyloid formation by human amylin 20-29. Biochemistry. 1999;38: 1811–1818. doi:10.1021/bi981658g

[28] Van Horssen J, Wesseling P, Van Den Heuvel LPWJ, De Waal RMW, Verbeek MM. Heparan sulphate proteoglycans in Alzheimer's disease and amyloid-related disorders. Lancet Neurol. 2003;Aug;2(8):482–492. doi:10.1016/S1474-4422(03)00484-8

[29] Clark A, Wells CA, Buley ID, Cruickshank JK, Vanhegan RI, Matthews DR, et al. Islet amyloid, increased A-cells, reduced B-cells and exocrine fibrosis: quantitative changes in the pancreas in type 2 diabetes. Diabetes Res. 1988;9: 151–159.

[30] Howard Jr. CF. Longitudinal studies on the development of diabetes in individual Macaca nigra. Diabetologia. 1986;29: 301–306.

[31] Green JD, Goldsbury C, Kistler J, Cooper GJS, Aebi U. Human amylin oligomer growth and fibril elongation define two distinct phases in amyloid formation. J Biol Chem. 2004;279: 12206–12212. doi:10.1074/jbc.M312452200

[32] Lorenzo a, Razzaboni B, Weir GC, Yankner B a. Pancreatic islet cell toxicity of amylin associated with type-2 diabetes mellitus. Nature. 1994;368: 756–760. doi: 10.1038/368756a0

[33] Makin OS, Serpell LC. Structural characterisation of islet amyloid polypeptide fibrils. J Mol Biol. 2004;335: 1279–1288. doi:10.1016/j.jmb.2003.11.048

[34] Bailey J, Potter KJ, Verchere CB, Edelstein-Keshet L, Coombs D. Reverse engineering an amyloid aggregation pathway with dimensional analysis and scaling. Phys Biol. 2011;Dec;8(6) 066009. doi:10.1088/1478-3975/8/6/066009

[35] Abedini A, Schmidt AM. Mechanisms of islet amyloidosis toxicity in type 2 diabetes. FEBS Lett. 2013;Apr 17;587(8):1119–1127. doi:10.1016/j.febslet.2013.01.017

[36] Soty M, Visa M, Soriano S, Carmona MDC, Nadal Á, Novials A. Involvement of ATP-sensitive potassium (K(ATP)) channels in the loss of beta-cell function induced by human islet amyloid polypeptide. J Biol Chem. 2011;286: 40857–40866. doi:10.1074/jbc.M111.232801

[37] Masters SL, Dunne A, Subramanian SL, Hull RL, Tannahill GM, Sharp FA, et al. Activation of the NLRP3 inflammasome by islet amyloid polypeptide provides a mechanism for enhanced IL-1β in type 2 diabetes. Nat Immunol. 2010;11: 897–904. doi: 10.1038/ni.1935

[38] Westwell-Roper C, Dai DL, Soukhatcheva G, Potter KJ, van Rooijen N, Ehses JA, et al. IL-1 Blockade attenuates islet amyloid polypeptide-induced proinflammatory cytokine release and pancreaticislet graft dysfunction. J Immunol. 2011;187: 2755–2765. doi: 10.4049/jimmunol.1002854

[39] Huang CJ, Lin CY, Haataja L, Gurlo T, Butler AE, Rizza RA, et al. High expression rates of human islet amyloid polypeptide induce endoplasmic reticulum stress mediated beta-cell apoptosis, a characteristic of humans with type 2 but not type 1 diabetes. Diabetes. 2007;56: 2016–2027. doi:10.2337/db07-0197

[40] Casas S, Gomis R, Gribble FM, Altirriba J, Knuutila S, Novials A. Impairment of the ubiquitin-proteasome pathway is a downstream endoplasmic reticulum stress response induced by extracellular human islet amyloid polypeptide and contributes to pancreatic beta-cell apoptosis. Diabetes. 2007;56: 2284–2294. doi:10.2337/db07-0178

[41] Potter KJ, Scrocchi LA, Warnock GL, Ao Z, Younker MA, Rosenberg L, et al. Amyloid inhibitors enhance survival of cultured human islets. Biochim Biophys Acta Gen Subj. 2009;1790: 566–574. doi:10.1016/j.bbagen.2009.02.013

[42] Feng Y, Wang X ping, Yang S gao, Wang Y jiong, Zhang X, Du X ting, et al. Resveratrol inhibits beta-amyloid oligomeric cytotoxicity but does not prevent oligomer formation. Neurotoxicology. 2009;30: 986–995. doi:10.1016/j.neuro.2009.08.013

[43] Meng F, Abedini A, Plesner A, Verchere CB, Raleigh DP. The Flavanol (-)-epigallocatechin 3-gallate inhibits amyloid formation by islet amyloid polypeptide, disaggregates amyloid fibrils, and protects cultured cells against IAPP-induced toxicity. Biochemistry. 2010;49: 8127–8133. doi:10.1021/bi100939a

[44] La Porte SL, Bollini SS, Lanz TA, Abdiche YN, Rusnak AS, Ho WH, et al. Structural basis of C-terminal β-Amyloid peptide binding by the antibody ponezumab for the treatment of Alzheimer's disease. J Mol Biol. 2012;421: 525–536. doi:10.1016/j.jmb.2011.11.047

[45] Cheng B, Gong H, Xiao H, Petersen RB, Zheng L, Huang K. Inhibiting toxic aggregation of amyloidogenic proteins: a therapeutic strategy for protein misfolding diseases. Biochim Biophys Acta. 2013;Oct;1830(10): 4860–4871. doi:10.1016/j.bbagen.2013.06.029

[46] N. Wijesekara, R. Ahrens, L. Wu, K. Ha, Y. Liu MBW andP. EF. Islet amyloid inhibitors improve glucose homeostasis in a transgenic mouse model of type 2 diabetesle. Diabetes Obes Metab. 2015;17: 1003–1006.

[47] Sommer T, Wolf DH. Endoplasmic reticulum degradation: reverse protein flow of no return. FASEB J. 1997;11: 1227–1233. doi:0892-6638/97/0011-1227

[48] Bukau B, Horwich AL. The Hsp70 and Hsp60 chaperone machines. Cell. 1998;Feb 6;92(3):351–366. doi:10.1016/S0092-8674(00)80928-9

[49] Nishikawa SI, Brodsky JL, Nakatsukasa K. Roles of molecular chaperones in endoplasmic reticulum (ER) quality control and ER-associated degradation (ERAD). J. Biochem. 2005;May;137(5):551–555. doi:10.1093/jb/mvi068

[50] Hatahet F, Ruddock LW. Protein disulfide isomerase: a critical evaluation of its function in disulfide bond formation. Antioxid Redox Signal. 2009;11: 2807–2850. doi:10.1089/ars.2009.2466

[51] Dobson CM. Protein folding and disease: a view from the first Horizon Symposium. Nat Rev Drug Discovery. 2003;Feb;2(2):154–160. doi:10.1038/nrd1013

[52] Rajan SS, Srinivasan V, Balasubramanyam M, Tatu U. Endoplasmic reticulum (ER) stress & diabetes. Indian J Med Res. 2007;Mar;125(3):411–424. doi:10.1007/s12291-010-0022-1

[53] Meusser B, Hirsch C, Jarosch E, Sommer T. ERAD: the long road to destruction. Nat Cell Biol. 2005;7: 766–772. doi:10.1038/ncb0805-766

[54] Bertolotti A, Zhang Y, Hendershot LM, Harding HP, Ron D. Dynamic interaction of BiP and ER stress transducers in the unfolded-protein response. Nat Cell Biol. 2000;2: 326–332.

[55] Hetz C, Chevet E, Harding HP. Targeting the unfolded protein response in disease. Nat Rev Drug Discov. 2013;12: 703–19. doi:10.1038/nrd3976

[56] Eizirik DL, Cardozo AK, Cnop M. The role for endoplasmic reticulum stress in diabetes mellitus. Endocr Rev. 2008;Feb;29(1):42–61. doi:10.1210/er.2007-0015

[57] Nadanaka S, Okada T, Yoshida H, Mori K. Role of disulfide bridges formed in the luminal domain of ATF6 in sensing endoplasmic reticulum stress. Mol Cell Biol. 2007;27: 1027–1043. doi:10.1128/MCB.00408-06

[58] Shen J, Chen X, Hendershot L, Prywes R. ER stress regulation of ATF6 localization by dissociation of BiP/GRP78 binding and unmasking of Golgi localization signals. Dev Cell. 2002;3: 99–111. doi:10.1016/S1534-5807(02)00203-4

[59] Oslowski CM, Hara T, O'Sullivan-Murphy B, Kanekura K, Lu S, Hara M, et al. Thioredoxin-interacting protein mediates ER stress-induced β cell death through initiation of the inflammasome. Cell Metab. 2012;16: 265–273. doi:10.1016/j.cmet.2012.07.005

[60] Hotamisligil GS. Endoplasmic reticulum stress and the inflammatory basis of metabolic disease. Cell. 2010;Mar 19;140(6):900–917. doi:10.1016/j.cell.2010.02.034

[61] Oyadomari S, Mori M. Roles of CHOP/GADD153 in endoplasmic reticulum stress. Cell Death Differ. 2004;11: 381–389. doi:10.1038/sj.cdd.4401373

[62] Morishima N, Nakanishi K, Takenouchi H, Shibata T, Yasuhiko Y. An endoplasmic reticulum stress-specific caspase cascade in apoptosis. Cytochrome c-independent activation of caspase-9 by caspase-12. J Biol Chem. 2002;277: 34287–34294. doi:10.1074/jbc.M204973200

[63] Potter KJ, Abedini A, Marek P, Klimek AM, Butterworth S, Driscoll M, et al. Islet amyloid deposition limits the viability of human islet grafts but not porcine islet grafts. Proc Natl Acad Sci USA. 2010;107: 4305–4310. doi:10.1073/pnas.0909024107

[64] Andersson A, Bohman S, Borg LA, Paulsson JF, Schultz SW, Westermark GT, et al. Amyloid deposition in transplanted human pancreatic islets: a conceivable cause of their long-term failure. Exp Diabetes Res. 2008;2008: 562985. doi:10.1155/2008/562985

[65] Casas S, Novials A, Reimann F, Gomis R, Gribble FM. Calcium elevation in mouse pancreatic beta cells evoked by extracellular human islet amyloid polypeptide involves activation of the mechanosensitive ion channel TRPV4. Diabetologia. 2008;51: 2252–2262. doi:10.1007/s00125-008-1111-z

[66] Hull RL, Zraika S, Udayasankar J, Aston-Mourney K, Subramanian SL, Kahn SE. Amyloid formation in human IAPP transgenic mouse islets and pancreas, and human pancreas, is not associated with endoplasmic reticulum stress. Diabetologia. 2009;52: 1102–1111. doi:10.1007/s00125-009-1329-4

[67] Montane J, Cadavez L, Novials A. Stress and the inflammatory process: a major cause of pancreatic cell death in type 2 diabetes. Diabetes Metab Syndr Obes. 2014;Feb 3;7:25–34. doi:10.2147/DMSO.S37649

[68] Lanuza-Masdeu J, Isabel Arévalo M, Vila C, Barberà A, Gomis R, Caelles C. In vivo jnk activation in pancreatic β-cells leads to glucose intolerance caused by insulin resistance in pancreas. Diabetes. 2013;62: 2308–2317. doi:10.2337/db12-1097

[69] Kaneto H, Matsuoka T, Nakatani Y, Kawamori D, Matsuhisa M, Yamasaki Y. Oxidative stress and the JNK pathway in diabetes. Curr Diabetes Rev. 2005;1: 65–72. doi:10.2174/1573399052952613

[70] Urano F, Wang X, Bertolotti a, Zhang Y, Chung P, Harding HP, et al. Coupling of stress in the ER to activation of JNK protein kinases by transmembrane protein kinase IRE1. Science. 2000;287: 664–666. doi:10.1126/science.287.5453.664

[71] Deng J, Lu PD, Zhang Y, Scheuner D, Kaufman RJ, Sonenberg N, et al. Translational repression mediates activation of nuclear factor kappa B by phosphorylated translation initiation factor 2. Mol Cell Biol. 2004;24: 10161–10168. doi:10.1128/MCB.24.23.10161-10168.2004

[72] Yamazaki H, Hiramatsu N, Hayakawa K, Tagawa Y, Okamura M, Ogata R, et al. Activation of the Akt-NF-kappaB pathway by subtilase cytotoxin through the ATF6 branch of the unfolded protein response. J Immunol. 2009;183: 1480–1487. doi:10.4049/jimmunol.0900017

[73] Marselli L, Dotta F, Piro S, Santangelo C, Masini M, Lupi R, et al. Th2 cytokines have a partial, direct protective effect on the function and survival of isolated human islets exposed to combined proinflammatory and Th1 cytokines. J Clin Endocrinol Metab. 2001;86: 4974–4978. doi:10.1210/jc.86.10.4974

[74] Wu JJ, Chen X, Cao XC, Baker MS, Kaufman DB. Cytokine-induced metabolic dysfunction of MIN6 beta cells is nitric oxide independent. J Surg Res. 2001;101: 190–195. doi:10.1006/jsre.2001.6285

[75] Ehses JA, Perren A, Eppler E, Ribaux P, Pospisilik JA, Maor-Cahn R, et al. Increased number of islet-associated macrophages in type 2 diabetes. Diabetes. 2007;56: 2356–2370. doi:10.2337/db06-1650

[76] Zhou R, Yazdi AS, Menu P, Tschopp J. A role for mitochondria in NLRP3 inflammasome activation. Nature. 2011;469: 221–225. doi:10.1038/nature09663

[77] Montane J. Stress and the inflammatory process: a major cause of pancreatic cell death in type PubMed Commons. Diabetes Metab Syndr Obes. 2014;Feb 3;7:25–34. 24520198. doi: 10.2147/DMSO.S37649

[78] Zhang S, Liu J, MacGibbon G, Dragunow M, Cooper GJS. Increased expression and activation of c-Jun contributes to human amylin-induced apoptosis in pancreatic islet β-cells. J Mol Biol. 2002;324: 271–285. doi:10.1016/S0022-2836(02)01044-6

[79] Saafi EL, Konarkowska B, Zhang S, Kistler J, Cooper GJ. Ultrastructural evidence that apoptosis is the mechanism by which human amylin evokes death in RINm5F pancreatic islet beta-cells. Cell Biol Int. 2001;25: 339–50. doi:10.1006/cbir.2000.0643

[80] Macgibbon GA, Cooper GJS, Dragunow M. Acute application of human amylin, unlike beta-amyloid peptides, kills undifferentiated pc12 cells by apoptosis. Neuroreport. 1997;8: 3945–3949.

[81] Konarkowska B, Aitken JF, Kistler J, Zhang S, Cooper GJS. The aggregation potential of human amylin determines its cytotoxicity towards islet◎beta-cells. FEBS J. 2006;273: 3614–3624. doi:10.1111/j.1742-4658.2006.05367.x

[82] Goldsbury C, Goldie K, Pellaud J, Seelig J, Frey P, Müller SA, et al. Amyloid fibril formation from full-length and fragments of amylin. J Struct Biol. 2000;130: 352–362. doi:10.1006/jsbi.2000.4268

[83] Aitken JF, Loomes KM, Scott DW, Reddy S, Phillips ARJ, Prijic G, et al. Tetracycline treatment retards the onset and slows the progression of diabetes in human amylin/islet amyloid polypeptide transgenic mice. Diabetes. 2010;59: 161–171. doi:10.2337/db09-0548

[84] O'Brien TD, Butler PC, Kreutter DK, Kane LA, Eberhardt NL. Human islet amyloid polypeptide expression in COS-1 cells. A model of intracellular amyloidogenesis. Am J Pathol. 1995;147: 609–616.

[85] Hiddinga HJ, Eberhardt NL. Intracellular amyloidogenesis by human islet amyloid polypeptide induces apoptosis in COS-1 cells. Am J Pathol. 1999;154: 1077–1088. doi:10.1016/S0002-9440(10)65360-6

[86] Lopest DHJ, Colin C, Degaki TL, De Sousa AC V, Vieira MNN, Sebollela A, et al. Amyloidogenicity and cytotoxicity of recombinant mature human islet amyloid polypeptide (rhIAPP). J Biol Chem. 2004;279: 42803–42810. doi:10.1074/jbc.M406108200

[87] Jyoti S, Satendra S, Sushma S, Anjana T, Shashi S. Antistressor activity of *Ocimum sanctum* (Tulsi) against experimentally induced oxidative stress in rabbits. Methods Find Exp Clin Pharmacol. 2007;29: 411–416. doi:1118135 [pii]\r10.1358/mf.2007.29.6.1118135

[88] Marzban L, Rhodes CJ, Steiner DF, Haataja L, Halban PA, Verchere CB. Impaired NH2-terminal processing of human proislet amyloid polypeptide by the prohormone convertase PC2 leads to amyloid formation and cell death. Diabetes. 2006;55: 2192–2201. doi:10.2337/db05-1566

[89] Cadavez L, Montane J, Alcarraz-Vizán G, Visa M, Vidal-Fàbrega L, Servitja JM, et al. Chaperones ameliorate beta cell dysfunction associated with human islet amyloid polypeptide overexpression. PLoS One. 2014;9: 1–11. doi:10.1371/journal.pone.0101797

[90] Montane J, de Pablo S, Obach M, Cadavez L, Castaño C, Alcarraz-Vizán G, et al. Protein disulfide isomerase ameliorates β-cell dysfunction in pancreatic islets overexpressing

human islet amyloid polypeptide. Mol Cell Endocrinol. 2016;420: 57–65. doi:10.1016/j.mce.2015.11.018

[91] Matveyenko A V, Butler PC. Islet amyloid polypeptide (IAPP) transgenic rodents as models for type 2 diabetes. ILAR J. 2006;47: 225–233.

[92] Couce M, Kane L a, O'Brien TD, Charlesworth J, Soeller W, McNeish J, et al. Treatment with growth hormone and dexamethasone in mice transgenic for human islet amyloid polypeptide causes islet amyloidosis and beta-cell dysfunction. Diabetes. 1996;45: 1094–1101.

[93] Soeller WC, Janson J, Hart SE, Parker JC, Carty MD, Stevenson RW, et al. Islet amyloid-associated diabetes in obese A(vy)/a mice expressing human islet amyloid polypeptide. Diabetes. 1998;47: 743–750. doi:10.2337/diabetes.47.5.743

[94] Butler AE, Jang J, Gurlo T, Carty MD, Soeller WC, Butler PC. Diabetes due to a progressive defect in β-cell mass in rats transgenic for human islet amyloid polypeptide (HIP rat): a new model for type 2 diabetes. Diabetes. 2004;53: 1509–1516. doi:10.2337/diabetes.53.6.1509

Chapter 11

Proteasome Inhibitors to Treat AL Amyloidosis

James J. Driscoll and Saulius Girnius

Additional information is available at the end of the chapter

http://dx.doi.org/10.5772/63467

Abstract

Amyloidoses represent a highly heterogeneous group of diseases characterized by the abnormal production and accumulation of abnormal, insoluble amyloid proteins in various tissues leading to organ dysfunction. Light-chain (AL) amyloidosis is the most common form of systemic amyloidosis and is characterized by extracellular deposition of pathologic insoluble fibrillar proteins in organs and tissues. Primary systemic AL amyloidosis (AL) arises from the production of abnormal immunoglobulins (Igs) by clonal plasma cells, such as those associated with the plasma cell dyscrasia multiple myeloma (MM). AL amyloidosis can affect a wide range of organs, most commonly the kidneys, and consequently presents with a range of symptoms. Currently, the most effective treatment is autologous bone marrow transplants with stem cell rescue, but many patients are too weak to tolerate this approach and are ineligible. Novel therapeutic strategies recently used include forms of chemotherapy and targeted therapy similar to those used to treat MM. As a single agent, the proteasome inhibitor bortezomib has notable activity in selected populations of patients with relapsed AL. Here, we discuss recent advances using proteasome inhibitors to improve the outcome of AL amyloidosis patients.

Keywords: Amyloid, light chain, plasma cell, proteasome inhibitor, bortezomib

1. Introduction

Light-chain amyloidosis (AL) is a dyscrasia of clonal origin that results in amyloid fibril deposition within vital organs leading to their progressive dysfunction and ultimately death. The precise molecular events that lead to AL amyloidosis are poorly understood and treatment options based upon the biology of disease that improve patient survival are limited. AL amyloidosis is frequently a challenge to diagnose because of its broad spectrum of symptoms. Clinical manifestations include nephrotic-range proteinuria, hepatomegaly, congestive heart failure (CHF), and autonomic and sensory neuropathy. Diagnostic advances include development of a serum-free light-chain assay, cardiac magnetic resonance imaging (MRI), and serologic cardiac biomarkers. Treatment advances include the inclusion of the proteasome inhibitor bortezomib. Here, we discuss current and emerging treatment strategies, many focused on proteasome inhibitors, that have evolved or are evolving to prolong survival and preserve organ function in patients with this disease. Finally, we discuss emerging strategies designed to eradicate the clonal cell of origin that may provide further clinical benefit for AL amyloidosis patients.

2. Targeting the ubiquitin + proteasome system in AL amyloidosis

Protein degradation is a highly complex, temporally controlled, highly regulated process that maintains proteostasis in eukaryotic cells [1–5]. In normal and transformed cells, protein degradation pathways fulfill an essential role to maintain many critical pro-survival pathways [1]. Studies by Schoenheimer [1] in the 1930s described the dynamic turnover of individual cellular proteins. Subsequently, it was shown that protein half-lives required energy, in the form of ATP, and that the half-lives of individual proteins varied widely within mammalian cells[2]. Previously, the lysosome had been considered the central site of intracellular proteolysis [3]. Discovery of the small polypeptide protein ubiquitin (Ub) followed as well as experiments demonstrating that Ub is covalently conjugated to target proteins to direct their proteasomal degradation then greatly advanced understanding protein degradation (**Figure 1**) [4, 5]. Ub is covalently linked to protein targets in three sequential steps to target proteins to direct their rapid, ATP-dependent proteasomal degradation. In the first step, Ub is activated by an enzyme referred to as E1. Ub is then transferred from E1 to an E2 Ub-conjugating enzyme, and an isopeptide bond is formed between a lysine residue on the substrate target and the carboxy-terminus glycine of the Ub moiety. E3 Ub protein ligases then recognize Ub-conjugated target proteins [4, 5].

The vast majority of intracellular proteins are degraded by proteasomes in eukaryotic cells. The 26S proteasome is high-molecular-weight, ATP-dependent structure that consists of a 20S catalytic core particle (CP) capped at the ends by 19S regulatory particles (RP) (**Figure 2**) [6–10]. The proteasome serves as the catalytic core of the Ub-proteasome system (UPS) to degrade short-lived and denatured proteins and was the first component of the Ub-proteasome pathway to be targeted therapeutically. Bortezomib is a selective, boron-containing reversible inhibitor of the proteasome that induces apoptosis in a number of different cancer cells. Bortezomib is a potent small molecule that binds reversibly to the proteasome β-5 subunit to inhibit the chymotryptic-like (Ct-L) activity (**Figure 3**). The anti-tumor effect of bortezomib was evident in a multitude of cell lines and xenograft models from different cancer types [11–15], including malignant plasma cells. Bortezomib has demonstrated substantial benefit in monotherapy or in combinations that induce chemo- or radiosensitization [11]. Federal Drug Administration (FDA)-approval of bortezomib (Velcade, Millennium-Takeda Oncology Co., Cambridge, MA) represented a major advance in the treatment of MM [11, 12].

Bortezomib is the first proteasome inhibitor to change the natural history of a hematologic malignancy. However, clinical efficacy in the treatment of solid tumors has not been achieved.

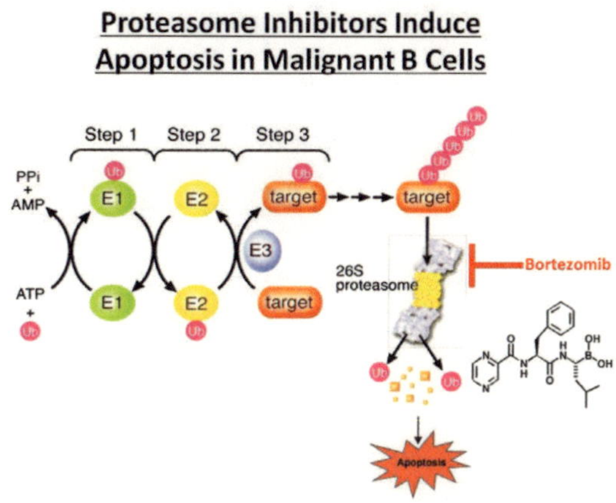

Figure 1. Schematic representation of the Ub + proteasome system. The UPS pathway for protein degradation in eukaryotic cells comprises: (1) a series of enzymes [E1, activation; E2, conjugation; E3, ligation] that covalently modify proteins with a polyubiquitin tag for recognition and targeted degradation and (2) the 26S proteasome, a 2 MDa multi-catalytic enzyme complex that hydrolyzes the polyubiquitin-tagged proteins into short polypeptides, typically seven to nine amino acids in length. The proteasome degrades unwanted proteins by recognizing specific polyubiquitin tags covalently attached to these proteins. Inhibition of the proteasome catalytic core by bortezomib leads to the unwanted accumulation of ubiquitinated proteins and culminates in apoptosis.

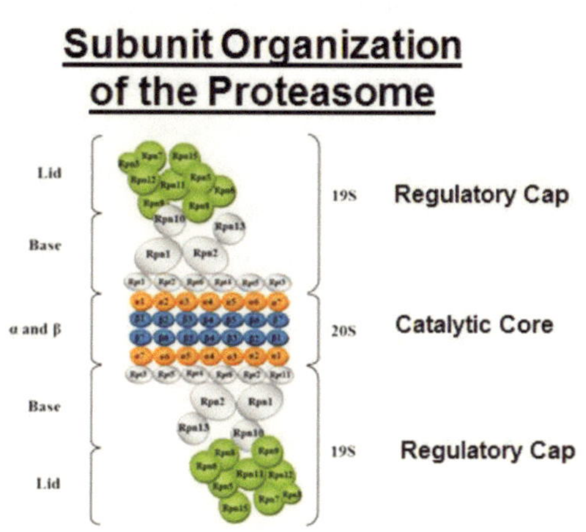

Figure 2. Subunit organization of the 26S proteasome. The 26S proteasome is a eukaryotic ATP-dependent, dumbbell-shaped protease complex with a molecular mass of approximately 2000 kDa. It consists of a central 20S proteasome, functioning as a catalytic machine, and two large V-shaped terminal modules, having possible regulatory roles, composed of multiple subunits of 25–110 kDa attached to the central portion in opposite orientations. Shown are the 20S proteasome catalytic particles (CP) and the 19S regulatory particles (RP). The 19S regulator is bound to either one or both ends of the 20S proteasome and stimulates hydrolytic activity of the 20S proteasome. The 19S RP enables ATP-dependent degradation of ubiquitinated proteins and supports elevated peptidase activity but not ubiquitin-conjugate degradation.

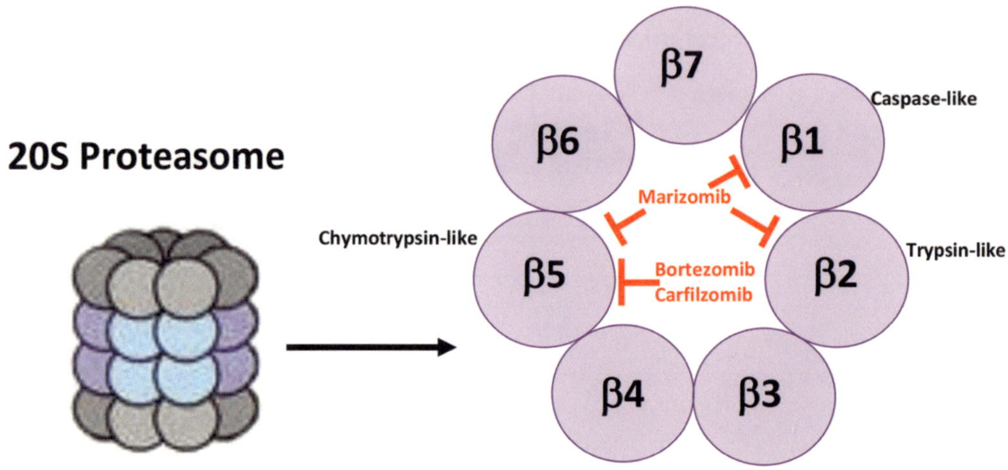

Figure 3. The 20S proteasome CP houses three pairs of catalytically active subunits, β1, β2, and β5, that exhibit protein substrate cleavage preferences referred to as caspase-like (C-L), trypsin-like (T-L), and chymotrypsin-like (CT-L), respectively, and which work in concert to degrade protein substrates. Substrate hydrolysis by the 20S CP commences with recognition of amino acid side chains by sequential binding pockets proximal to the proteolytic active site. Bortezomib forms a reversible, non-covalent adduct at the active site of the β-5 subunit. Carfilzomib has irreversible binding properties for the same active site of the β-5 subunit. Marizomib is a β-lactone-γ-lactam that binds slowly with sustained inhibition of the proteasome β-1, β-2, and β-5 active sites.

The aim of current treatment strategies for AL is to inhibit production of insoluble amyloidogenic immunoglobulin light-chain fragments and ultimately restore organ function [16–18]. AL and MM are both clonal plasma cell dyscrasias and, therefore, AL treatment is typically based on therapies that have shown efficacy in MM [19, 20]. The depth of hematologic response and complete response (CR) has been linked with improved organ function in AL patients and improved overall survival (OS) in MM [21–23]. Intensive therapy with high-dose melphalan and stem cell transplantation has been shown to be highly effective in AL, but a risk-adapted strategy may be needed to reduce mortality and toxicity [24, 25]. In addition, similar to MM, side effects with treatment are evident and drug resistance emerges even in patients that do respond initially.

Second-generation proteasome inhibitors offer a number of potential advantages over bortezomib. The newer proteasome inhibitors may provide improved target specificity, safety, tolerability, and the capacity to overcome bortezomib resistance (**Table 1**). Second-generation proteasome inhibitors include the recently FDA-approved epoxyketone carfilzomib [26], and agents in clinical development that include ONX-0912 [27], Ixazomib (Ninlaro) [28] (Millennium-Takeda), Marizomib [29] (NPI-0052), and CEP-18870 [30] (Cephalon). In contrast to bortezomib, carfilzomib is an irreversible proteasome inhibitor. Ixazomib is an orally bioavailable reversible proteasome inhibitor that is immediately hydrolyzed to its active form, MLN2238 after conversion in aqueous solutions. Ixazomib binds preferentially to the proteasome β-5 active site to inhibit the chymotrypsin-like activity. Ixazomib and CEP-18770 are reversible inhibitors of the proteasome Ct-L activity that exhibit inhibitory activity comparable to bortezomib. The differences improved anti-tumor activity.

Inhibitor	Structural Class	Inhibitor Type inhibited	Activity	Stage of Development	Route of administration
Bortezomib (Millennium)	Peptide- boronic acid	R	Ct-L	FDA-approved Immuno	IV
Carfilzomib (Onyx)	Tetrapeptide epoxyketone	I	Ct-L	FDA-approved	IV
MLN9708 (Millennium	Peptide boronic acid	R	Ct-L	Phase I	IV/po
Marizomib (Nereus)	β-lactone- γ-lactam	I	Ct-L, Tryptic, Caspase-like	Phase Ib	IV
ONX-0912 (Onyx)	Peptide epoxyketone	R	Ct-L	Phase I	IV/po
Cep-18870 (Cephalon)	Peptide- >boronic acid	R	Ct-L	Phase I–III	IV/po

R = reversible, I = irreversible; Ct-L = chymotryptic-like; Immuno = immunoproteasome, IV = intravenous; po = oral

Table 1. Agents to target the proteolytic activities within the proteasome complex.

Carfilzomib is a tetrapeptide epoxyketone that also irreversibly inhibits the Ct-L activity of proteasomes [31–36]. Carfilzomib yields a more sustained inhibition compared to bortezomib and has been shown to promote cell death in bortezomib-resistant cells. ONX-0912 is an orally bioavailable analog of carfilzomib that has been investigated in early phase trials to study the effect on solid tumors. ONX-0912 irreversibly inhibits β-5 activity and in xenograft models was shown to reduce tumor growth and prolong survival. ONX-0914 is an immunoproteasome-specific inhibitor with potential to treat both cancers and autoimmune diseases. Marizomib (NPI-0052) irreversibly inhibits the β-5 subunit and is a natural β-lactone derived from *Salinospora tropica.* Marizomib inhibits the major catalytic activities (Ct-L, tryptic-like, and caspase-like) of proteasomes which may yield a long-term benefit to preclude resistance (**Figure 3**). Thus, the benefit of second-generation proteasome inhibitors may be due to their ability to act as irreversible inhibitors and to inhibit multiple active sites within the proteasome.

3. Clinical evaluation of proteasome inhibitors for AL amyloidosis treatment

Intensive therapy with high-dose melphalan (a chemotherapy drug belonging to the class of nitrogen mustard alkylating agents) and stem cell transplantation (SCT) have been combined as a regimen (MEL-SCT) and used as an effective therapy in AL amyloidosis. MEL-SCT is used as a risk-adapted approach that is necessary to minimize treatment-related mortality

(TRM). Therefore, up to 82% of persons with AL amyloidosis may be ineligible for MEL-SCT based upon age, performance status, and severity of cardiac involvement. Wechalekar et al. [37] reported preliminary observations with bortezomib and demonstrated its effectiveness in a heavily pre-treated population, with an 80% hematologic overall response (OR) rate, including 15% hematologic CR rates. A subsequent phase I/II study of single agent bortezomib in relapsed/refractory aL amyloidosis showed excellent tolerance to both once- and twice-weekly [38]. Importantly, the median time to response in the twice-weekly arm was only 0.7 months. One-year hematologic response rates were 72.2 and 74.6%, one-year response rates were 93.8 and 84.0%, and one-third of patients exhibited a CR. The median OS was 61.1 months [39]. Rates of neuropathy were as high as 35% in the twice-weekly, with 9% rate of discontinuation and 6% rate of dose reductions.

Deregulating the ubiquitin-proteasome pathway may affect the heart, causing plaque instability, altered intracellular signal transduction resulting in decreased myocardial cytoprotection, desensitization of adrenergic receptors, and accumulation of unfolded proteins impairing cardiac function [40]. Although cardiac toxicity was described in small series, case reports, and clinical trials, subsequent meta-analysis did not support an increase in cardiotoxicity in multiple myeloma (MM) [41]. Early sudden death has been described in amyloid cardiomyopathy in persons treated with bortezomib. The Greek and UK groups demonstrated increased rates of early cardiac death in those treated with bortezomib, when compared to lenalidomide [42, 43]. However, sudden death is not uncommon in advanced amyloid cardiomyopathy. Since bortezomib typically has a shorter time to hematologic response, it is used more frequently than lenalidomide in advanced cardiac amyloidosis. Therefore, increased rates of sudden death may be related to patient selection, rather than a class effect from proteasome inhibitors.

Since bortezomib demonstrated such great promise, several studies explored the clinical efficacy in triplets, including cyclophosphamide, bortezomib, and dexamethasone (CyBorD). These retrospective studies reported on 17 and 43 patients, with hematologic response rates of 81–94% and hematologic CR rates of 39.5–71.5% [44, 45]. At least half of the patients had symptomatic cardiac involvement and many had a cardiac-specific response. However, a retrospective study from the UK demonstrated poorer outcomes than the two aforementioned studies [46]. Of 230 patients, a hematologic response rate was 60%, which decreased to 42% in those with advanced cardiac stage III patients. Cardiac response was achieved in only 17% of patients. Unfortunately, CyBorD is associated with grade 3 and grade 4 toxicities in 50% of patients.

Bortezomib has been combined with melphalan and dexamethasone, possibly with more promising outcomes than CyBorD (**Table 2**). A prospective, multi-center phase II trial of bortezomib, melphalan, and dexamethasone (VMD) in newly diagnosed or relapsed AL amyloidosis showed hematologic response rates of 94%, with CR of 38%. However, this was a small trial and 52% of patients required dose reduction despite an excellent performance status, questioning whether such an impressive response can be replicated off trial [47]. A subsequent phase I trial demonstrated improved safety and greater tolerability [48]. Using prospectively collected data, the Pavia group demonstrated higher response rates with VMD, when compared to CyBorD (p=0.033) or melphalan/dexamethasone alone ($p = 0.010$) [49]. While the exposure to upfront bortezomib is associated with longer OS, a difference between CyBorD and VMD could not be detected. A bortezomib/dexamethasone backbone is necessary in persons ineligible for melphalan-stem cell transplantation (MEL-SCT), and it is not clear whether melphalan or cyclophosphamide should be added. The addition of melphalan is supported with more prospective data, but higher cumulative doses are associated with leukemia, and melphalan should be avoided in persons who are borderline candidates for autologous stem cell transplantation.

Regimen	Type of Study	Patients	Population Size	ORR (%)	CR (%)	Dose Adjustment/ discontinuation (%)
BD[36]	Retrospective	R/R	18	94	44	61
BD[27]	Retrospective	R/R	20	80	15	40
BD[43]	Retrospective	ND	18	81	47	
BD[43]	Retrospective	R/R	76	68	20	
BD[28]	Phase I/II	R/R	70	69	37.5	53
CyBorD[34]	Retrospective	ND	17	94	71	
CyBorD[35]	Retrospective	ND, R/R	43	81	42	
CyBorD[36]	Retrospective	ND	230	60	23	
VMD[37]	Phase I/II	ND, R/R	30	94	38	52
VMD[38]	Phase I/II		9			
ID[40]	Phase I	R/R	22	53	11	
KD[41]	Phase I	R/R	12	77	0	

AL = light chain; ORR = overall response rate; CR = hematologic complete response; BD = bortezomib/dexamethasone; ND = newly diagnosed; CyBorD = cyclophosphamide/bortezomib/dexamethasone; VMD= bortezomib/melphalan/dexamethasone; ID= ixazomib/dexamethasone; KD= carfilzomib/dexamethasone

Table 2. Proteasome inhibitors used in treatment regimens for AL amyloidosis.

The use of ixazomib in a phase I study in relapsed/refractory AL amyloidosis was reported only in abstract form [50]. Of the 22 patients enrolled, 11 patients were previously treated with bortezomib and 15 with cardiac involvement. Seventy-seven percent were able to reach maximum-tolerated dose. A hematologic response was obtained in 53%, including 11% CR. An organ-specific cardiac response was seen in three of nine patients. The 2-year OS was 57%, up to 85% in proteasome inhibitor naïve patients. Tourmaline-AL1, a phase III trial for ixazomib/dexamethasone vs. physician's choice is currently ongoing and accruing patients.

Carfilzomib is another second-generation proteasome inhibitor that is being investigated as a potential treatment in AL amyloidosis. A phase I dose escalation study of carfilzomib in AL amyloidosis in a bortezomib-exposed population enrolled 12 patients [51]. A hematologic OR rate of 77% was reported and no dose-related toxicity was noted in carfilzomib doses as high as 36 mg/m^2. However, three significant cardiac events were noted, including ventricular tachycardia, grade 4 restrictive cardiomyopathy, and a grade 3 drop in the left ventricular ejection fraction. Although promising, second-generation proteasome inhibitors may not provide significant long-term benefit and overcome therapeutic resistance in refractory patients. Numerous mechanisms of resistance have been proposed, for example, mutations of PSMB5, upregulation of other proteasome subunits, alterations of gene and protein expression in stress response pathways, induction of autophagy, and an increase in anti-apoptotic pathways as well as multidrug resistance pathways. Hence, a number of novel therapeutic strategies for AL amyloidosis are under development [52, 53]. Currently, treatment choices remain highly individualized and are dependent on a careful assessment of performance status and organ function.

4. Targeting the clonal cell of origin as a treatment strategy for AL amyloidosis

The incidence of AL amyloidosis is similar to that of Hodgkin's lymphoma and chronic myelogenous leukemia (CML). Approximately 5–12 individuals/million/year are affected, although autopsy studies suggest a higher incidence. Amyloidosis is a monoclonal plasma cell disorder in which the secreted monoclonal Ig protein forms insoluble fibrillar deposits in one or more organs. In nearly all cases, the deposits contain Ig light (L) chains or L-chain fragments. AL is related to both MM and monoclonal gammopathy of undetermined significance (MGUS), a pre-malignant condition that nearly uniformly precedes MM. These monoclonal plasma cell disorders are categorized according to the total body burden of monoclonal plasma cells. When this burden is large, the diagnostic criteria for MM are fulfilled; when this burden is lower, MGUS is diagnosed. The plasma cell burden is typically low at 5–10%, and in ~10–15% of patients, AL amyloidosis occurs in association with MM.

5. Concluding remarks

While targeting proteostasis is a highly effective strategy to treat plasma cell dyscrasias such as AL, more effective agents are needed to improve organ dysfunction and advance patients to SCT. Moreover, similar to MM, high-risk forms of disease exist which do not respond to bortezomib and for those that do respond drug resistance eventually emerges. While the explosion of novel agents with activity in MM holds promise for the care of patients with AL amyloidosis, a commitment specifically to the clinical investigation of AL amyloidosis is needed to improve patient outcomes. Therefore, there is an urgent and unmet need for more effective therapeutic agents based upon the biology of the disease that increase patient survival.

http://dx.doi.org/10.5772/63467

Author details

James J. Driscoll[1,2*] and Saulius Girnius[1,2]

*Address all correspondence to: driscojs@uc.edu

1 The Vontz Center for Molecular Studies, University of Cincinnati College of Medicine, Cincinnati, OH, USA

2 Division of Hematology and Oncology, University of Cincinnati College of Medicine, Cincinnati, OH, USA

References

[1] Schoenheimer R. The dynamic state of body constituents. Harvard University Press. Cambridge, MA; 1942.

[2] Simpson MV. The release of labeled amino acids from proteins in liver slices. J. Biol. Chem. 1953;201:143–54.

[3] De Duve C, Gianetto R, Appelmans F, Wattiaux R. Enzymic content of the mitochondria fraction. Nature (London). 1953;172:1143–44.

[4] Ciechanover A, Hod Y, Hershko A. A heat-stable polypeptide component of an ATP-dependent proteolytic system from reticulocytes. Biochem. Biophys. Res. Common. 1978;81:1100–05.

[5] Ciechanover A. From the lysosome to ubiquitin and the proteasome. Nat. Rev. Mol. Cell Biol. 2005;6:79–86.

[6] Eytan E, Ganoth D, Armon T, Hershko A. ATP-dependent incorporation of 20S protease into the 26S complex that degrades proteins conjugated to ubiquitin. Proc. Natl. Acad. Sci. USA. 1989;86:7751–55.

[7] Driscoll J, Goldberg AL. The proteasome (multicatalytic protease) is a component of the 1500-kDa proteolytic complex which degrades ubiquitin-conjugated proteins. J. Biol. Chem. 1990;265:4789–92.

[8] Brown MG, Driscoll J, Monaco JJ. Structural and serological similarity of MHC-linked LMP and proteasome (multicatalytic proteinase) complexes. Nature. 1991;353:355–57.

[9] Driscoll J, Brown MG, Finley D, Monaco JJ. MHC-linked LMP gene products specifically alter peptidase activities of the proteasome. Nature. 1993;365:262–64.

[10] Ciechanover A, Hershko A, Rose I. 7 May 2016; http://www.nobelprize.org/nobel_prizes/chemistry/laureates/2004

[11] Chen D, Dou QP. The ubiquitin-proteasome system as a prospective molecular target for cancer treatment and prevention. Curr. Protein Pept. Sci. 2010;11(6):459–70.

[12] Orlowski RZ, Kuhn DJ. Proteasome inhibitors in cancer therapy: lessons from the first decade. Clin. Cancer Res. 2008;15;14(6):1649-57.

[13] Nawrocki ST, Bruns CJ, Harbison MT, et al. Effects of the proteasome inhibitor PS-341 on apoptosis and angiogenesis in orthotopic human pancreatic tumor xenografts. Mol. Cancer Ther. 2002;1:1243–53.

[14] Williams S, Pettaway C, Song R. Differential effects of the proteasome inhibitor bortezomib on apoptosis and angiogenesis in human prostate tumor xenografts. Mol. Cancer Ther. 2003;2:835–43.

[15] Hideshima T, Richardson P, Chauhan D, et al. The proteasome inhibitor PS-341 inhibits growth, induces apoptosis, and overcomes drug resistance in human multiple myeloma cells. Cancer Res. 2006;61:3071–76.

[16] Reece DE, Hegenbart U, Sanchorawala V, Merlini G, Palladini G, Blade J et al. Efficacy and safety of once-weekly and twice-weekly bortezomib in patients with relapsed systemic AL amyloidosis: results of a phase 1/2 study. Blood. 2011;118(4):865–73.

[17] Comenzo RL. Managing systemic light-chain amyloidosis. J. Natl. Compr. Cancer Netw. 2007;5(2):179–87.

[18] Guidelines Working Group of UK MM Forum, British Committee for Standards in Hematology of the British Society for Haematology. Guidelines on the diagnosis and management of AL amyloidosis. Br. J. Haematol. 2004;125(6):681–700.

[19] Falk RH, Comenzo RL, Skinner M. The systemic amyloidoses. N. Engl. J. Med. 1997;337(13):898–909.

[20] Rosen PJ, Gordon M, Lee PN, Sausville E, Papadopoulos KP, Wong AF, J Clin Oncol 27:15s, 2009 (suppl; abstr 3515).

[21] Merlini G, Palladini G. Amyloidosis: is a cure possible? Ann. Oncol. 2008;19(suppl 4):iv63–66.

[22] Gertz MA, Lacy MQ, Dispenzieri A, et al. Effect of hematologic response on outcome of patients undergoing transplantation for primary amyloidosis: importance of achieving a complete response. Haematologica. 2007;92(10):1415–18.

[23] Jaccard A, Moreau P, Leblond V, et al. High-dose melphalan versus melphalan plus dexamethasone for AL amyloidosis. N. Engl. J. Med. 2007; 357(11):1083–93.

[24] Skinner M, Sanchorawala V, Seldin DC, et al. High-dose melphalan and autologous stem-cell transplantation in patients with AL amyloidosis: an 8-year study. Ann. Intern. Med. 2004; 140(2):85–93.

[25] Gertz MA, Lacy MQ, Dispenzieri A. Myeloablative chemotherapy with stem cell rescue for the treatment of primary systemic amyloidosis: a status report. Bone Marrow Transpl. 2000;25(5):465–70.

[26] Kupperman E, et al., Cancer Res. Phase II results of Study PX-171-007: a phase Ib/II study of carfilzomib (CFZ), a selective proteasome inhibitor, in patients with selected advanced metastatic solid tumors. ASCO. 7 May 2016; Abstract 3515.

[27] Development: ONX 0914 (PR-957). www.onyx-pharm.com/view.cfm/679/ONX-0914

[28] Rodler ET, Infante JR, Siu LL. First-in-human, phase I dose-escalation study of investigational drug MLN9708, a second-generation proteasome inhibitor, in advanced nonhematologic malignancies. J. Clin. Oncol. 2010;28:15s(suppl):abstr 3071.

[29] Groll M, Huber R, Potts BC. Crystal structures of salinosporamide A (NPI-0052) and B (NPI-0047) in complex with the 20S proteasome reveal important consequences of β-lactone ring opening and a mechanism for irreversible binding. J. Am. Chem. Soc. 2006;128:5136–41.

[30] Piva R, Ruggeri B, Williams M, et al. CEP-18770: a novel, orally active proteasome inhibitor with a tumor-selective pharmacologic profile competitive with bortezomib. Blood. 2008;111(5):2765–75.

[31] Dick, LR, Fleming, PE. Building on bortezomib: second-generation proteasome inhibitors as anti-cancer therapy. Drug Discov. Today. 2010;15:243–49.

[32] Papadopoulos KP, Burris HA, 3rd, Gordon M, et al. A phase I/II study of carfilzomib 2-10-min infusion in patients with advanced solid tumors. Cancer chemotherapy and pharmacology. 2013 Oct;72(4):861–8.

[33] Demo SD, Kirk CJ, Aujay MA, et al. Antitumor activity of PR-171, a novel irreversible inhibitor of the proteasome. Cancer Res. 2007;67(13):6383–91.

[34] Min CK, Lee SE, Yahng SA, et al. The impact of novel therapeutic agents before and after frontline autologous stem cell transplantation in patients with multiple myeloma. Blood Res. 2013 48(3):198–205.

[35] Yaqub S, Ballester G, Ballester O. Frontline therapy for multiple myeloma: a concise review of the evidence based on randomized clinical trials. Cancer Invest. 2013;31(8): 529–37.

[36] De la Puente P., Azab Ak. Contemporary drug therapies for multiple myeloma. Drugs Today. 2013;49(9):563–73.

[37] Wechalekar AD, Lachmann HJ, Offer M, Hawkins PN, Gillmore JD. Efficacy of bortezomib in systemic AL amyloidosis with relapsed/refractory clonal disease. Haematologica. 2008;93(2):295–98.

[38] Reece DE, Hegenbart U, Sanchorawala V, et al. Efficacy and safety of once-weekly and twice-weekly bortezomib in patients with relapsed systemic AL amyloidosis: results of a phase 1/2 study. Blood. 2011;118(4):865–73.

[39] Reece DE, Hegenbart U, Sanchorawala V, et al. Long-term follow-up from a phase 1/2 study of single-agent bortezomib in relapsed systemic AL amyloidosis. Blood. 2014;124(16):2498–506.

[40] Orciuolo E, Buda G, Cecconi N, et al. Unexpected cardiotoxicity in haematological bortezomib treated patients. Br. J. Haematol. 2007;138(3):396–97.

[41] Xiao Y, Yin J, Wei J, Shang Z. Incidence and risk of cardiotoxicity associated with bortezomib in the treatment of cancer: a systematic review and meta-analysis. PLoS One. 2014;9(1):e87671.

[42] Kastritis E. Outcomes of primary systemic light chain (AL) amyloidosis in patients treated upfront with bortezomib of lenalidomide and the importance of risk adapted strategies. XIVth International Symposium on Amyloidosis. Indianapolis, IN; 2014.

[43] Wechalekar AD. Characterisitcs and outcomes of 714 patients with systemic AL amyloidosis – analysis of prospective study (ALChemy Study). XIVth International Symposium of Amyloidosis. Indianapolis, IN; 2014.

[44] Mikhael JR, Schuster SR, Jimenez-Zepeda VH, et al. Cyclophosphamide-bortezomib-dexamethasone (CyBorD) produces rapid and complete hematologic response in patients with AL amyloidosis. Blood. 2012;119(19):4391–94.

[45] Venner CP, Lane T, Foard D, et al. Cyclophosphamide, bortezomib, and dexamethasone therapy in AL amyloidosis is associated with high clonal response rates and prolonged progression-free survival. Blood. 2012;119(19):4387–90.

[46] Palladini G, Sachchithanantham S, Milani P, et al. A European collaborative study of cyclophosphamide, bortezomib, and dexamethasone in upfront treatment of systemic AL amyloidosis. Blood. 2015;126(5):612–15.

[47] Zonder J. Melphalan and dexamethasone plus bortezomib induces hematologic and organ responses in AL-amyloidosis with tolerable neurotoxicity. American Society of Hematology. New Orleans, LA; 2009.

[48] Shimazaki C, Fuchida S, Suzuki K, et al. Phase 1 study of bortezomib in combination with melphalan and dexamethasone in Japanese patients with relapsed AL amyloidosis. Int. J. Hematol. 2016;103(1):79–85.

[49] Palladini G, Milani P, Riva E, et al: Accurate risk stratification identifies patients with AL amyloidosis benefiting most from upfront bortezomib combinations: A study of treatment outcomes in 984 patients. 57th American Society of Hematology Annual Meeting and Exposition. Orlando, FL, December 5-8, 2015 (abstr 190).

[50] Merlini G. Long-term outcome of a Phase 1 study of the investigational oral proteasome inhibitor (PI) ixazomib at the recommended phase 3 dose (RP3D) in patients (Pts)

with relapsed or refractory systemic light-chain (AL) amyloidosis (RRAL). American Society of Hematology. San Francisco, CA; 2014.

[51] AD C. A phase I dose-escalation study of Carfilzomib in patients with previously-treated systemic light-chain (AL) amyloidosis. American Society of Hematology. San Francisco, CA; 2014.

[52] Kastritis E, Anagnostopoulos A, Roussou M, et al. Treatment of light chain (AL) amyloidosis with the combination of bortezomib and dexamethasone. Haematologica. 2007;92(10):1351–58.

[53] Kastritis E, Wechalekar AD, Dimopoulos MA, et al. Bortezomib with or without dexamethasone in primary systemic (light chain) amyloidosis. J. Clin. Oncol. 2010;28(6): 1031–37.

Chapter 12

Amyloid Nephropathy: A Practical Diagnostic Approach and Review on Pathogenesis

Paisit Paueksakon

Additional information is available at the end of the chapter

http://dx.doi.org/10.5772/64083

Abstract

Amyloidosis comprises a group of protein-folding disorders in which extracellular deposits share unique Congo red staining properties and fibrillary ultrastructural appearance. These fibrillary deposits ultimately cause tissue destruction and progressive disease. Amyloidosis can be either systemic affecting multiple organs or localized. Renal involvement by amyloidosis (amyloid nephropathy) is a frequent manifestation of systemic amyloidosis. Immunofluorescence, immunohistochemistry (IHC), and more recently laser microdissection and mass spectrometry (LMD/MS) are important techniques in typing of amyloid nephropathy. This in-depth review discusses practical diagnostic approach and pathogenesis of amyloid nephropathy and includes discussion of treatment and prognosis.

Keywords: amyloid nephropathy, light microscopy, immunofluorescence, immunohistochemistry, electron microscopy, proteomics

1. Introduction

Amyloidosis comprises a group of protein-folding disorders in which extracellular deposits share unique Congo red staining properties and fibrillary ultrastructural appearance [1]. These fibrillary deposits ultimately cause tissue destruction and progressive disease. Amyloid consists of randomly arranged, nonbranching fibrils that measure 8–12 nm in diameter [1]. Amyloidosis is a rare group of diseases, with an estimated prevalence of 1: 60,000 [2]. In the USA and Europe, amyloidosis derived from immunoglobulin (Ig) light chain (AL) secondary to plasma cell dyscrasia is the most prevalent form, followed by reactive AA amyloidosis (AA) derived from serum amyloid A (SAA), which is typically associated with chronic inflammatory conditions. This is in contrast to developing countries in Africa and Middle East of Asia, where AA is much more common than AL [3–5]. Leukocyte chemotactic factor 2 amyloidosis (ALECT2), derived from leukocyte chemotactic factor 2 protein (LECT2), is newly recognized as a common type of amyloid, with unknown etiology [6]. Familial amyloidosis is diagnosed with increasing frequency with the use of new immunohistochemical studies and mass spectrometry [7]. Amyloidosis can be either systemic affecting multiple organs or localized. Renal disease is a frequent manifestation of systemic amyloidosis with AL, previously called primary amyloidosis, the most common type involving the kidney.

2. Amyloid nephropathy

The types of amyloid are categorized by the chemical composition of the proteins. There are more than 25 precursor proteins identified as major proteins in amyloid deposition so far. A large study from the Mayo clinic [8] showed that among 474 patients with amyloid diagnosed by renal biopsies between 2007 and 2011, Ig-related amyloidosis (AIg) was the most common form involving the kidney (85.9%), followed by AA (7.0%), ALECT2 (2.7%), fibrinogen A α chain amyloidosis (AFib) (1.3%), apolipoprotein AI amyloidosis (AApo AI), apolipoprotein AII amyloidosis (AApo AII), or apolipoprotein AIV amyloidosis (AApo AIV) (0.6%), AA/light and heavy chain amyloidosis (AHL) (0.2%), and unclassified amyloidosis (2.3%). AIg in most cases is derived from fragments of monoclonal light-chain protein (AL). However, in rare cases, AIg is derived from truncated Ig heavy chain and light chain (AHL) or isolated truncated Ig heavy chain [8, 9]. AIg is associated with B-cell lymphoproliferative disorders including multiple myeloma and plasma cell dyscrasia, B-cell lymphoma, and Waldenström's macroglobulinemia [8]. In contrast, AA is characterized by tissue deposition of serum amyloid A protein, which is derived from an acute-phase reactant protein synthesized by the liver [10]. AA is seen in conditions associated with chronic inflammation including rheumatoid arthritis, ankylosing spondylitis, chronic draining infections (i.e., osteomyelitis, chronic skin infections including decubitus ulcers, bronchiectasis, and chronic sinusitis), Crohn disease, tuberculosis, and familial Mediterranean fever (FMF) [10]. Familial amyloidosis comprises another group of amyloid that is now being diagnosed more frequently and includes amyloid derived from transthyretins (TTR) [11], fibrinogen [12], lysozyme (Lys) [13], gelsolin (Gel) [14], Apo AI [15], Apo AII [16], and Apo AIV [17]. ALECT2 nephropathy was first described in 2008 [6, 18]. LECT2 is a chemotactic factor for neutrophils and has other physiologic functions, including cell proliferation, immunomodulation, repair after injury, tumor suppression, and glucose metabolism [6, 18]. ALECT2 is now the third most common type of amyloid nephropathy in the USA and accounts for 2.5–2.7% of amyloid nephropathy cases [6, 18]. ALECT2 involves mainly in the kidney and liver but rarely involve other organs such as spleen, adrenal, and myocardium [6, 18]. Type and precursor protein of amyloid nephropathy are summarized in **Table 1**.

Amyloid precursor protein	Amyloid type
Restricted light chain (lambda or kappa)	AL
Ig heavy chain	AH
Ig heavy and light chain	AHL
Serum amyloid associated protein (SAA)	AA
Leukocyte chemotactic factor type 2 (LECT2)	ALECT2
Fibrinogen A-α chain	AFib
Transthyretin (TTR)	ATTR
Apolipoprotein A-I	AApo AI
Apolipoprotein A-II	AApo AII
Apolipoprotein A-IV	AApo AIV
Gelsolin	AGel
Lysozyme	ALys

Table 1. Type and precursor protein of amyloid nephropathy.

3. Clinical features

The clinical features of patients with amyloidosis vary, depending on the varying predilection of different types of amyloid for specific organ involvement. As described above, renal involvement is a frequent manifestation of amyloidosis, more often in AIg nephropathy, AA nephropathy, and some forms of familial amyloidosis [10, 12]. Amyloid nephropathy of any type is more common in men than in women [8]. A large retrospective review of patients with amyloidosis evaluated from 1981 to 1992 at the Mayo Clinic in Rochester, Minnesota, revealed 1315 patients, including 918 patients with AL amyloidosis (69.8%). Of these, 474 patients had new-onset AL amyloidosis, including 69% men and 31% women with median age of 64 years [19]. At the time of diagnosis, about 17% of AL patients had either multiple myeloma or smoldering myeloma and about 16% had history of monoclonal gammopathy of undetermined significance (MGUS). On presentation, about 51% of men and 47% of women had renal failure, and about 73% of patients had proteinuria. The median 24-h urine protein was 1.2 g/d and in the patients with full nephrotic syndrome, about a quarter of patients, the mean 24-h urine protein excretion was 7.0 g/d. Serum protein electrophoresis (SPEP) revealed a monoclonal protein in about 48% of patients and when serum immunoelectrophoresis was tested the percentage increased to about 72%. A monoclonal light chain was detected in about 73% of the patients by urine immunoelectrophoresis or immunofixation, including about 68% with lambda and about 32% with kappa. Overall, about 89% of the patients with AL amyloidosis showed a serum or urine monoclonal spike (M spike).

Patients with AA nephropathy usually present at younger age than AL patients, whereas ALECT2 is more common in older patients. ALECT2 nephropathy mainly affects patients of

Hispanic or Mexican origin and rarely affects Caucasian patients, whereas AL and AA do not show evident ethnic differences [6, 18]. As in AL amyloid, proteinuria is also the most common clinical presentation in AA, ALECT2, and familial amyloid nephropathy [8]. Extrarenal manifestations of amyloidosis include congestive heart failure caused by myocardial infiltration by amyloid, orthostatic hypotension, bladder dysfunction, and dysesthesias caused by amyloid infiltration into autonomic and peripheral nerves, lymphadenopathy, hepatomegaly, splenomegaly, and macroglossia [18, 20]. The treatment and prognosis of amyloid nephropathy will be discussed below.

4. Molecular mechanisms and pathogenesis of amyloidosis

Misfolding of extracellular proteins has a prominent role in the molecular mechanisms and pathogenesis of amyloidosis [21, 22]. The misfolded proteins are highly prone to self-aggregation. There are different mechanisms of formation of pathologic misfolded proteins [22]. The first is based on intrinsic propensity of the protein to assume pathologic conformation, which becomes more evident with aging. Examples of these mechanisms are evident when molecularly normal transthyretin misfolds in patients with senile systemic amyloidosis [22]. The second way is due to alteration of the normal protein sequence, as seen with the replacement of a single amino acid in protein, e.g., in AL and familial amyloidosis [22]. Only a small portion of Ig light chains is amyloidogenic; thus, AL nephropathy occurs only in about 12–15% of the patients with multiple myeloma [23]. The amyloid fibrils in amyloid nephropathy consist of either intact light chains containing the variable and constant domains or solely the variable domains, which contains the N-terminus portion of the light-chain molecule. The VλVI subgroup of the light chain preferentially leads to amyloid formation in patients with AL nephropathy [23, 24]. Therefore, it appears that germ line sequences, which enhanced near the N-terminus of the lambda light chain and in the VλVI of the light chain may be prone to mutations that generate amyloidogenic light chains. These altered proteins lead to destabilization of light chain and increase the likelihood of fibril formation [25]. In familial amyloidosis, such as Transthyretin-related hereditary amyloidosis (ATTR) and Lysozyme-related amyloidosis (ALys), the substitution of a single amino acid transforms a normal protein into an amyloidogenic protein [26, 27]. The unstable protein produced by amino acid substitution may allow the protein to precipitate when stimulated by the local physicochemical milieu, such as local surface pH, electric field, and hydration forces on the cellular surfaces [22]. A third mechanism contributing to amyloid formation is proteolytic remodeling of the protein precursor, as seen in Alzheimer's disease, in which the fibrils are composed of proteolytic fragments of 39–43 residues derived from 753-residue β-amyloid precursor protein (APP) [28]. This type of amyloid does not affect the kidney. In addition, excessive concentration of amyloidogenic protein due to unregulated production of high local concentration can promote amyloidosis [29]. When the protein precursor reaches a critical point of local concentration, it triggers fibril formation. This mechanism is enhanced further by environmental physicochemical factors and interaction with extracellular matrix. This mechanism may occur in AA amyloidosis associated with chronic inflammatory conditions or familial Mediterranean fever [30]. The excessive concentration of amyloidogenic protein may also be caused by decrease in clearance from the body; e.g., Beta-2 microglobulin associated amyloidosis (Aβ2M) develops in end-stage renal disease patients who received long-term dialysis because of ineffective clearance of β2M from circulation during dialysis or due to inability of the body to destroy the accumulation by natural mechanism [31]. Regardless of mechanism of misfolding, the misfolded proteins are prone to self-aggregate, generating protofilaments that interact to form fibrils [22].

In AL nephropathy, amyloid formation in the kidney first begins in the mesangium. The specific uptake of light-chain protein by mesangial cells underlies the predominant kidney tropism and is an important step in amyloid fibril formation. There are several factors that might promote or decelerate amyloid deposition in glomeruli, including the negative ion charge and the high concentration of glycosaminoglycan of the glomerular basement membranes with the presence of enzyme proteases that could render protein amyloidogenic [32]. Mesangial cells are modified smooth muscle cells, which have phagocytic activity [33]. Upon interaction with light-chain proteins, the light-chain proteins are avidly internalized and delivered to the primary lysosomes where the amyloid fibrils are primarily formed [34]. During this process, the mesangial cells transform into a macrophage phenotype with prominent primary lysosomes, making them more capable of processing of internalized amyloidogenic light-chain proteins and fibril formation [34]. The amyloid deposition within the mesangium further stimulates metalloproteinase enzymes, causing mesangial matrix degradation, inhibiting transforming growth factor β (TGF-β) and thus impairing mesangial matrix repair [33, 35] and increasing apoptosis, finally leading to significant mesangiolysis and replacement of the mesangial area by amyloid deposits [36]. These changes result in the absence of mesangial argyrophilia and significant mesangial cell deletion in the advanced stage of glomerular amyloidosis [34].

LECT2 has multiple functions including as a cytokine involved in chemotaxis of neutrophils and a growth factor involved in cell proliferation and regulation of repair after injury, immunomodulation, tumor suppression, and glucose metabolism [37]. The pathogenesis of ALECT2 is not well understood, but may be due to increased synthesis of LECT2 by hepatocytes or secondary to hepatocellular damage or involve interference, possible due to genetic defect, in the LECT2 catabolism or LECT2 transportation, which may give rise to local LECT2 tissue concentration and finally lead to amyloid fibril formation [6, 18, 37].

The normal plasma protein serum amyloid P component (SAP), a glycoprotein that belongs to the pentraxin family, independently binds to fibrils in all types of amyloid and contributes to pathogenesis of amyloidosis [38]. SAP is highly protected against proteolysis, and a binding of SAP to amyloid fibrils in vitro protect them from proteolytic enzymes and degradation by phagocytic cells. Moreover, SAP is a stubborn glycoprotein that can persist within human amyloid deposits for prolonged periods and is completely unmodified with respect to circulating SAP [38]. It is suggested that SAP may contribute to the failure to clear amyloid deposition in vivo, leading to tissue architecture destruction and organ dysfunction.

Furthermore, amyloid can be deposited in multiple organs, and this tendency might depend on several physicochemical factors, such as high concentration of local protein, low pH, presence of proteolytic processing, and seeding of protofilaments [22]. The amyloid deposits cause tissue architecture destruction, presumed to cause organ dysfunction [22]. Furthermore, the amyloidogenic precursor proteins, folding intermediates, and protofilaments have toxicities independent of the amyloid deposits and these toxicities can also contribute to disease manifestations [39].

5. Gross findings

Postmortem examination of patients with amyloidosis generally shows enlarged kidneys, unlike other causes of chronic kidney disease (CKD) where kidneys are small and shrunken. In addition, cut surfaces of kidney in patients with amyloid nephropathy are pale, firm, waxy, and flat [38] (**Figure 1a**), which are different from the normal kidney or the kidney in the patients with CKD (**Figure 1b**), which bulges slightly causing in slight curvature of the cut surfaces.

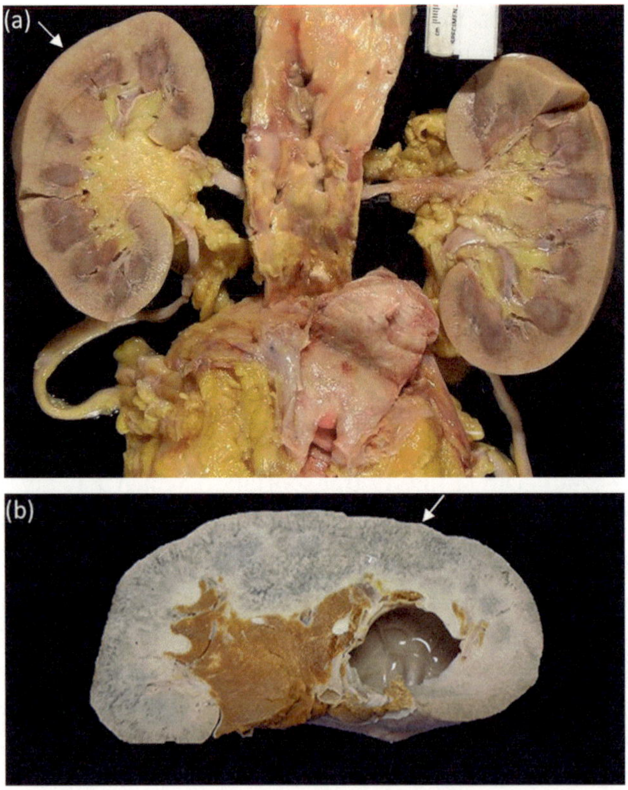

Figure 1. At autopsy of a patient with amyloid nephropathy, the kidney is enlarged and pale with waxy and flat cut surface (a, arrow), which is different from the kidney in a patient with chronic kidney disease with a simple cyst, which bulges slightly (arrow) resulting in slight curvature of the cut surfaces (b).

http://dx.doi.org/10.5772/64083

6. Histologic diagnosis and identification of amyloid

6.1. Light microscopy

The light microscopic (LM) findings of amyloidosis are identical regardless of the type of amyloid. Glomerular amyloid deposition begins with progressive accumulation of acellular amorphous eosinophilic material (cotton candy appearance) on hematoxylin and eosin (H&E)-stained sections (**Figure 2**) that appear pale with the periodic acid Schiff (PAS) stain (**Figure 3a** and **b**). In the advanced stage, the mesangial matrix is extensively replaced by acellular amorphous material exhibiting uniform expansion with compression of the capillary spaces and occasional nodular formation, resembling diabetic nephropathy or monoclonal immunoglobulin deposition disease. The nodular pattern is seen more frequently in AA nephropathy. The amyloid deposits are paler on PAS stain than the Kimmelstiel-Wilson nodules in diabetic nephropathy, or deposits in light-chain deposition disease or fibrillary glomerulonephritis. Further, fibrillary glomerulonephritis typically is proliferative, with increased cellularity seen by light microscopy. The amyloid deposits stain weakly or are negative with Jones methenamine silver stain (JMS) and appear as negative defects in the expanded mesangium and thick glomerular basement membranes (**Figure 4a** and **b**). Occasionally, there is a focal parallel alignment of amyloid fibrils in the subepithelial zone that results in focal capillary wall spikes, which are best visualized by JMS (**Figure 5**). These spikes are focal, closely clustered, and longer than the typical spikes of membranous nephropathy. The focal clusters of spikes may resemble feathers, so-called feathery spikes. Amyloid feathery spikes are more common in AL than AA or familial amyloidosis [7]. Rarely crescent formation can be seen in both AA and AL [7], indicating glomerular basement membrane breaks, the injury that triggers crescent formation, can occur. Vascular involvement by amyloidosis is common, frequently involving arteriolar walls, followed by arteries, peritubular capillaries, and veins. In rare cases, particularly in AL or in ATTR nephropathy, the vessels are the only part in the kidney where amyloid is demonstrated. Interstitial amyloid deposition is seen in about 50% of cases but is present in most cases of ALECT2 nephropathy (**Figure 6**). Glomerular involvement is not extensive in ALECT2 and apolipoprotein AI (AApo AI/), AII (AApoAII), and AIV (AApoAIV) nephropathy in comparison with other types of amyloid. In addition, the histology of AFib nephropathy is very characteristic, showing glomerular enlargement with near-total replacement of the glomeruli by amyloid, with little or no vascular or interstitial involvement [10]. Special IF and immunohistochemistry (IHC) together with mass spectrometry analyses are typically used to identify the type of amyloid (see below). However, potassium permanganate treatment prior to Congo red staining has been used to distinguish between AA and AL nephropathy: after this treatment, birefringent Congo red staining is lost by AA but retained by AL. This technique is not commonly used and has been replaced by more specific SAA immunohistochemistry (IHC).

Amyloid is defined by its tinctorial characteristics, which include Congo red positivity (orange, salmon pink, or pale rose staining, **Figure 7**). The Congo red stain gives apple-green or traffic light green birefringence under polarized light (**Figure 8**). The mesangial expansion can be focal and may be segmental, global, or even nodular. However, the degree of proteinuria does not correlate with the amount of amyloid deposition; as a result, cases with early amyloidosis with scant and segmental amyloid deposition can be mistakenly diagnosed as minimal change disease if no Congo red stain, immunofluorescence (IF) and electron microscopy (EM) is performed. To demonstrate small amounts of amyloid deposits in tissue sections, it is recommended that the sections be cut thicker than normal (6 μm, instead of customary 2 μm) [40]. Proper detection of apple green birefringence depends on the intensity of the transmitted light and, thus, a strong light source is strongly suggested to maximize results. In early amyloidosis with small amounts of amyloid, it might be difficult to demonstrate Congo red positivity. Therefore, an alternative way of identifying a small amount of amyloid deposits by Congo red stain is to place the stained section under fluorescent light; amyloid then is bright red [41] (**Figure 9**). Of note, false positivity may result from overstaining, and this technique is not specific for amyloid. Thus, amyloid must be confirmed by apple green polarization, immunofluorescence, IHC, and/or electron microscopy. An alternative option to demonstrate amyloid deposits in cases with no paraffin embedded tissue available is to perform Congo red stain on frozen tissue (**Figure 10**). This technique is more sensitive than a Congo red stain performed on paraffin embedded tissue from our experience. Of note, positive controls should then, of course, also be performed on frozen tissues.

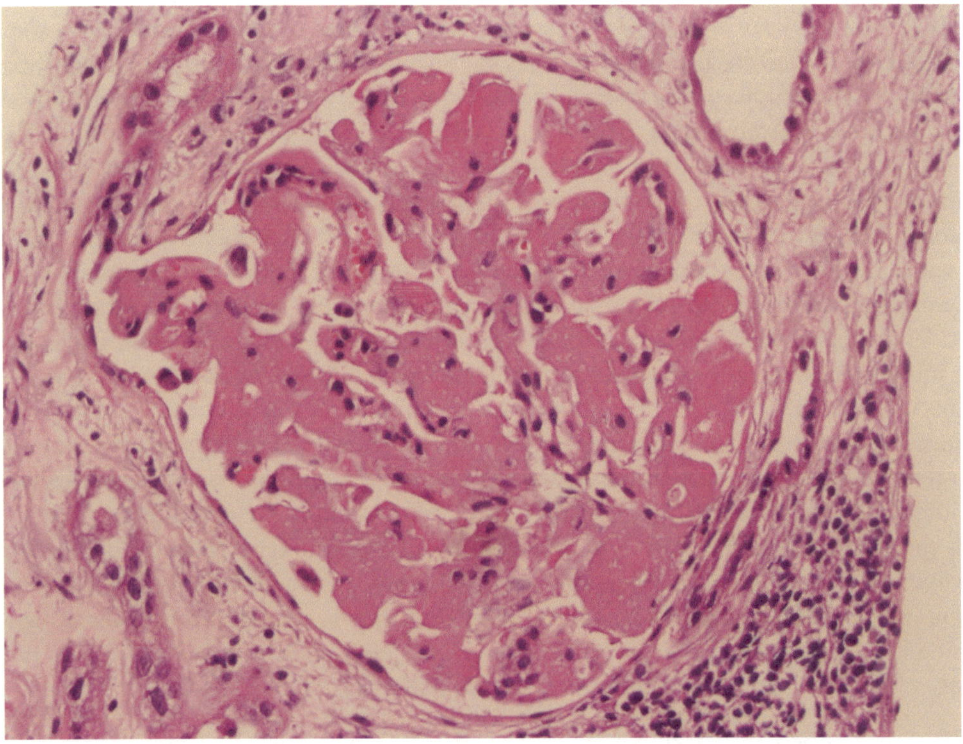

Figure 2. In amyloid nephropathy, there is extensive mesangial expansion by amorphous eosinophilic acellular material ("cotton candy" appearance), which segmentally extends to the glomerular capillary loops (H&E stain, original magnification ×400).

http://dx.doi.org/10.5772/64083

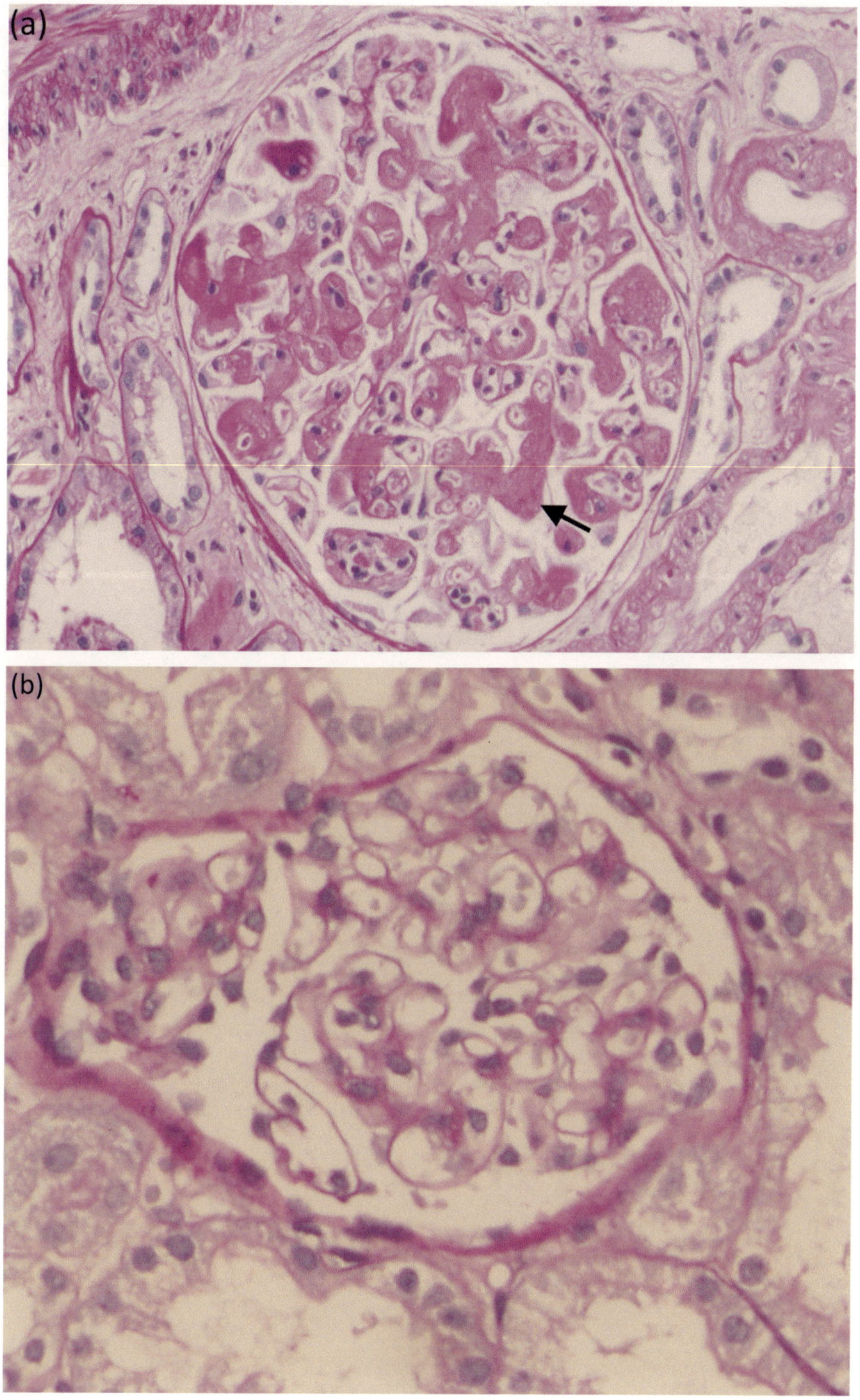

Figure 3. In amyloid nephropathy (a), mesangial areas are globally expanded by weak PAS positive acellular deposits (arrow) in comparison to a glomerulus (b) in normal kidney biopsy (PAS stain, original magnification ×400).

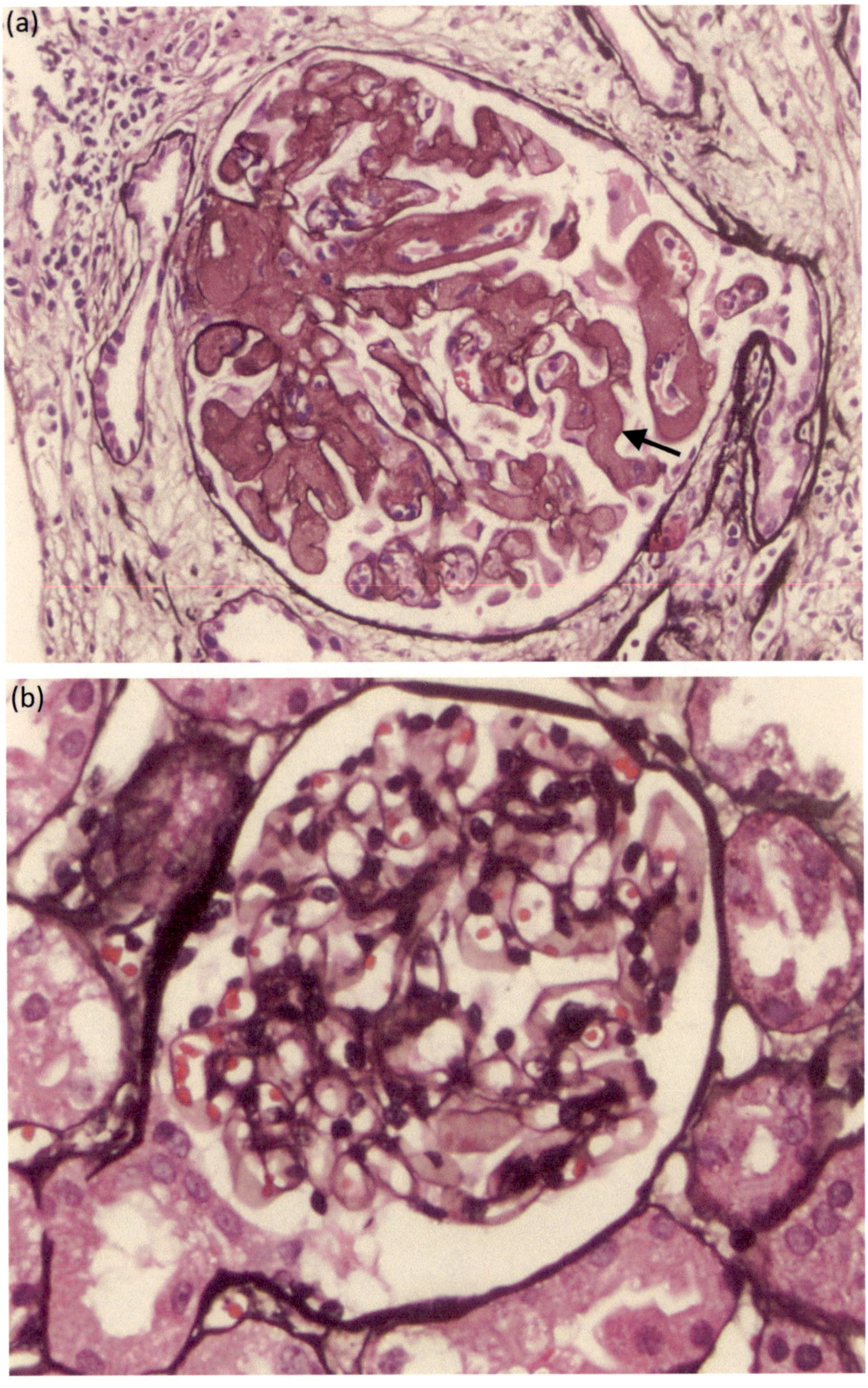

Figure 4. In amyloid nephropathy (a), mesangial amyloid deposits are nonargyrophilic (silver negative, arrow) in comparison with a glomerulus in the normal kidney biopsy (silver positive, b) (JMS stain, original magnification ×400).

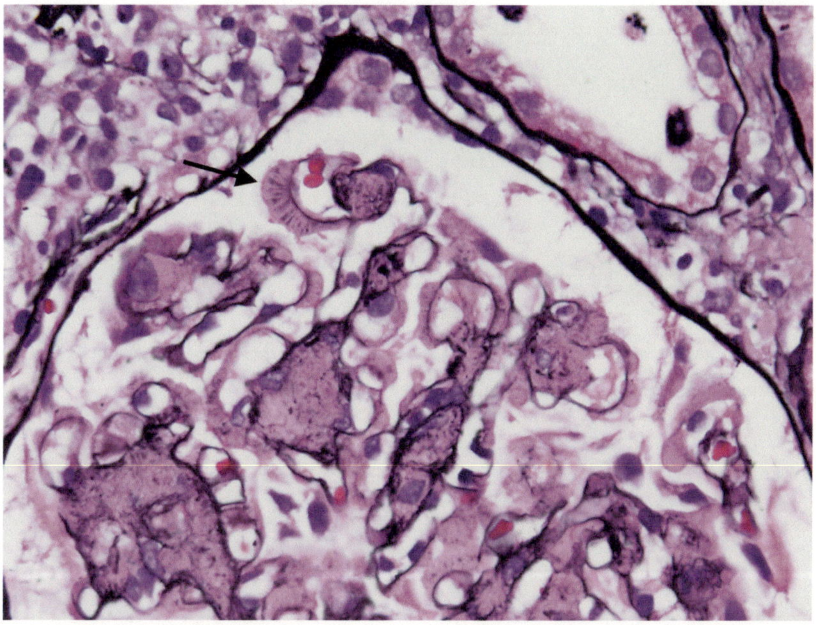

Figure 5. Feathery spikes (arrow) are a characteristic features of amyloid nephropathy seen on JMS, and are seen more frequently in AIg than other forms of amyloid nephropathy (JMS stain, original magnification ×400).

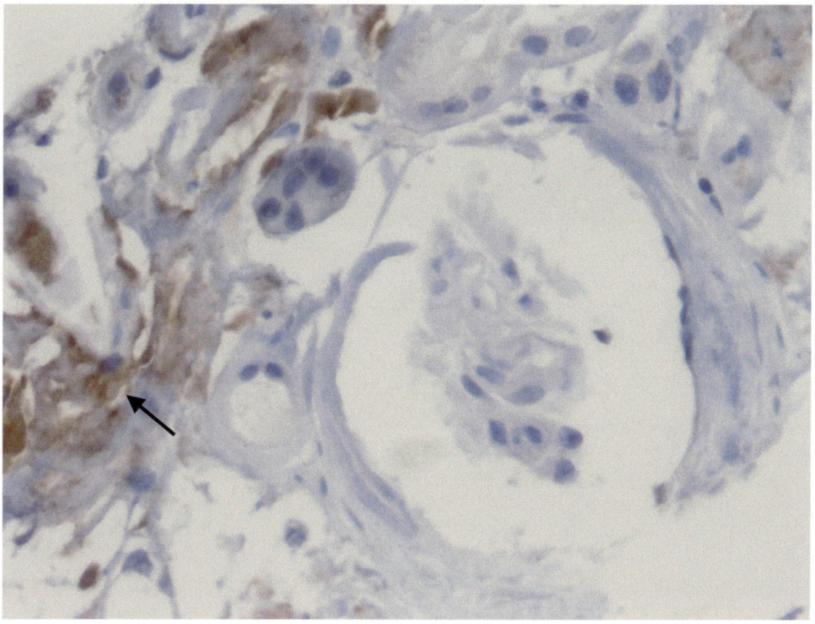

Figure 6. ALECT2 amyloid nephropathy with intense interstitial amyloid (arrow) seen by immunohistochemistry staining (anti-LECT2 IHC, original magnification ×400).

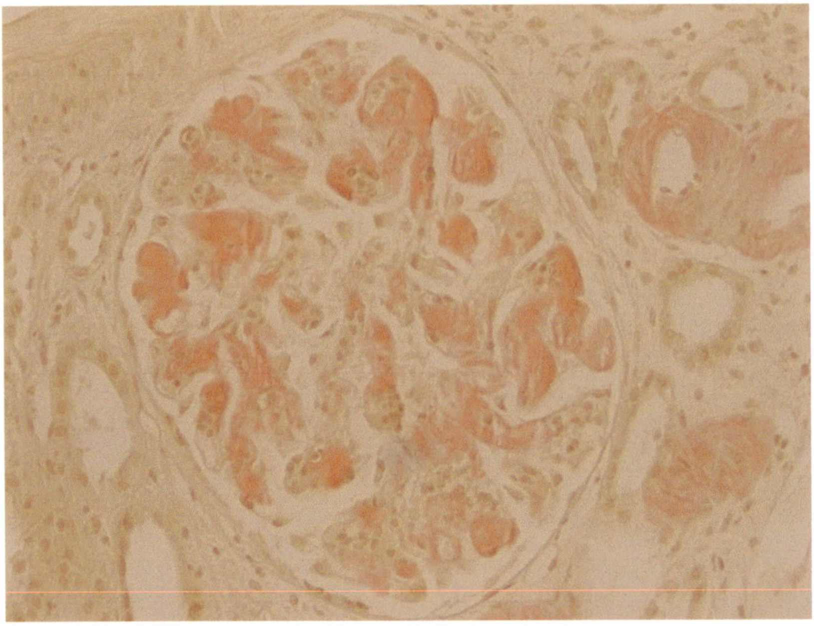

Figure 7. Congo red positive mesangial deposits of amyloid with orange or salmon pink staining (Congo red stain, original magnification ×400).

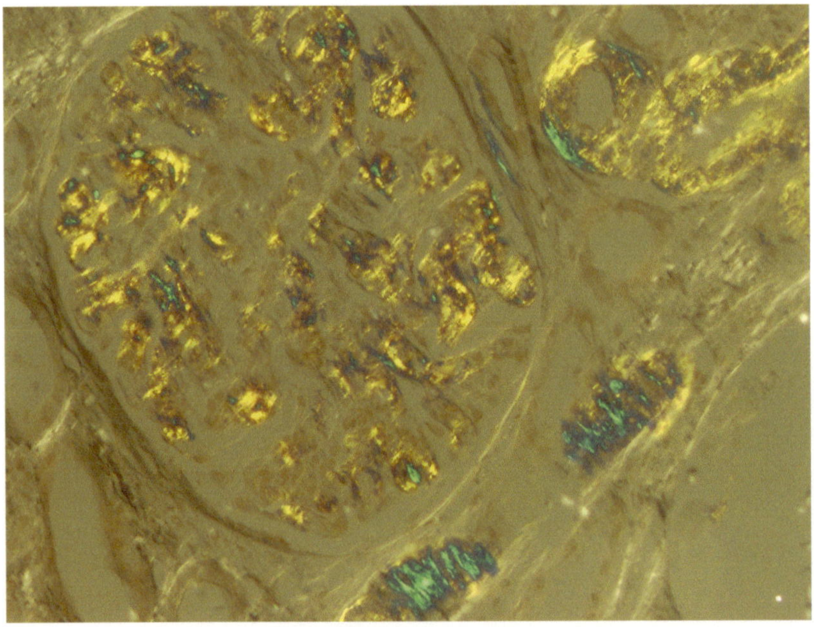

Figure 8. Amyloid deposits with characteristic apple green birefringence when viewed by polarized light (Congo red stain, original magnification ×400).

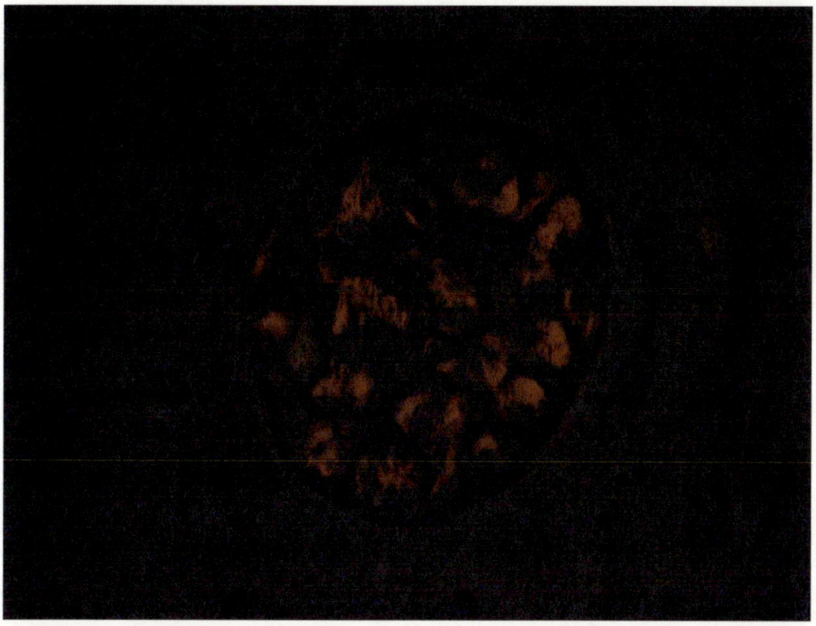

Figure 9. A small amount of amyloid deposits can be detected by placing the Congo red stained section under fluorescent light (Congo red stain, original magnification ×400).

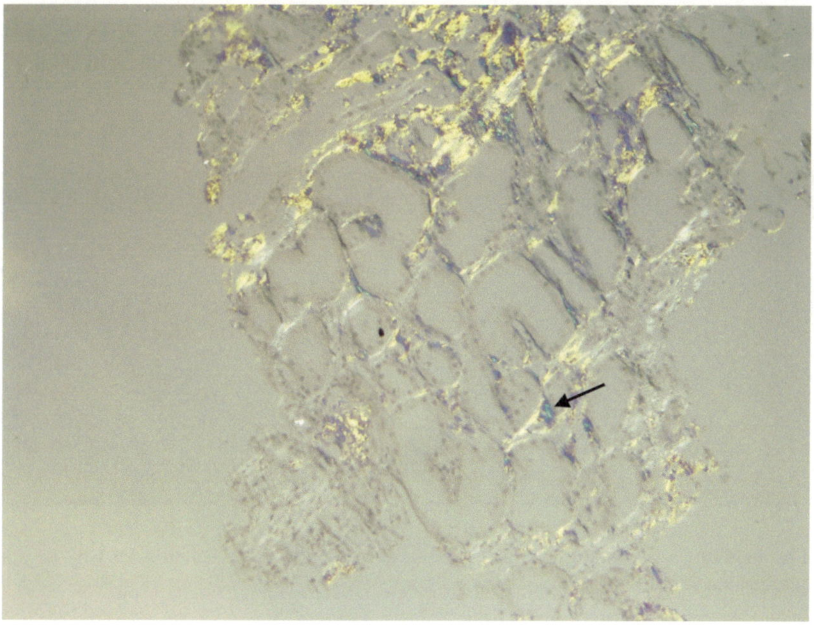

Figure 10. Congo red stain performed on frozen tissue with green birefringence (arrow) when viewed by polarized light (Congo red stain, original magnification ×400).

Thioflavin T is an additional sensitive but nonspecific fluorescent stain for amyloid, which is activated by blue light to emit yellow green fluorescence staining upon binding to amyloid [42]. This test is more sensitive than Congo red in detecting a small amount of amyloid deposits. However, due to lack of specificity, it must be confirmed by Congo red apple green birefringence, IF, IHC, and/or EM.

AL amyloid nephropathy may coexist with other manifestations of the monoclonal protein, such as light-chain cast nephropathy, light-chain proximal tubulopathy, and rarely monoclonal immunoglobulin deposition disease. Any amyloid type may have coexisting other conditions in the kidney biopsy, such as acute tubular necrosis, diabetic nephropathy, thin basement membrane lesion, or arterionephrosclerosis.

6.2. Immunofluorescence microscopy

Immunofluorescence (IF) microscopy or immunohistochemistry is crucial for confirming the presence and for typing of amyloid nephropathy. IF is useful for detection of amyloid derived from Ig light and heavy chains. Amyloid deposits have a distinctive smudgy appearance of staining (**Figure 11a**). Restriction for light chain, either kappa or more commonly lambda, or for heavy-chain determents (γ or μ) must be demonstrated, in association with Congo red positivity, for a diagnosis of AIg amyloidosis. Therefore, IF staining for kappa and lambda should be routinely performed on all native renal biopsies. The findings of strong staining for a monoclonal Ig light chain with negativity for Ig heavy chains is diagnostic of AL nephropathy (**Figure 11a** and **b**). About 75% of AL nephropathy cases are due to monoclonal lambda deposits. The diagnosis of AH nephropathy is based on the presence of strong staining for a single Ig heavy chain with negativity for kappa and lambda light chains (**Figure 12**). AHL nephropathy shows intense staining for Ig heavy chain and a single Ig light chain (**Figure 13a** and **b**).

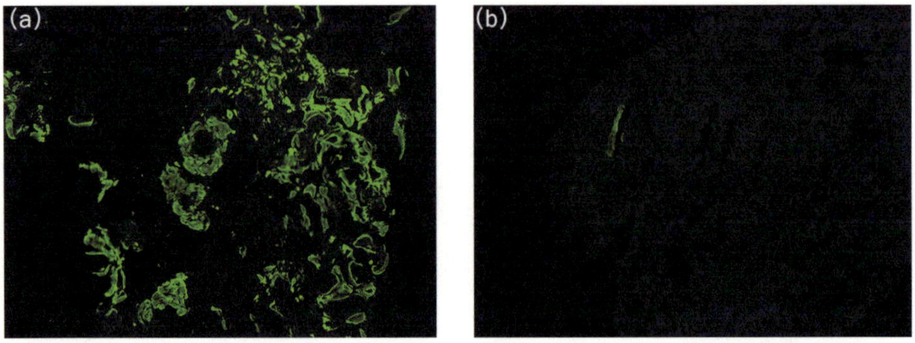

Figure 11. AL nephropathy with smudgy mesangial, vascular, and interstitial staining for lambda (a) and negative kappa (b) (IF, original magnification ×400).

In addition to specific staining for proteins that comprise the amyloid, amyloid deposits often have low levels of nonspecific trapping with several reagent antibodies, including Ig and complements (**Figure 14a** and **b**). This varies, with different reagent antibodies and different

http://dx.doi.org/10.5772/64083

specimens, and is more common with AA nephropathy than AL nephropathy. The basis for this low level of staining is not well understood, but may result from charge interaction between the amyloid and the reagent antibodies, contamination with serum proteins, and/or humoral reaction directed against amyloid fibrils. These low levels of nonspecific trapping sometime render the distinction between AA nephropathy and AL/AH/AHL nephropathy difficult. About 21% of AA nephropathy cases from a study by Nasr et al. [8] could not be diagnosed with certainty by IF and needed confirmation of amyloid type by mass spectrometry.

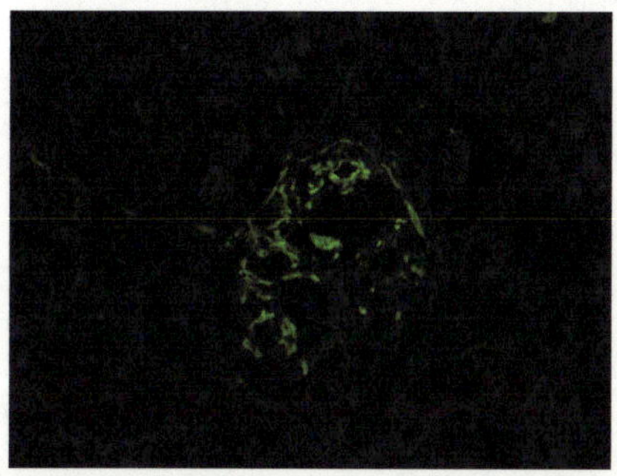

Figure 12. AH nephropathy. Intense glomerular staining for IgG heavy chain. Kappa and lambda are negative (IF, original magnification ×400).

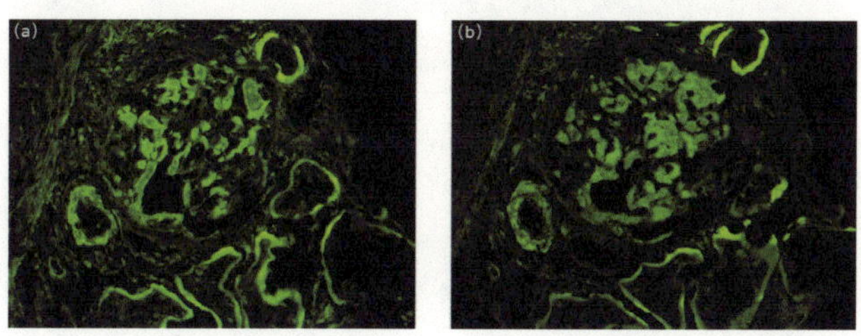

Figure 13. AHL nephropathy. Intense glomerular, vascular and tubular basement membrane staining for IgG heavy chain (a) and lambda light chain (b). Kappa is negative (IF, original magnification ×400).

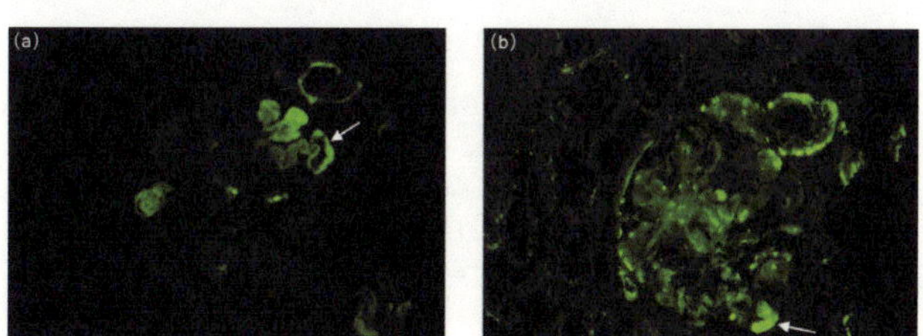

Figure 14. Low level of non-specific staining for Immunoglobulin M (IgM) (a, arrow) and complement 3 (C3) (b, arrow) in AA nephropathy (IF, original magnification ×400).

6.3. Electron microscopy

Transmission electron microscopy (TEM) is helpful in confirming the diagnosis of amyloidosis, but it is not helpful in determining the type of amyloid. At low magnification, amyloid deposits have a characteristic cottony appearance (**Figure 15**) that should alert the pathologist to investigate at higher magnification the possibility of amyloidosis. At high magnification, amyloid is composed of randomly arranged, elongated fibrils that measure 8–12 nm in diameter (**Figure 16**). Amyloid fibrils are associated with smaller, round structures, namely, amyloid p component. The fibrils are extracellular and located near mesangial cells in glomeruli and myocytes in the media of vessel walls in amyloid nephropathy. The amyloid

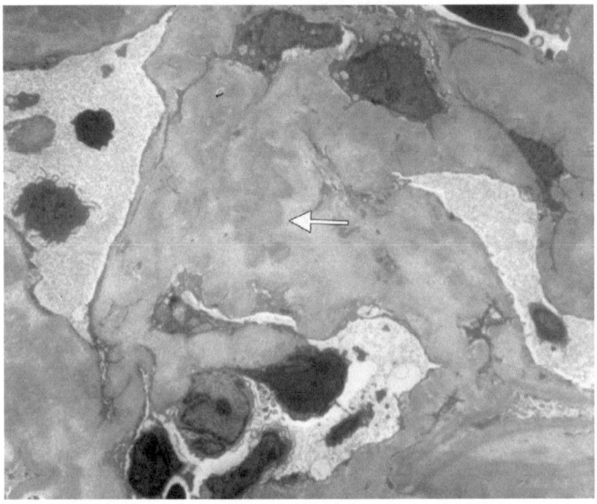

Figure 15. Extensive expansion of the mesangium by amyloid, which shows lumpy cottony appearance (arrow) on low power electron microscopy (transmission electron microscopy (TEM), original magnification, ×5600).

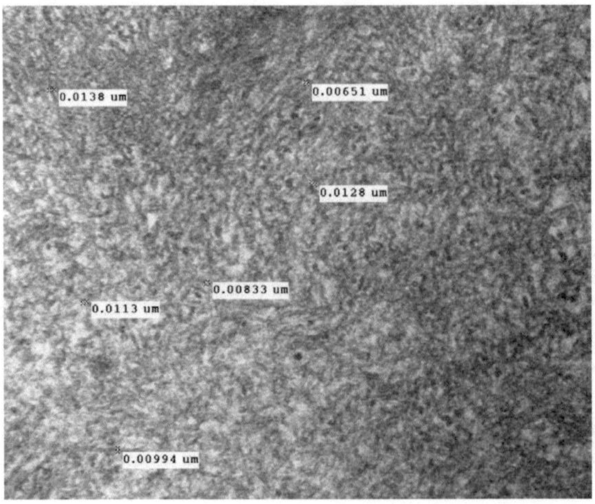

Figure 16. AL nephropathy. Amyloid fibrils replacing normal mesangium. Typical amyloid fibrils are randomly arranged, nonbranching and measure 8–12 nm in diameter (TEM, original magnification, ×14,000).

http://dx.doi.org/10.5772/64083

fibrils may extend into the capillary walls and thus, foot process effacement is commonly seen in the segments of glomerular basement membranes overlying amyloid deposits. The podocyte cytoplasm adjacent to the amyloid deposits often shows condensation of actin cytoskeleton. When amyloid deposits extend into the subepithelial zone, the fibrils usually show parallel alignment (**Figure 17**). This is the basis for the JMS-positive feathery spikes that may be seen by light microscopy (LM).

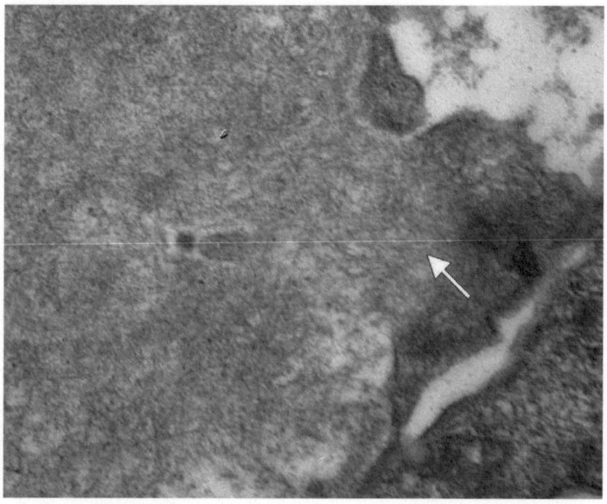

Figure 17. Alignment of amyloid fibrils (arrow) in the subepithelial zone of a glomerular basement membrane. This is the basis for the JMS-positive feathery spikes that may be seen by LM (TEM, original magnification, ×5600).

6.4. Differential diagnosis

The differential diagnosis and distinction from other glomerular diseases are summarized in **Table 2**. By LM, the differential diagnosis includes any disease process that induces accumulation of acellular eosinophilic material in glomeruli, blood vessels, and interstitium. Accumulations of collagenous matrix, as in Kimmelstiel-Wilson nodules in diabetic nephropathy or sclerosis secondary to chronic immune complex glomerulonephritis or hypertensive nephrosclerosis, usually can be readily distinguished from amyloid by routine staining. As mentioned earlier, amyloid stains weakly with PAS and very little or negative with JMS, whereas sclerotic matrix is strongly PAS and JMS positive. Extensive glomerular deposits present in immune complex glomerulonephritis, fibrillary glomerulonephritis, immunotactoid glomerulopathy, and collagenofibrotic glomerulopathy may mimic amyloidosis on H&E stained sections; however, special stains, IHC, and EM demonstrate the distinctive features of each of these diseases. The Congo red stain is then necessary to confirm the diagnosis of amyloid nephropathy.

Light-chain deposition disease (LCDD) shares monoclonal immunoglobulin light-chain staining with AL nephropathy, but the pattern of staining is much different. LCDD typically has a more diffuse and regular distribution of staining that appears linear or ribbon-like along glomerular and tubular basement membranes. The expanded mesangium also shows globular staining in LCDD, in contrast to AL nephropathy, which typically shows a smudgy pattern of lambda or kappa light-chain staining with fuzzy border in the mesangium or along glomerular basement membranes, but no ribbon-like tubular basement membrane deposits.

Differential diagnosis	**Congo red stain**	**LM**	**IF**	**EM**
Light-chain deposition disease	Negative	Deposition of PAS positive and argyrophilic material in mesangium with occasional nodular formation	Diffuse intense staining of single light chain (more often kappa) along tubular and/or glomerular basement membranes (ribbon-like), involving mesangium (globular), and blood vessels	Finely granular (punctate) or amorphous electron dense deposits along the inner aspect of glomerular basement membranes and outer aspect of tubular basement membranes
Light- and heavy-chain deposition disease	Negative	Deposition of PAS positive and argyrophilic material in mesangium with occasional nodular formation, more mesangial hypercellularity	Diffuse intense staining of single Ig heavy chain (more often IgG) and a single light chain along tubular and/or glomerular basement membranes (ribbon-like), involving mesangium (globular), and blood vessels	Finely granular (punctate) or amorphous electron dense deposits along the inner aspect of glomerular basement membranes and outer aspect of tubular basement membranes, occasional immune complex-type deposits, or rarely no electron deposits detected
Heavy-chain deposition disease	Negative	Deposition of PAS positive and argyrophilic material in mesangium with occasional nodular formation, more mesangial hypercellularity	Diffuse intense staining of single Ig heavy chain (more IgG3) along tubular and/or glomerular basement membranes (ribbon-like), involving mesangium (globular), and blood vessels, no kappa or lambda staining	Finely granular (punctate) or amorphous electron dense deposits along the inner aspect of glomerular basement membranes and outer aspect of tubular basement membranes, occasional immune complex-type deposits, or rarely no electron deposits detected
Fibrillary GN	Negative	Deposition of PAS positive and nonargyrophilic in mesangium and occasionally along glomerular basement membranes	Smudgy staining for IgG (more often IgG4), C3, kappa, and lambda in mesangium and along capillary loops, about 10% show restriction of light-chain staining	Randomly arranged nonbranching fibrils size of 12-27 nm in diameter within mesangium, along outer aspect of glomerular basement membranes, and rarely along tubular basement membranes
Immunotactoid glomerulopathy	Negative	Deposition of PAS positive and nonargyrophilic in	Smudgy staining for IgG (more often IgG1), C3, with light chain	Microtubular or cylindrical structure with hollow cores with a size from 20 to 90 nm in

http://dx.doi.org/10.5772/64083

Differential diagnosis	Congo red stain	LM	IF	EM
		mesangium and occasionally along glomerular basement membranes	restriction (more kappa), staining in mesangium and capillary loops	diameter, arranged in parallel arrays, predominantly present in mesangium and subepithelial zone
Diabetic nephropathy	Negative	Accumulation of PAS positive and argyrophilic glycosylate products, Kimmelstiel-Wilson nodules, prominent glomerular basement membranes	Linear accentuation of IgG and albumin along glomerular and tubular basement membranes	Diabetic fibrillosis with branching fibrils with a size of 10–25 nm in diameter in mesangium, thickened glomerular basement membranes
Collagenofibrotic glomerulopathy	Negative	Increase in mesangial matrix, argyrophilic, PAS positive material with intense blue staining on Masson trichrome stain	Negative staining	curved and frayed, sometimes worm-like of comma-shaped fibers with transverse band structure with periodicity of 43–65 nm when sectioned transversely
Fibronectin glomerulopathy	Negative	Mesangial matrix accumulation of nonargyrophilic material with bright red staining on Masson trichrome stain	May have nonspecific staining for IgG, IgM, and C3	Granular to fibrillary substructures with a size of 14–16 nm in diameter

Table 2. Histologic differential diagnosis of amyloid nephropathy.

By EM, the differential diagnosis includes other renal diseases that have deposits containing organized fibrillary or microtubular substructures, including fibrillary glomerulonephritis, immunotactoid glomerulopathy, and collagenofibrotic glomerulopathy. Fibrillary glomerulonephritis is characterized by glomerular deposits composed of randomly arranged, nonbranching fibrils that usually are 12–27 nm in diameter (**Figure 18**). The diagnosis of amyloidosis is unlikely if fibrils are larger than 20 nm. Immunotactoid glomerulopathy has organized microtubular substructures with hollow cores, measuring 20–90 nm (**Figure 19**). Collagenofibrotic glomerulopathy shows collagen fibrils deposited predominantly in the mesangium but sometimes can extend to subendothelial zone. The collagen fibrils appear curved and often frayed with periodicity of 43–65 nm. In diabetic fibrillosis, the fibrils are 10–25 nm, negative for Congo red and Thioflavin T. These fibrils tend to be shorter and more often aligned in parallel, slightly curved, and sometimes are oriented at right angles to mesangial cell surfaces, and may touch plasma membranes (**Figure 20**). Of note, the presence of diabetic fibrillosis in diabetic nephropathy does not appear to have any specific clinical connotations because a patient with this disorder behaves similarly clinically to those without fibrils [36]. For each of the above conditions with substructure of material by EM, IF and light microscopic appearances, and negative Congo red stain, allow distinction from amyloidosis.

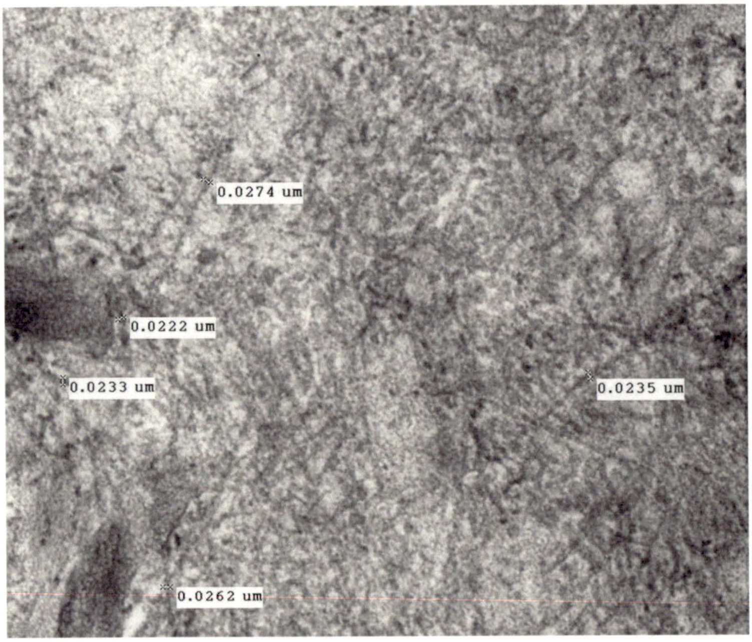

Figure 18. Fibrillary glomerulonephritis with randomly arranged nonbranching fibrils that measure 12–27 nm in diameter (TEM, original magnification, ×14,000).

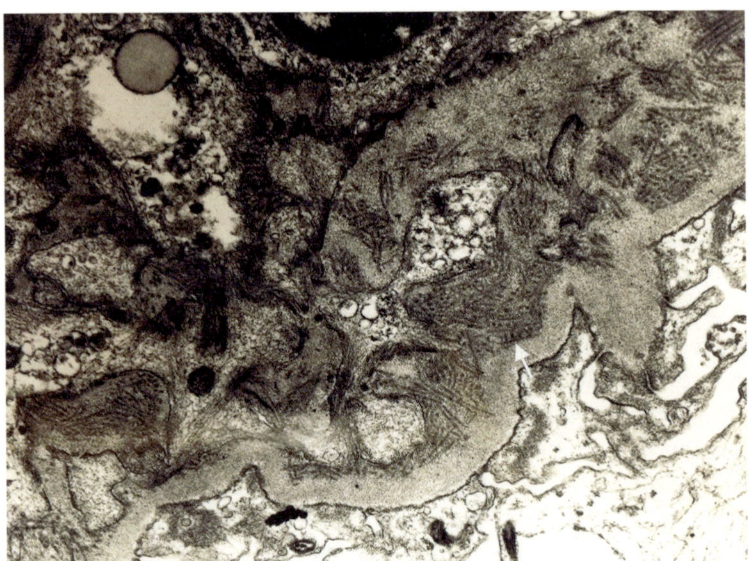

Figure 19. Immunotactoid glomerulopathy. Replacement of mesangial matrix by microtubular substructures (arrow) with hollow cores that measure 20–90 nm in diameter (TEM, original magnification, ×14, 000).

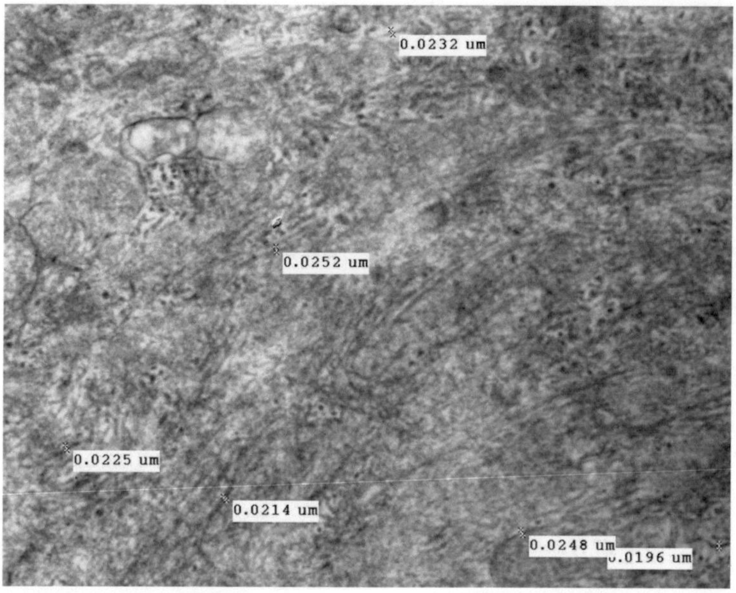

Figure 20. Diabetic fibrillosis. Replacement of mesangial matrix by short nonbranching fibrils that measure 10–25 nm in diameter. These fibrils tend to be more often aligned in parallel, slightly curved, and sometimes are oriented at right angles to mesangial cell surfaces (TEM, original magnification, ×14,000).

6.5. Typing of amyloid does matter

Amyloid typing is absolutely crucial for clinical management in order to avoid misdiagnosis and inappropriate, potentially harmful treatment, to assess prognosis and to offer genetic counseling if relevant. The classification is based on the nature of amyloid precursor plasma proteins. The initial step is IF, which is an important technique for AL typing. In AL nephropathy, there is restriction for either kappa or lambda light chain. In AH nephropathy, the deposits stain only a single subclass of Ig heavy chain, whereas a single heavy-chain and a single light-chain stain positive in AHL nephropathy. In cases where no frozen tissue is available, IF can be performed on paraffin embedded tissue by a pronase-digested technique. The paraffin-embedded tissue pronase-digested technique has less sensitivity than frozen tissue IF. Thus, negative IF staining for Ig light chains or heavy chain does not completely rule out AL nephropathy, AH nephropathy, or AHL nephropathy, as some monoclonal proteins may be mutated and not recognized by commercial antibodies. However, a negative IF study does typically suggest another type of amyloid nephropathy and requires further exploration by other modalities to diagnose the type of amyloid.

Current diagnostic methods, such as IHC technique using antibody-based amyloid typing, have limited ability to detect the full spectrum of amyloid forming proteins. Although IHC can be performed using commercially available antibodies against amyloid of the classes AL, AH, AA, AFib, ATTR, AApo AI, and Aβ2M [10], of these antibodies, serum amyloid A (SAA) IHC on paraffin-embedded tissue is the most extensively used and is considered the gold standard technique for diagnosing AA (**Figure 21**). AA IHC reveals a pattern of distribution matching that seen by LM. From our study, IHC on paraffin-embedded tissue for LECT2 is sensitive; however, it is not entirely specific for ALECT2 [41]. It is recommended that the diagnosis of ALECT2 nephropathy should be confirmed by mass spectrometry analysis of renal tissues when the staining pattern shows equivocal Intensity [41].

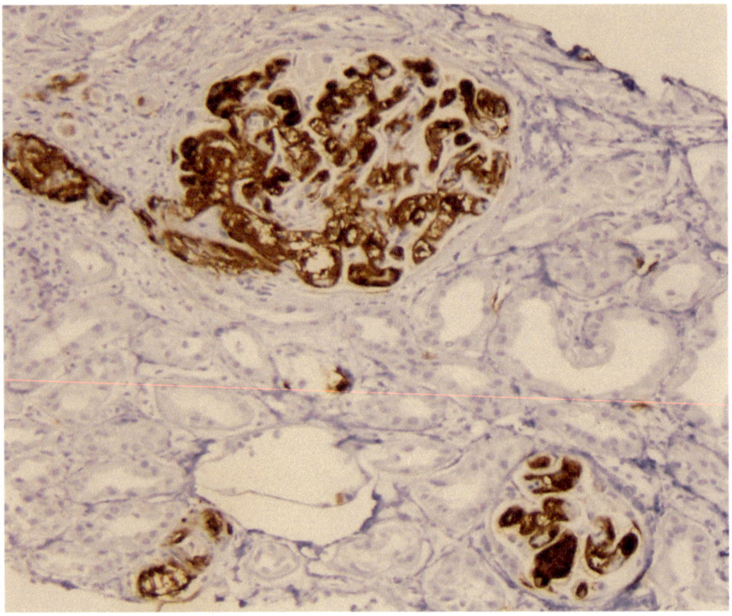

Figure 21. AA nephropathy with intense glomerular and vascular staining for SAA IHC (anti-SAA IHC, original magnification ×200).

In spite of the availability of IF and IHC, there are multiple drawbacks of these methods, such as sensitivity and specificity of commercial antibodies that are designed against only nonmutated proteins. Mutant proteins and proteins with conformational changes might be less reactive to commercial antibodies [39]. For example, in 7–35% of the AL nephropathy cases, the amyloid deposits were negative for both kappa and lambda IF staining on frozen tissue [7]. Therefore, be aware that a negative staining for light- and/or heavy-chain IF does not exclude AIg nephropathy. Of note, rare cases of amyloid nephropathy show more than one type of amyloid protein, leading to difficulty in typing. The drawbacks of these techniques may be solved by mass spectrometry, which is discussed below.

6.6. Proteomics

The direct technique of amyloid demonstration is based on proteomic analysis using laser microdissection/mass spectrometry (LMD/MS), which has the capability for identification of the many different proteins [43]. This technique has a high sensitivity and specificity and solves many of the problems presented by other techniques [44].

LMD/MS has proved to be useful to determine the nature and type of the amyloid precursor protein in cases that could not be typed by routine IHC panels [45, 46]. The major advantage of LMD/MS over conventional IHC techniques in typing of amyloid is that LMD/MS is a single test that can identify and type the amyloid protein, in contrast to IHC that may require several antibodies staining multiple sections [47]. Furthermore, LMD/MS is performed from paraffin-embedded tissue and requires no special treatment. The common indications for LMD/MS in amyloid nephropathy include amyloid type confirmation, insufficient tissue sample for IF or IHC studies but with remaining tissue in paraffin block, difficult cases on routine renal biopsy studies such as heavy-chain amyloidosis and familial and hereditary forms of amyloidosis [17, 48, 49]. The diagnosis of amyloidosis at the proteomic level using LMD/MS is purely based on the presence of large spectra of proteins, which have amyloidogenic properties, in addition to apolipoprotein E (Apo E) and SAP that are commonly present in all types of amyloid [40]. Therefore, in AA nephropathy, large spectra numbers of serum amyloid-associated protein along with Apo E and SAP are present. In contrast, in ALECT2 and AGel nephropathy, large spectra numbers of LECT2 and gelsolin are present along with Apo E and SAP.

LMD/MS has been very helpful in achieving amyloid typing from formalin-fixed paraffin-embedded tissue. LMD/MS has also been critical for the typing of cases with limited antibody reactivity and in the discovery of new protein types of amyloid. From a study by Said et al., the type of amyloid in 16% of amyloid nephropathy cases could not have been typed without LMD/MS [8]. In spite of these major advantages, LMD/MS also has a few drawbacks. As mentioned above, identification of amyloid proteins is purely based on the presence of large spectra for proteins, which have amyloidogenic properties within the analyzed sample. In a case of focal amyloidosis, a small amount of amyloid deposit may be obscured by Apo E, SAP, and various serum proteins. Furthermore, the observed peptide fragmentation data must be matched to known protein sequences that are available in the public data base, and thus, unknown protein sequences due to certain germ line polymorphisms or somatic mutations, may not be identified. Despite these drawbacks, the number of cases of amyloid with undetermined type has markedly decreased with use of this technique to 7%, with 3% of the sample insufficient for analysis [7, 8, 50]

6.7. Treatment and prognosis

The goal of current treatment approaches for AIg nephropathy is to eradicate the clone of plasma cells that produce amyloidogenic monoclonal light chains, Ig heavy chain, and Ig heavy and light chain. Patients with AIg nephropathy are usually treated with chemotherapeutic regimens appropriate for B-cell or plasma cell neoplasm. Melphalan-dexamethasone-bortezomib is commonly used as frontline regimen for patients with Stages I and II cardiac involvement [51]. Patients with Stage III cardiac involvement or advanced chronic kidney disease (CKD) patients are generally treated with cyclophosphamide-bortezomib-dexamethasone [51, 52], which showed overall 81.4% hematologic response [53]. High-dose intravenous melphalan followed by autologous stem cell transplantation (HDM/ASCT) to support bone marrow recovery has emerged as the most likely to eradicate the clonal plasma cells [39].

Experiences from several treatment centers has suggested that 25–50% of patients who undergo such treatment have complete hematologic response, indicating that there is no evidence of ongoing production of monoclonal light chains, Ig heavy chain, or Ig heavy chain and light chain [52–54]. HDM/ASCT is generally offered to patients with Stages I or II cardiac involvement patients who have glomerular filtration rate (GFR) ≥ 30 mL/min in the absence of advanced other organ involvement [54–56].

Treatment of the underlying chronic inflammatory diseases, such as immunosuppressive agents for rheumatoid arthritis and inflammatory bowel diseases is beneficial in patients with AA nephropathy. The basis of modern treatment in AA nephropathy is still reduction of SAA production. Additionally, steroids and cytotoxic drugs, treatment with monoclonal antibodies against cytokines, particularly tumor necrotic factors (TNF) and interleukin-6 (IL-6), are effective in many cases [57]. This approach of treatment is targeted not only at amyloid fibrils themselves but also at messengers in the acute-phase response. Other therapies, such as antisense oligonucleotides, have been suggested to specifically lower the expression of SAA in the liver [57]. AA nephropathy caused by familial Mediterranean fever responds to colchicine [58]. In familial amyloidosis, including AFib, ATTR, and AApo AI, in which the liver is the source of precursor protein, patients are treated with liver transplantation [57]. A novel drug, R-1-[6-[R-2carboxy-pyrrolidin-1-yl]-6-oxo-hexanoyl]pyrrolidine-2-carboxylic acid is a competitive inhibitor of SAP binding to amyloid fibrils [59, 60]. This palindromic compound also cross-links and dimerizes SAP molecules, leading to their very rapid clearance by the liver, and hence produces a marked reduction in human SAP in the circulation [61]. This mechanism of drug action potently removes SAP from the deposits of amyloid in human tissue and may provide a new therapeutic approach to AA amyloidosis and diseases associated with local amyloid deposition, including Alzheimer's disease [61].

The prognosis for patients with AL nephropathy is generally poor and depends on systemic organ involvement, but survival can be prolonged with treatment [62, 63]. Patients with AL nephropathy have a median overall survival of 1–2 years [62, 63]. Patients with AA nephropathy have a better prognosis than those with AL nephropathy with the median survival varies between 2 and 10 years [13, 64]. In AL nephropathy and AA nephropathy, cardiac involvement is an independent negative predictive factor of patient survival [13]. Patients with AA, AH, AHL, AFib, and ALECT2 nephropathy have longer overall survival compared with AL nephropathy, largely because of a lower rate of cardiac involvement [13, 65, 66]. The mean survival for AFib is 15 years [10], and the median survival for ALECT nephropathy is 62 months [66].

In AL nephropathy, kidney transplantation is ideally performed after production of amyloidogenic light-chain proteins has been eradicated. Kidney transplantation for systemic AL patients has a relative good outcome with 1- and 5-year patient survival of 75% and 67% and median graft survival of 5.8 years [67–69]. However, amyloidosis may recur in kidney transplants, depending on the amyloid type and progression of the underlying disease. In a large series from the UK, among 246 patients with AL nephropathy with renal failure, only 10% received kidney transplants [69], and of these, amyloidosis recurred in 28%; however, no graft was lost due to recurrent AL amyloidosis [67]. Patient survival was best among patients who had achieved partial remission before kidney transplantation (8.9 years). In a French series of 59 recipients with AA amyloidosis, recurrence was documented in 14% at a median of 10 years posttransplant and was often associated with nephrotic range proteinuria [70]. Among 10 recipients with hereditary AFib amyloidosis who received kidney transplantation only, recurrent AFib amyloidosis was detected in 70% and median graft survival was 7.3 years [69]. In contrast, no recurrence was detected in the nine patients who received combined kidney and liver transplantation, but the mean renal graft survival was 6.4 years [62]. Hereditary AApo I amyloidosis has recurred in 30% who received kidney transplantation only, and of these, one graft was lost to recurrent AApo I amyloidosis [68]. There is no effective therapy for ALECT2 nephropathy [37]. Because the precursor protein in ALECT2 is nonmutant, liver transplantation is likely ineffective [26]. Kidney transplantation has been suggested as a treatment option for ALECT2 nephropathy patients with advanced renal failure [35]. Although the disease may recur in about 20% of allografts, no graft was lost to recurrent ALECT2 nephropathy [69]. Possible future therapies for ALECT2 nephropathy include reducing the supply of LECT2 (e.g., inhibiting the Wnt/β-catenin signal pathway), inhibiting amyloid fibril formation by blocking the binding of glycoaminoglycans to amyloid fibrils, promoting clearance of amyloid by immunotherapy, and promoting amyloid regression by SAP-targeted therapy.

Acknowledgements

The author thanks Dr. Agnes Fogo and Dr. Mark Lusco for their helpful advice.

Author details

Paisit Paueksakon

Address all correspondence to: paisit.paueksakon@vanderbilt.edu

Department of Pathology, Microbiology, and Immunology, Vanderbilt University Medical Center, Nashville, TN, USA

References

[1] Kisilevsky R. Amyloid and amyloidoses: differences, common themes, and practical considerations. Mod Pathol. 1991; 4(4): 514–8.

[2] Thornton C. Amyloid disease. An autopsy review of the decades 1937–46 and 1961–70. Ulster Med J. 1983; 52(1): 31–4.

[3] Tuglular S, Yalcinkaya F, Paydas S, Oner A, Utas C, Bozfakioglu S, Ataman R, Akpolat T, Ok E, Sen S, Düsünsel R, Evrenkaya R, Akoglu E. A retrospective analysis for aetiology and clinical findings of 287 secondary amyloidosis cases in Turkey. Nephrol Dial Transplant. 2002; 17(11): 2003–5.

[4] Ensari C, Ensari A, Tümer N, Ertug E. Clinicopathological and epidemiological analysis of amyloidosis in Turkish patients. Nephrol Dial Transplant. 2005; 20(8): 1721–5.

[5] Lekpa FK, Ndongo S, Pouye A, Tiendrebeogo JW, Ndao AC, Ka MM, Diop TM. Amyloidosis in sub-Saharan Africa. Med Sante Trop. 2012; 22(3): 275–8.

[6] Larsen CP, Walker PD, Weiss DT, Solomon A. Prevalence and morphology of leukocyte chemotactic factor 2-associated amyloid in renal biopsies. Kidney Int. 2010 77: 816–819.

[7] Sethi S, Vrana JA, Theis JD, Dogan A. Mass spectrometry based proteomics in the diagnosis of kidney disease. Curr Opin Nephrol Hypertens. 2013; 22(3):273–80.

[8] Said SM, Sethi S, Valeri AM, Leung N, Cornell LD, Fidler ME, Herrera Hernandez L, Vrana JA, Theis JD, Quint PS, Dogan A, Nasr SH. Renal amyloidosis: origin and clinicopathologic correlations of 474 recent cases. Clin J Am Soc Nephrol. 2013; 8(9): 1515–23.

[9] Manabe S, Hatano M, Yazaki M, Nitta K, Nagata M. Renal AH amyloidosis associated with a truncated immunoglobulin heavy chain undetectable by immunostaining. Am J Kidney Dis. 2015; 66(6): 1095–100.

[10] Markowitz GS. Dysproteinemia and the kidney. Adv Anat Pathol. 2004; 11(1): 49–63.

[11] von Hutten H, Mihatsch M, Lobeck H, Rudolph B, Eriksson M, Röcken C. Prevalence and origin of amyloid in kidney biopsies. Am J Surg Pathol. 2009; 33: 1198–1205.

[12] Gillmore JD, Lachmann HJ, Rowczenio D, Gilbertson JA, Zeng CH, Liu ZH, Li LS, Wechalekar A, Hawkins PN. Diagnosis, pathogenesis, treatment, and prognosis of hereditary fibrinogen A alpha-chain amyloidosis. J Am Soc Nephrol. 2009; 20(2): 444–51.

[13] Bergesio F, Ciciani AM, Manganaro M, Palladini G, Santostefano M, Brugnano R, Di Palma AM, Gallo M, Rosati A, Tosi PL, Salvadori M.; Immunopathology Group of the Italian Society of Nephrology. Renal involvement in systemic amyloidosis: an Italian collaborative study on survival and renal outcome. Nephrol Dial Transplant. 2008; 23(3): 941–51.

[14] Sethi S, Thesis JD, Quint P, Maierhofer W, Kurtin PJ, Dogan A, Highsmith EW Jr. Renal amyloidosis associated with a novel sequence variant of gelsolin. Am J Kidney Dis. 2013; 1: 161–166.

[15] Soutar AK, Hawkins PN, Vigushin DM, Tennent GA, Booth SE, Hutton T, Nguyen O, Totty NF, Feest TG, Hsuan JJ, et al. Apolipoprotein AI mutation Arg-60 causes autosomal dominant amyloidosis. Proc Natl Acad Sci U S A. 1992; 89(16): 7389–93.

[16] Yazaki M, Liepnieks JJ, Yamashita T, Guenther B, Skinner M, Benson MD. Renal amyloidosis caused by a novel stop-codon mutation in the apolipoprotein A-II gene. Kidney Int. 2001; 60(5): 1658–65.

[17] Sethi S, Theis JD, Shiller SM, Nast CC, Harrison D, Rennke HG, Vrana JA, Dogan A. Medullary amyloidosis associated with apolipoprotein A-IV deposition. Kidney Int. 2012; 81(2): 201–6.

[18] Benson MD, James S, Scott K, Liepnieks JJ, Kluve-Beckerman B. Leukocyte chemotactic factor 2: a novel renal amyloid protein. Kidney Int. 2008 Jul;74(2):218–22.

[19] Kyle RA, Gertz MA. Primary systemic amyloidosis: clinical and laboratory features in 474 cases. Semin Hematol. 1995; 32(1): 45–59.

[20] Fu J, Seldin DC, Berk JL, Sun F, O'Hara C, Cui H, Sanchorawala V. Lymphadenopathy as a manifestation of amyloidosis: a case series. Amyloid. 2014; 21(4): 256–60.

[21] Loo D, Mollee PN, Renaut P, Hill MM. Proteomics in molecular diagnosis: typing of amyloidosis. J Biomed Biotechnol. 2011; 754109.

[22] Merlini G, Bellotti V. Molecular mechanisms of amyloidosis. N Engl J Med. 2003;349(6): 583–96.

[23] Ozaki S, Abe M, Wolfenbarger D, Weiss DT, Solomon A. Preferential expression of human lambda-light-chain variable-region subgroups in multiple myeloma, AL amyloidosis, and Waldenström's macroglobulinemia. Clin Immunol Immunopathol. 1994; 71(2): 183–9.

[24] Solomon A, Frangione B, Franklin EC. Bence Jones proteins and light chains of immunoglobulins. Preferential association of the V lambda VI subgroup of human light chains with amyloidosis AL (lambda). J Clin Invest. 1982; 70(2): 453–60.

[25] Hurle MR, Helms LR, Li L, Chan W, Wetzel R. A role for destabilizing amino acid replacements in light-chain amyloidosis. Proc Natl Acad Sci U S A. 1994; 91(12): 5446–50.

[26] McCutchen SL, Lai Z, Miroy GJ, Kelly JW, Colón W. Comparison of lethal and nonlethal transthyretin variants and their relationship to amyloid disease. Biochemistry. 1995; 34(41): 13527–36.

[27] Booth DR, Sunde M, Bellotti V, Robinson CV, Hutchinson WL, Fraser PE, Hawkins PN, Dobson CM, Radford SE, Blake CC, Pepys MB. Instability, unfolding and aggregation of human lysozyme variants underlying amyloid fibrillogenesis. Nature. 1997; 385(6619): 787–93.

[28] Hardy J, Selkoe DJ. The amyloid hypothesis of Alzheimer's disease: progress and problems on the road to therapeutics. Science. 2002; 297(5580): 353–6.

[29] McLaurin J, Yang D, Yip CM, Fraser PE. Review: modulating factors in amyloid-beta fibril formation. Struct Biol. 2000; 130(2–3): 259–70.

[30] Kisilevsky R, Manley PN. Acute-phase serum amyloid A: perspectives on its physiological and pathological roles. Amyloid. 2012;19 (1): 5–14.

[31] Verdone G, Corazza A, Viglino P, Pettirossi F, Giorgetti S, Mangione P, Andreola A, Stoppini M, Bellotti V, Esposito G. The solution structure of human beta2-microglobulin reveals the prodromes of its amyloid transition. Protein Sci. 2002; 11(3): 487–99.

[32] Scholefield Z, Yates EA, Wayne G, Amour A, McDowell W, Turnbull JE. Heparan sulfate regulates amyloid precursor protein processing by BACE1, the Alzheimer's beta-secretase. J Cell Biol. 2003; 163(1): 97–107.

[33] Ding Y, Kim JK, Kim SI, Na HJ, Jun SY, Lee SJ, Choi ME. TGF-{beta}1 protects against mesangial cell apoptosis via induction of autophagy. J Biol Chem. 2010; 285(48): 37909–19.

[34] Teng J, Russell WJ, Gu X, Cardelli J, Jones ML, Herrera GA. Different types of glomerulopathic light chains interact with mesangial cells using a common receptor but exhibit different intracellular trafficking patterns. Lab Invest. 2004; 84(4): 440–51.

[35] Teng J, Turbat-Herrera EA, Herrera GA. Extrusion of amyloid fibrils to the extracellular space in experimental mesangial AL-amyloidosis: transmission and scanning electron microscopy studies and correlation with renal biopsy observations. Ultrastruct Pathol. 2014;38(2):104–15.

[36] Herrera GA, Turbat-Herrera EA. Renal diseases with organized deposits: an algorithmic approach to classification and clinicopathologic diagnosis. Arch Pathol Lab Med. 2010; 134(4): 512–31.

[37] Nasr SH, Dogan A, Larsen CP. Leukocyte cell-derived chemotaxin 2-associated amyloidosis: a recently recognized disease with distinct clinicopathologic characteristics. Clin J Am Soc Nephrol. 2015; 10(11): 2084–93.

[38] Richards DB, Cookson LM, Berges AC, Barton SV, Lane T, Ritter JM, Fontana M, Moon JC, Pinzani M, Gillmore JD, Hawkins PN, Pepys MB. Therapeutic clearance of amyloid by antibodies to serum amyloid P component. N Engl J Med. 2015; 373(12): 1106–14.

[39] Dember LM. Amyloidosis-associated kidney disease. J Am Soc Nephrol. 2006; 17(12): 3458–71.

[40] Dikman SH, Churg J, Kahn T. Morphologic and clinical correlates in renal amyloidosis. Hum Pathol. 1981; 12(2): 160–9.

[41] Elghetany MT, Saleem A, Barr K. The Congo red stain revisited. Ann Clin Lab Sci. 1989; 19(3) :190–5.

[42] Westermark GT, Johnson KH, Westermark P. Staining methods for identification of amyloid in tissue. Methods Enzymol. 1999; 309: 3–25.

[43] Paueksakon P, Fogo AB, Sethi S. Leukocyte chemotactic factor 2 amyloidosis cannot be reliably diagnosed by immunohistochemical staining. Hum Pathol. 2014; 45(7): 1445–50.

[44] Leung N, Nasr SH, Sethi S. How I treat amyloidosis: the importance of accurate diagnosis and amyloid typing. Blood. 2012; 120(16): 3206–13.

[45] Sethi S, Vrana JA, Theis JD, Leung N, Sethi A, Nasr SH, Fervenza FC, Cornell LD, Fidler ME, Dogan A. Laser microdissection and mass spectrometry-based proteomics aids the diagnosis and typing of renal amyloidosis. Kidney Int. 2012; 82(2): 226–34.

[46] Vrana JA, Gamez JD, Madden BJ, Theis JD, Bergen HR 3rd, Dogan A. Classification of amyloidosis by laser microdissection and mass spectrometry-based proteomic analysis in clinical biopsy specimens. Blood. 2009; 114(24): 4957–9.

[47] Murphy CL, Wang S, Williams T, Weiss DT, Solomon A. Characterization of systemic amyloid deposits by mass spectrometry. Methods Enzymol. 2006; 412: 48–62.

[48] Murphy CL, Eulitz M, Hrncic R, Sletten K, Westermark P, Williams T, Macy SD, Wooliver C, Wall J, Weiss DT, Solomon A. Chemical typing of amyloid protein contained in formalin-fixed paraffin-embedded biopsy specimens. Am J Clin Pathol. 2001; 116(1): 135–42.

[49] Sethi S, Theis JD, Leung N, Dispenzieri A, Nasr SH, Fidler ME, Cornell LD, Gamez JD, Vrana JA, Dogan A. Mass spectrometry-based proteomic diagnosis of renal immunoglobulin heavy chain amyloidosis. Clin J Am Soc Nephrol. 2010; 5(12): 2180–7.

[50] Dogan A, Theis JD, Vrana JA. Mass spectrometry based proteomics for classification of amyloidosis. Mayo Clinic experience. In: Hazenberg BP, Bijzet J, van Gameren II, et al., eds. XIIIth International Symposium on Amyloidosis. Groningen: UMCG. 2013;183–185.

[51] Kastritis E, Dimopoulos MA. Recent advances in the management of AL amyloidosis. Br J Haematol. 2016; 172(2): 170–86.

[52] Rannigan L, Gibbs SD, Pinney JH, Whelan CJ, Lachmann HJ, Gillmore JD, Hawkins PN, Wechalekar AD. Cyclophosphamide, bortezomib, and dexamethasone therapy in AL amyloidosis is associated with high clonal response rates and prolonged progression-free survival. Blood. 2012; 119(19): 4387–90.

[53] Venner CP, Lane T, Foard D, Rannigan L, Gibbs SD, Pinney JH, Whelan CJ, Lachmann HJ, Gillmore JD, Hawkins PN, Wechalekar AD. Cyclophosphamide, bortezomib, and dexamethasone therapy in AL amyloidosis is associated with high clonal response rates and prolonged progression-free survival. Blood. 2012; 119(19):4387–90.

[54] Skinner M, Sanchorawala V, Seldin DC, Dember LM, Falk RH, Berk JL, Anderson JJ, O'Hara C, Finn KT, Libbey CA, Wiesman J, Quillen K, Swan N, Wright DG. High-dose

melphalan and autologous stem-cell transplantation in patients with AL amyloidosis: an 8-year study. Ann Intern Med. 2004; 140(2): 85–93.

[55] Gertz MA, Lacy MQ, Dispenzieri A, Gastineau DA, Chen MG, Ansell SM, Inwards DJ, Micallef IN, Tefferi A, Litzow MR. Stem cell transplantation for the management of primary systemic amyloidosis. Am J Med. 2002; 113(7): 549–55.

[56] Moreau P, Leblond V, Bourquelot P, Facon T, Huynh A, Caillot D, Hermine O, Attal M, Hamidou M, Nedellec G, Ferrant A, Audhuy B, Bataille R, Milpied N, Harousseau JL. Prognostic factors for survival and response after high-dose therapy and autologous stem cell transplantation in systemic AL amyloidosis: a report on 21 patients. Br J Haematol. 1998; 101(4):766–9.

[57] Westermark GT, Fändrich M, Westermark P. AA amyloidosis: pathogenesis and targeted therapy. Annu Rev Pathol. 2015; 10: 321–44.

[58] Meneses CF, Egües CA, Uriarte M, Belzunegui J, Rezola M. Colchicine use in isolated renal AA amyloidosis. Reumatol Clin. 2015; 11(4): 242–3.

[59] Sahota T, Berges A, Barton S, Cookson L, Zamuner S, Richards D. Target mediated drug disposition model of CPHPC in patients with systemic amyloidosis. CPT Pharmacom Syst Pharmacol. 2015; 4(2): e15.

[60] Kolstoe SE, Mangione PP, Bellotti V, Taylor GW, Tennent GA, Deroo S, Morrison AJ, Cobb AJ, Coyne A, McCammon MG, Warner TD, Mitchell J, Gill R, Smith MD, Ley SV, Robinson CV, Wood SP, Pepys MB. Trapping of palindromic ligands within native transthyretin prevents amyloid formation. Proc Natl Acad Sci U S A. 2010; 107(47): 20483–8.

[61] Pepys MB, Herbert J, Hutchinson WL, Tennent GA, Lachmann HJ, Gallimore JR, Lovat LB, Bartfai T, Alanine A, Hertel C, Hoffmann T, Jakob-Roetne R, Norcross RD, Kemp JA, Yamamura K, Suzuki M, Taylor GW, Murray S, Thompson D, Purvis A, Kolstoe S, Wood SP, Hawkins PN. Targeted pharmacological depletion of serum amyloid P component for treatment of human amyloidosis. Nature. 2002; 417(6886): 254–9.

[62] Kyle RA, Linos A, Beard CM, Linke RP, Gertz MA, O'Fallon WM, Kurland LT. Incidence and natural history of primary systemic amyloidosis in Olmsted County, Minnesota, 1950 through 1989. Blood. 1992; 79(7): 1817–22.

[63] Falk RH, Comenzo RL, Skinner M. The systemic amyloidoses. N Engl J Med. 1997; 337(13): 898–909.

[64] Gillmore JD, Hawkins PN, Pepys MB. Amyloidosis: a review of recent diagnostic and therapeutic developments. Br J Haematol. 1997; 99(2): 245–56.

[65] Nasr SH, Said SM, Valeri AM, Sethi S, Fidler ME, Cornell LD, Gertz MA, Dispenzieri A, Buadi FK, Vrana JA, Theis JD, Dogan A, Leung N. The diagnosis and characteristics of renal heavy-chain and heavy/light-chain amyloidosis and their comparison with renal light-chain amyloidosis. Kidney Int. 2013; 83(3): 463–70.

[66] Said SM, Sethi S, Valeri AM, Chang A, Nast CC, Krahl L,Molloy P, Barry M, Fidler ME, Cornell LD, Leung N, Vrana JA, Theis JD, Dogan A, Nasr SH. Characterization and outcomes of renal leukocyte chemotactic factor 2-associated amyloidosis. Kidney Int. 2014; 86(2): 370–7.

[67] Sattianayagam PT, Gibbs SD, Pinney JH, Wechalekar AD, Lachmann HJ, Whelan CJ, Gilbertson JA, Hawkins PN, Gillmore JD. Solid organ transplantation in AL amyloidosis. Am J Transplant. 2010; 10(9): 2124–31.

[68] Herrmann SM, Gertz MA, Stegall MD, Dispenzieri A, Cosio FC, Kumar S, Lacy MQ, Dean PG, Prieto M, Zeldenrust SR, Buadi FK, Russell SJ, Nyberg SL, Hayman SR, Dingli D, Fervenza FC, Leung N. Long-term outcomes of patients with light chain amyloidosis (AL) after renal transplantation with or without stem cell transplantation. Nephrol Dial Transplant. 2011; 26(6): 2032–6.

[69] Pinney JH, Lachmann HJ, Sattianayagam PT, Gibbs SD, Wechalekar AD, Venner CP, Whelan CJ, Gilbertson JA, Rowczenio D, Hawkins PN, Gillmore JD. Renal transplantation in systemic amyloidosis-importance of amyloid fibril type and precursor protein abundance. Am J Transplant. 2013; 13(2): 433–41.

[70] Kofman T, Grimbert P, Canouï-Poitrine F, Zuber J, Garrigue V, Mousson C, Frimat L, Kamar N, Couvrat G, Bouvier N, Albano L, Le Thuaut A, Pillebout E, Choukroun G, Couzi L, Peltier J, Mariat C, Delahousse M, Buchler M, Le Pogamp P, Bridoux F, Pouteil-Noble C, Lang P, Audard V. Renal transplantation in patients with AA amyloidosis nephropathy: results from a French multicenter study. Am J Transplant. 2011; 11(11): 2423–31.

Chapter 13

A Nanobody-Based Approach to Amyloid Diseases, the Gelsolin Case Study

Adriaan Verhelle and Jan Gettemans

Additional information is available at the end of the chapter

http://dx.doi.org/10.5772/63981

Abstract

Gelsolin amyloidosis (AGel) is an autosomal-dominant inherited disease caused by point mutations in the gelsolin gene. At the protein level, these mutations result in the loss of a Ca^{2+}-binding site, crucial for the correct folding and function. In the trans-Golgi network, this mutant plasma gelsolin is cleaved by furin, giving rise to a 68 kDa C-terminal fragment. When secreted in the extracellular matrix, this fragment undergoes proteolysis by MT1-MMP–like proteases, resulting in the production of 8 and 5 kDa amyloidogenic peptides. Nanobodies, the variable part of the heavy chain of heavy-chain antibodies, have been used as molecular chaperones for mutant plasma gelsolin and the 68 kDa C-terminal fragment in an attempt to inhibit their pathogenic proteolysis. Furthermore, these nanobodies have also been tested and applied as a ^{99m}Tc-based imaging agent in the gelsolin amyloidosis mouse model.

Keywords: AGel, Gelsolin, Nanobody, SPECT/CT, VHH, FAF

1. Introduction

Gelsolin amyloidosis is an autosomal-dominant inherited disease caused by a point mutation in the gelsolin gene; G640A and G640T are most common; G580A and C633A were more recently discovered [1–3]. At the protein level, these mutations result in the amino acid substitutions D187N, D187Y, G167R and N184K in gelsolin domain 2. Consequently, a Ca^{2+}-binding site, crucial for the correct folding and function, is lost. As a result, mutant plasma gelsolin (PG*) adopts an intermediate state between active and inactive, thereby negatively influencing the overall structural stability of the protein and exposing a cryptic, otherwise buried, furin cleavage site [4]. In the trans-Golgi network, this intermediate form of mutant plasma gelsolin is susceptible to furin cleavage, giving rise to a 68 kDa C-terminal fragment (C68) [5]. In its turn, C68 is cleaved by MT1-MMP–like proteases during secretion into the extracellular matrix. This MMP activity results in the formation of 8 and 5 kDa amyloidogenic peptides, which polymerize into mature amyloid fibrils [6]. Patients are generally heterozygous for the mutations and experience a triad of neurological, ophthalmological and dermatological symptoms starting from their thirties [7]. Given the importance of furin and MT1-MMP–like proteases in cell homeostasis, a classical small compound therapy targeting these proteases is unlikely to be successful. Moreover, the gain-of-toxicity nature of this disease rules out replacement gene therapy. In gelsolin amyloidosis, the mutant gelsolin gene still undergoes normal expression. Curing gelsolin amyloidosis through gene therapy would therefore require the deletion of the mutant gene from every single cell. This is (at the moment) not possible with the available gene therapy technology. Shielding the mutant gelsolin from furin and MT1-MMP–like proteases, however, proved to be a worthwhile approach to tackle this disease. One of that may be applicable to other similar amyloid diseases.

Using nanobodies, the variable part of the heavy chain of heavy-chain antibodies, two routes to address AGel have been explored. In a first approach, nanobodies, which partly protect C68 against MT1-MMP, were intraperitoneally injected in AGel mice [8]. In a second approach, a mouse model expressing Nb11 was developed [9]. Nb11 binds to mutant plasma gelsolin (PG*) and shields it from furin degradation. The mouse model secretes this nanobody in its bloodstream. These mice were crossed with AGel mice. During the secretion pathway, Nb11 encounters PG* in the trans-Golgi network. Both techniques resulted in a reduced deposition of amyloidogenic gelsolin.

The nanobodies binding to C68 are also capable of recognizing the 8 kDa amyloidogenic fragment. This characteristic was further explored to develop a ^{99m}Tc-based imaging agent.

2. Gelsolin amyloidosis

2.1. Discovery

In 1969, the Finnish ophthalmologist Jouko Meretoja [10] first described a new familial amyloidosis syndrome characterized by corneal dystrophy, cranial neuropathies and skin affliction. Over the years, this syndrome came to be known under many different names: Meretoja's disease, amyloid polyneuropathy type IV, gelsolin-related amyloidosis, familial amyloidosis of the Finnish type (FAF), corneal lattice dystrophy type II and gelsolin amyloidosis (AGel).

It was not until 1990 that the role of gelsolin in AGel was demonstrated. Two independent research groups had isolated and sequenced the amyloid fibrils from patient tissues [11, 12]. The fragments appeared to be an internal part of a gelsolin variant having an aspartate to asparagine mutation at position 187 of the primary structure of gelsolin. AGel therefore seemed to arise from an abnormal internal degradation from this gelsolin variant.

http://dx.doi.org/10.5772/63981

In the following years, the role of gelsolin, the genetic cause and pathogenic pathway were further elaborated. At the moment, there are four known mutations, which cause gelsolin-related amyloidosis: D187N, D187Y, G167R and the recently discovered N184K [1–3].

2.2. Biochemistry and genetics of gelsolin

The gelsolin superfamily of actin-binding proteins comprises gelsolin, villin, supervillin, advillin, villin-like protein, severin, fragmin CapG (gCap39) and flightless I [13–16]. These proteins are highly conserved in the animal kingdom, and all contain three or more prototypical 'gelsolin-like' domains. A 'gelsolin-like' domain consists of five or six beta-sheets packed between a long roughly parallel and a short roughly perpendicular alpha helix [17, 18].

Gelsolin was described in 1979 as a protein able to transform solid actin gels into a soluble solution: the gel-sol reaction, hence the name. Present in almost every human tissue, gelsolin is capable of binding, severing and capping actin filaments and plays a pivotal role in cytoskeletal homeostasis [19]. It comes in three isoforms, all derived from the same gelsolin gene located at chromosome 9q34. Alternative splicing gives rise to cytoplasmic gelsolin (CG, 82 kDa), plasma gelsolin (PG, 84 kDa) and gelsolin-3 (82 kDa). The first two are the main isoforms, with PG differing from CG by a 24 amino acid, N-terminal extension, which remains present after cleavage of the signal sequence, and the presence of a disulfide bond. The third variant has only been detected in brain oligodendrocytes, lungs and testis tissue and is characterized by 11 additional residues at the N-terminus [20].

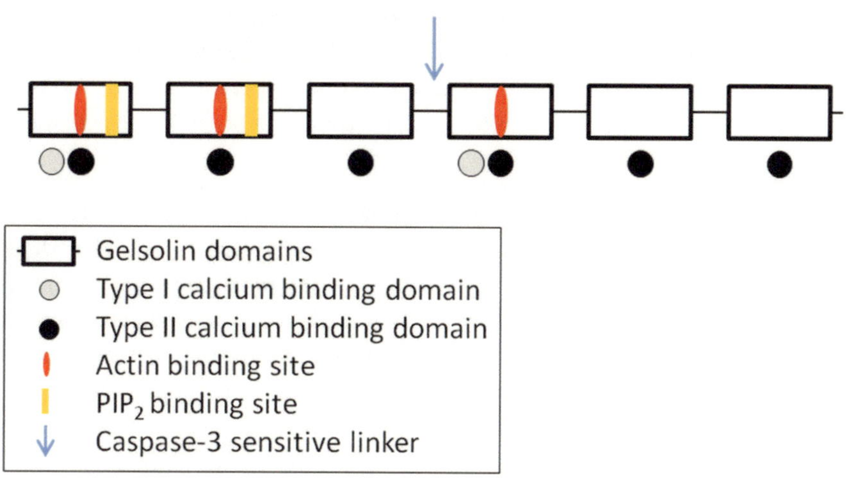

Figure 1. Schematic representation of gelsolin. Black boxes represent the six gelsolin domains. Calcium-binding sites (grey and black dots), actin-binding sites (red), PIP$_2$-binding sites (yellow) and caspase-3–sensitive linker (blue arrow) are indicated.

Gelsolin is composed of six domains (G1–6) of 120–130 amino acids which, in a calcium-free environment, are closely packed together. This inactive state is controlled by three latches: the tail latch, formed by the C-terminus and G2 domain, the G1–G3 latch and the G4–G6 latch [21].

Upon binding of calcium, the three latches open up and expose the actin-binding surfaces of domains 2, 1 and 4, respectively. Following this activation, gelsolin will bind and subsequently sever F-actin [4]. The sequence homology between G1–3 and G4–6 suggests that the protein arose from a gene triplication followed by a duplication [22]. The two homologous halves are connected through a caspase-3–sensitive linker (**Figure 1**). Overall, stability and function of gelsolin are regulated through Ca^{2+} and phosphatidylinositol 4,5-biphosphate (PIP_2). Each domain contains a Ca^{2+}-binding site, and G1 and G2 also have PIP_2-binding capacity (**Figure 1**) [14].

The G2 domain has two major foci of stability. First, there is the Ca^{2+}-binding pocket (Kd 650 nM) formed by residues D187, E209 and D259 [23]. Second, L166, Q164, N184 and D187 form cooperative hydrogen bonds with one another [18]. Mutation of any of these residues leads to a destabilization of G2 and consequently of gelsolin as a whole. This is actually what happens in AGel. Three out of four of the known mutations (D187N, D187Y and N184K) can be directly traced back to one of these two foci of stability. The fourth mutation, G167R, possibly has a destabilizing effect on hydrogen bonding as it is close to Q164. It should be noted that both the N184K and G167R mutations have only recently been discovered in two isolated patients and their kindred [2, 3]. The overall majority of patients carry the D187N/Y mutation, but it is nevertheless noteworthy to observe that these pathological mutations are all in G2 of gelsolin, pointing to this region as a gelsolin stability sensor.

Although the causative mutations of AGel are present in all three gelsolin isoforms, the plasma variant is the sole source of gelsolin amyloidogenic peptides [24]. As mentioned earlier, the overall stability of gelsolin is highly regulated by Ca^{2+} binding. The AGel mutant plasma gelsolin form can no longer properly bind Ca^{2+} through its G2 domain. Consequently, this aberrant variant gives rise to a structurally intermediate state between active and inactive. This exposes an otherwise internal inaccessible furin cleavage site (R-X-X-R) at the surface of gelsolin.

Furin is a membrane-bound member of the proprotein convertase family, active in the endosomal and lysosomal pathways. It shuttles between the trans-Golgi network and the cell surface while activating a wide range of serum proteins, hormones and receptors [25–27]. During secretion, PG naturally encounters furin without any consequence since wild-type gelsolin is already correctly folded due to high calcium levels in the ER/Golgi compartments. PG* on the other hand is susceptible to pathological furin processing due to its induced structural intermediate state. The scissile bond between R172 and A173 is cleaved, thereby releasing a 68 kDa C-terminal fragment [28]. During secretion, this aberrant C68 constitutes a substrate for MT1-MMP–like proteases present in the extracellular matrix. MT1-MMP–like proteases are members of the matrix metalloprotease family [29]. They play a pivotal role in protein degradation processes during embryonic development and tissue remodelling. Here, however, 8 kDa (AA 173–243) and 5 kDa (AA 173–225) gelsolin amyloidogenic peptides are generated (**Figure 2**). Over time, the 8 and 5 kDa fragments start to aggregate in a cross-beta sheet configuration, a hallmark of amyloid fibrils with the former being the major component of gelsolin amyloid in patients.

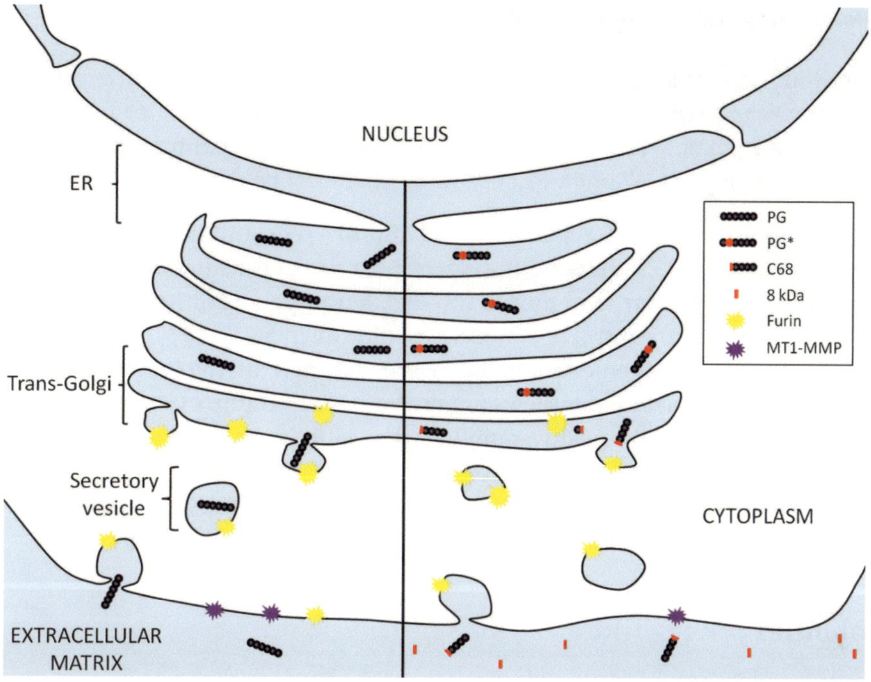

Figure 2. Molecular characteristics of AGel: non-pathological versus pathological plasma gelsolin processing. The left-hand side depicts the non-pathological synthesis and secretion of wild-type plasma gelsolin through the ER and Golgi-network. On the right hand, the mechanism for mutant plasma gelsolin is depicted. Furin cleaves PG* in the trans-Golgi network, thereby releasing a C68 fragment. During secretion, C68 is cleaved by MT1-MMP–like proteases, forming 8 and 5 kDa amyloidogenic fragments in the extracellular matrix.

2.3. Diagnosis and treatment

The clinical diagnosis of AGel most commonly starts with the detection of corneal lattice dystrophy [30]. Together with cutis laxis and bilateral facial pareses, it forms a triad of consistent features differentiating AGel from other amyloid disorders. The diagnosis can be easily confirmed using molecular genetics. In older or homozygous patients, renal amyloidosis, resulting in proteinuria, can also be a first clue [7].

No specific treatment is currently available. Only symptomatic treatments are being offered to improve the overall quality of life. Most important is good ophthalmological care ranging from eye drops to corneal transplantation. Next to that, aesthetic surgery is often needed to ameliorate the patients' overall confidence as the facial pareses and cutis laxis burden the patients with a constant droopy facial expression [31].

Although therapeutic strategies involving the inhibition of protease activity have been suggested, unwanted side effects are to be expected given the major physiological roles of furin and MT1-MMP [28, 29]. Tackling the problem the other way round, directly shielding PG* from degradation, may prove to be a more valuable route, as will be discussed later in this chapter.

2.4. A gelsolin amyloidosis mouse model

To further study the molecular aspects of the disease and to test the different therapeutic avenues, two animal models were set up. In a first attempt, the gene coding for the 8 kDa amyloidogenic fragment was successfully transferred into the genome of *Drosophila melanogaster*. Unfortunately, AGel amyloid deposition could not be detected [7].

As of 2009, a mouse model is available that faithfully recapitulates the entire proteolytic cascade of human PG* [32]. Following the electroporation of the human plasma GSN cDNA, carrying the D187N mutation, into mouse ES cells, a transgenic animal was obtained where gelsolin is expressed under control of a muscle creatine kinase (MCK) promoter. PG*, C68 and the 8 and 5 kDa amyloidogenic fragments were detected in the heart, skeletal muscle, diaphragm and skin. Plasma samples contain both full length PG* and C68. With age, increasing amounts of gelsolin-positive amyloid depositions can be seen in the endomysium. Eventually, the phenotype of old homozygous D187N mice starts to resemble sporadic inclusion body myositis (sIBM) with accompanied muscle weakness.

3. Nanobodies

3.1. Research and clinic applications of conventional antibodies

Since the introduction of hybridoma technology in 1975, monoclonal antibodies (mAb) have become an indispensable tool in fundamental research and all sorts of clinical applications [33]. The ability to mass produce antibodies against a plethora of proteins, carbohydrates, nucleic acids and haptens gave rise to molecular diagnostic tests, such as ELISA, Western blotting, immunohistochemistry (IHC) and immunofluorescence. Antibodies in the clinic are used in diagnostic applications by linkage to radioactive or fluorescent moieties. Furthermore, they are also being applied therapeutically, be it directly or as a route for drug delivery. As the applications became more and more sophisticated and diversified, the potential pitfalls of this technology also surfaced. First, the production of vast amounts of mAbs is very expensive. Second, the mAb format is hard to manipulate to obtain site-specific linkage to other molecules such as fluorophores and radioactive nuclides. Last but not least, mAb hold the potential of evoking an immune response rendering the therapy ineffective. This last hurdle has been addressed with the production of so-called humanized antibodies. These second-generation antibodies contain a humanized antigen-binding fragment (Fab). Third-generation antibodies go one step further and also include an engineered Fc domain to improve the therapeutic activity in patients, particularly in subpopulations expressing low affinity variants of the Fc receptor [34].

Conventional antibodies are comprised of 2 heavy chains and 2 light chains. This multichain nature is one of the major hurdles when trying to manipulate mAb. Attempts have been made to bypass this by producing mAb fragments such as antigen-binding fragments and single-chain variable fragments (scFv). The first, Fab, is composed of the variable and constant domain of a heavy chain, combined with the variable and constant domain of a light chain. The second,

http://dx.doi.org/10.5772/63981

scFv, only contains the variable parts of the heavy and light chain, but these are interconnected through a linker. Although these smaller formats ameliorated some of the problems posed by classical mAbs, their production still proved to be troublesome and the functionality of the original mAb was (partly) lost in some cases.

3.2. Discovery of nanobodies

By a stroke of luck in 1993, a new type of antibody was discovered in the blood of Camelus dromedarius [35]. These antibodies consist solely of two heavy chains; hence, they were named heavy-chain antibodies (HCAbs). Their paratope is no longer formed by a combination of a heavy and light chain variable fragment but consists exclusively of the variable fragment of a heavy chain. The single-domain nature of this paratope offered the natural solution for which researchers had been looking for. It has since been named variable domain of the heavy chain of heavy-chain antibodies, VHH in short or Nanobody® (www.ablynx.com) (**Figure 3**). Since their discovery, these HCAbs have been detected in the blood of all Camelidae family members, nurse sharks, wobbegongs and ratfish.

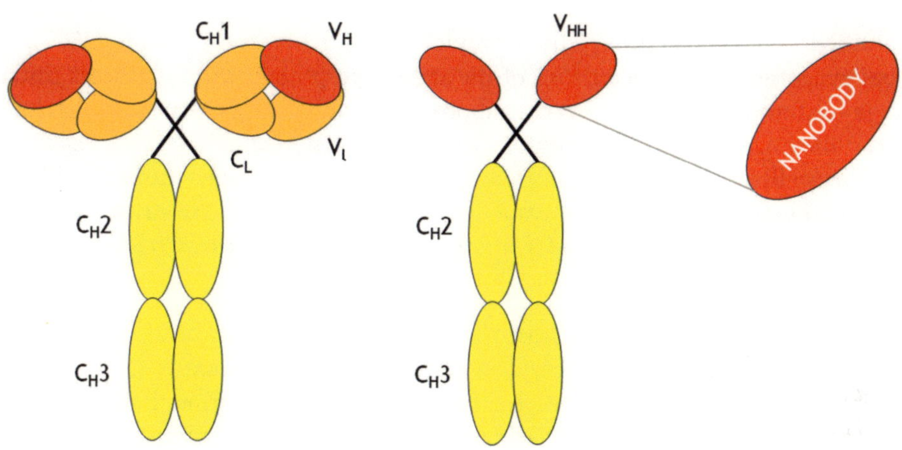

Figure 3. Schematic representation of a conventional antibody, heavy-chain antibody and a nanobody. A conventional antibody (left) consists of two heavy chains (C_H3, C_H2, C_H1 and V_H) and two light chains (C_L and V_l). Heavy-chain antibodies (middle) only consist of two heavy chains (C_H3, C_H2 and V_{HH}). A nanobody (right) corresponds with the variable part of the heavy chain of heavy-chain antibodies (V_{HH}).

3.3. Properties and production of nanobodies

The most important novelty about nanobodies was, and still is, the fact that they are the smallest, single-domain, natural, antigen-binding fragment available. Their complementary determining regions 3 (CDR3) sequences are on average longer (16–18 AA) compared those of regular human antibodies (12 AA). Not only does this compensate for the absence of a light chain, but it also allows the CDR3 to form protruding loops that are able to bind cryptic epitopes. The fact that they are encoded by a single short gene fragments allows easy and straightforward protein engineering, thereby overcoming one of the mayor hurdles of the multichain nature of conventional Abs. By the same token, it allows relatively easy production in bacteria and yeast cells. With yields of up to 40–70 mg/l, nanobodies can be produced at a fraction of the cost of mAbs. When produced, their high resistance towards chaotropic reagents or prolonged high temperatures and stability at high concentrations allows easy storage without any functionality loss.

3.4. Nanobody applications

Nanobodies, being small and stable, are ideal candidates for various research purposes, diagnostic or clinical applications. Equipped with a radionuclide, they can be applied as imaging tracers in a single-photon emission computed tomography (SPECT) or positron emission tomography (PET)-based set-up allowing in vivo visualization of tumours, artherosclerotic plaques and rheumatoid arthritis-associated inflammation sites [36–38]. Nanobodies are also capable of stabilizing proteins in a particular conformation and of minimizing structural flexibility. This has been nicely demonstrated in the case of human lysozyme amyloidosis, a hereditary systemic disease associated with at least seven amyloidogenic lysozyme variants [39, 40]. Aggregation of these lysozyme variants leads to the accumulation of amyloid in the extracellular matrix of several tissues and organs. Two nanobodies have been identified who, upon binding mutant amyloidogenic lysozyme (D67H and I56T), restored the global cooperativity characteristics of the wild-type protein through direct contact and long-range conformational effects. What's more, this stabilizing capacity can also be conducive to crystallizing proteins. β2-microglobulin–specific nanobodies have been shown to serve as efficient crystallization chaperones for transient intermediate species during fibrillation [41]. This type of antibody chaperone co-crystallization was also used to unravel the structure of the G protein-coupled receptor β-2 adrenergic receptor (β2AR), research which received the 2012 Nobel Prize in Chemistry [42].

Another major field where the potential use of nanobodies is currently being explored is amyloidosis. In Alzheimer's research, nanobodies have been found which inhibit beta-secretase 1 (BACE1) activity, the first step in amyloid beta formation, both in vitro and in vivo [43]. Alternatively, nanobodies could also be raised against amyloid precursor protein (APP) to protect it from BACE1 degradation, as direct inhibition of the enzyme could evoke unwanted side effects. We present here the case of gelsolin amyloidosis where this approach has proven successful both in vitro and in vivo. The remainder of this chapter will focus on the obtained results, current status and future prospects regarding this AGel research arena.

4. Extracellular targeting of the AGel pathological pathway

Consecutive aberrant cleavage of PG* by furin and MT1-MMP–like proteases leads to the production of amyloidogenic fragments which eventually polymerize into fibrils, causing gelsolin amyloidosis pathology. But these two proteases are active in different compartments. Indeed, whereas furin is active in the (intracellular) ER-Golgi compartments, MT1-MMP is inserted in the plasma membrane and oriented to the extracellular environment. This has far-reaching consequences in terms of molecular therapeutic avenues that should be followed when gelsolin has to be protected from cleavage by either of these proteases. As the second cleavage step occurs in the extracellular matrix, we reasoned that it might be possible to block this process by intraperitoneal administration of C68 chaperone nanobodies [8].

A dromedary was simultaneously immunized with the G2 domain and the 8 kDa fragment of PG*. Phage panning was also performed with both gelsolin fragments. This yielded three different nanobodies, termed FAF Nb1-3. All three bind to PG, PG*, C68 and the 8 kDa peptide

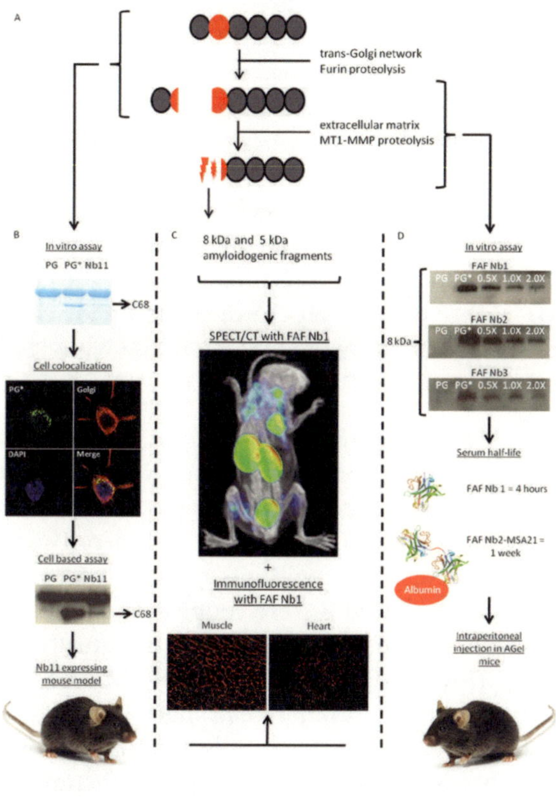

Figure 4. Overview of different nanobody-based strategies to diagnose and to counter amyloidogenesis in transgenic mice. A, Schematic representation of the steps leading from mutant plasma gelsolin to the 8 and 5 kDa amyloidogenic fragments. B (upper panel), Gelsolin Nb11 reduces C68 formation in vitro—lane 1: PG incubated with furin, lane 2: PG* incubated with furin and lane 3: PG* incubated with furin and Nb11. B (second panel), Nb11 co-localizes with mutant gelsolin in the secretory pathway of HEK293T cells. B (third panel), **Nb 11** decreases C68 formation in HEK293T cells: lane 1: medium from cells transfected with PG, lane 2: medium from cells transfected with PG* and lane 3: medium from cells transfected with PG* and Nb11. This led to designing the Nb11-expressing mouse model. C, Representative images obtained with ^{99m}Tc-labeled FAF Nb1 in 9-month-old AGel mice. The heart and front and hind leg muscles show a clear signal (blue). Kidneys and bladder signal represents unbound nanobody which is cleared through the urinary system (green and red). FAF Nb1 can also be used as a primary antibody to stain amyloidogenic gelsolin build-up in AGel mice tissue (lower panel). D (upper panel), FAF Nb1-3 partly inhibits C68 proteolysis in vitro. For each nanobody, from left till right, after incubation with MT1-MMP: PG, PG*, PG* + 0.5, 1.0 and 2.0 X FAF Nb. Numbers indicate the Nb/PG* molar ratios. D (middle panel), Linkage with the albumin-binding MSA21 nanobody increases serum half-life from 4 h to more than 1 week (middle panel). D (lower panel), In vivo analysis was performed through intraperitoneal injection in AGel mice.

when tested through immunoprecipitation on crude bacterial lysates, but they did not cross-react with CapG, a protein that is structurally related to gelsolin. Unlike gelsolin, CapG is only capable of capping actin filaments but does not sever. It is the member of the gelsolin superfamily most closely resembling gelsolin. It possesses 49% identity with the N-terminal half of gelsolin.

The hypothesis was that if one of these FAF nanobodies bound to C68 in the vicinity of the MT1-MMP cleavage site or an important docking area, it would be able to (at least partly) inhibit the production of the 8 kDa fragments. This was indeed confirmed by in vitro experiments. C68 was preincubated with one of the three FAF Nbs after which MT1-MMP was added to the mixture. Formation of the 8 kDa fragment could be followed by Western blotting, and this showed a 70–80% reduction in the presence of a FAF nanobody, attesting to their ability to indirectly prevent MT1-MMP activity on gelsolin (**Figure 4A** and **D**). Nb13, a nanobody that binds to the linker between gelsolin domains 4 and 5, did not show the same effect. Furthermore, the FAF Nbs had no effect on the proteolysis of collagen, another substrate of MT1-MMP. Therefore, it was concluded that a nanobody can be used as a chaperone to prevent degradation of a structural protein by an enzyme without directly inhibiting the activity of the enzyme. In doing so, potential side effects may be prevented. Whether the observed effects are due to a direct inhibition of MT1-MMP docking on C68 or shielding the cleavage site or rather due to an indirect structural affect caused by the binding of the Nb with C68 still remains to be clarified. A crystal structure of MT1-MMP bound to C68 would bring clarity in this matter.

While these results were promising at first, a new caveat presented itself when considering that nanobodies, because of their small size, are characterized by rapid blood clearance. This could impede their use as a therapeutic in vivo. Indeed, although their small size is mostly advantageous, when used as a therapeutic, it is rather a burden. Thus, it seemed necessary to increase their half-life in the circulation as this will improve their probability of binding C68 gelsolin. To achieve this goal, FAF Nb1-3 were coupled to the albumin-binding nanobody MSA21 through a short Gly-Ser linker. This linkage did not greatly affect the binding affinity between the Nb and C68 (FAF2 = Kd: $8.4 \times 10^{-7} \pm 4.7 \times 10^{-8}$ M, FAF2-MSA21 = Kd: $5.4 \times 10^{-7} \pm 0.6 \times 10^{-7}$ M, determined by isothermal titration calorimetry). The bispecific FAF2-MSA21 Nb binds albumin in the bloodstream, and the formation of this larger complex should extend the half-life, resulting in a higher efficiency of the FAF Nb1-3 therapeutic intervention. Serum analysis of injected mice confirmed this assumption. While the monovalent FAF Nb1-3 were no longer detectable after 4 h, the bispecific format could still be clearly visualized up until one week post-injection (**Figure 4D**). Additionally, the linkage between FAFNb1-3 and MSA21 did not offset the MT1-MMP–inhibiting potential in vitro. Hence, all requirements were fulfilled to test their effect in vivo.

The in vitro results were validated using the available AGel mouse model. Over a period of 12 weeks, mice were weekly injected with 100 μg of either FAF Nb1, FAF Nb2-MSA21 or phosphate-buffered saline (PBS). The trial started at the age of 4 weeks, and the nanobodies used were the ones which performed best during the in vitro set-up. End-stage analysis consisted of immunohistochemistry (IHC) and ex vivo muscle contractility measurements. IHC revealed a decrease in amyloidogenic gelsolin staining for FAF Nb1 of 15% and FAF Nb2-

MSA21 of 30%. Both results were statistically significant. The difference between both nanobody formats shows that a longer half-life is definitely desirable in a therapeutic approach such as this. The reduction seen with IHC in the FAF Nb2-MSA21–treated mice translated into improved muscle contractility and relaxation speed function in the extensor digitorum longus (EDL). Therefore, these nanobodies are endowed with a therapeutic quality. It should be noted that the FAF Nbs display an intermediate affinity for their target. Although clear data in support of this contention are wanting, it seems likely that stronger binders might even have stronger effects in vivo. Further exploration of the FAF Nb2-MSA21 potential in human gelsolin amyloidosis patients requires two important modification to be made. Firstly, the MSA21 nanobody would have to be replaced by a human serum albumin binder. The longer serum half-life of human versus mouse albumin (19 days versus 35 h) may further lower the administration frequency. Secondly, although nanobodies are known for their low immunogenicity, humanizing their framework regions can further decrease the risk of an undesirable immune response during therapeutic intervention. More specifically, a universal humanized nanobody scaffold has already been proposed onto which all the CDR antigen-binding loops could be grafted [44].

5. Intracellular targeting of the AGel pathological pathway

Thanks to their excellent stability, nanobodies are also valuable compounds to be used as intrabodies. The reducing environment of the cytoplasm seems to have little effect on their functionality [45, 46]. As mentioned above, the FAF Nb approach significantly reduced AGel amyloid build-up in vivo, but it did not completely halt the 8 kDa peptide production. AGel pathogenesis is a two step process; a furin cleavage of mutant plasma gelsolin produces C68, which is then on its turn cleaved by MT1-MMP, thereby releasing 8 kDa amyloidogenic peptides. This opens the opportunity for a double-hit approach.

For that reason, we tested whether a different set of gelsolin nanobodies could be applied as a chaperone for gelsolin to divert furin activity in the same manner as we had implemented the FAF Nb1-3 towards C68 [9].

The nanobodies used in this study were not specifically designed for this purpose. Instead, they had been raised against wild-type gelsolin and characterized some time ago. Through in vitro epitope mapping experiments, Nb11 was shown to interact with the G2–G3 domains (N-terminal half), whereas Nb13 interacts with G4–G5 (C-terminal half). Furthermore, both nanobodies interact with different populations of gelsolin in cells. Indeed, Nb11 binds human gelsolin with high affinity (Kd = $3.65 \times 10^{-9} \pm 0.54 \times 10^{-9}$ M, determined by isothermal titration calorimetry), irrespective of whether calcium is present or not, whereas Nb13 strongly interacts with gelsolin (Kd = $9.26 \times 10^{-9} \pm 1.61 \times 10^{-9}$ M, determined by isothermal titration calorimetry), only when the latter is activated by calcium. Both nanobodies were further shown to act as reliable tracers of gelsolin in MCF-7 cells when expressed as intrabodies. Both gelsolin and nanobody are abundantly present in the cytoplasm of unstimulated MCF-7 cells, preventing straightforward assessment of their co-localization. However, when the cells were stimulated with epidermal growth factor (EGF), both endogenous gelsolin and the nanobodies extensively decorated membrane ruffles [47]. In view of the binding region of Nb11 in gelsolin, it was surmised that it could interfere with furin-mediated degradation. In analogy with the MT1-MMP study, these gelsolin nanobodies were incubated with PG*, and Western blotting showed that only Nb11 reduced furin cleavage of PG* by 34% when added in concentrations equimolar to PG* (**Figure 4A** and **B**).

This finding, however, does not guarantee that the same result will be obtained in mammalian cells. Plasma gelsolin will naturally travel through the secretory pathway, but simple expression of the nanobody will result in its cytoplasmic and nuclear localization in cells. Hence, the nanobody will not be able to protect gelsolin. For this reason, the nanobody was equipped with an ER signal peptide to ensure its secretion through the Golgi apparatus. Furin naturally resides in the Golgi apparatus, and the first step in the AGel pathology takes place in this compartment. By quantifying the amount of C68 that is secreted in the extracellular environment, it could be confirmed that Nb11 exerts a protective effect. The cell media from HEK cells transfected with PG* and Nb11 contained 80% less C68 compared to HEK cells solely transfected with PG* (**Figure 4B**).

Although nanobodies can, and are, currently being applied in research involving intracellular perturbation of protein-protein interactions, at the moment there is no efficient, fail proof method to introduce them into cells in a recombinant format. Therefore, to test whether the observed effect of Nb11 in vitro could be reproduced in vivo, a Nb11-expressing mouse model had to be created. To our knowledge, this is the first transgenic mammal that contains a therapeutic nanobody in its genome. The ER-directed Nb11 cDNA was cloned in the pROSA-DV2 vector, which targets the ROSA26 locus. This locus was identified in 1991 using gene-trap mutagenesis screening on embryonic stem cells. Thanks to its ubiquitous expression in both embryonic and adult tissues, over 130 knock-in mouse lines have been created using this cloning site. G4 ES cells were electroporated, and positive colonies were selected through Southern blotting. Next, cells were aggregated with Swiss inner cell mass cells. These blastocysts were transferred into pseudopregnant mice uteri, and the resulting chimeric offspring was backcrossed with wild-type C57BL/6 to check for germline transmission. Finally, these mice could then be crossed with a non-tissue specific Cre/lox-deleter mouse strain. This resulted in CAGG promoter-driven Nb11 expression, resulting in the first Nb11-expressing mice. Nb11 could be visualized and quantified in the serum through co-immunoprecipitation and Western blotting.

The newly developed Nb11 mouse model was crossed with AGel mice. Double positive offspring was evaluated at three distinct time points: 3, 6 and 9 months. Gastrocnemius muscle tissue was stained for AGel build-up. A costaining for laminin was used as an internal control and to discern any potential artefacts. The AGel staining was homogenous in every age group, allowing quantification. Compared to AGel mice or littermates not expressing Nb11, a reduction in AGel staining of 27 and 28%, respectively, could be detected at 3 and 9 months of age. For the group of 6 months, no significant reduction could be found. The reason for this is unclear. The group of 9-month-old mice was also subjected to a muscle performance evaluation. The extensor digitorum longus (EDL) muscle showed a strong attenuation of the typical decrease in contraction speed during the fatiguing protocol. This therapeutic effect was not mimicked by Nb13 that binds to another region in gelsolin (G4–G5 linker) and that had no effect on gelsolin degradation by furin. Neither Nb11 nor Nb13 showed any cross-reactivity with endogenous mouse gelsolin. Thus, Nb11 attenuates amyloid build-up by (partly) protecting gelsolin against degradation by furin. One might wonder why the reduction in AGel staining was not as high as expected, given that Nb11 is a strong binder (Kd ~ 5 nM) where calcium moreover has no effect on binding. One possibility involves the relative expression levels of gelsolin and Nb11. Western blotting with internal gelsolin and nanobody standards indicated that both are present at roughly equimolar levels. In the AGel mouse model, however, gelsolin is secreted from muscle, whereas nanobody expression is thought to be secreted from multiple organs, tissues and cells, because no tissue-specific promoter was used to drive expression of the nanobody. Therefore, the nanobody that was detected in the serum of these animals has multiple origins suggesting that its secretion from muscle is significantly lower as compared to gelsolin secretion. This contention however needs to be examined experimentally.

6. In vivo visualization of AGel build-up

AGel is a chronic, gain of toxicity, affliction. Accordingly, any therapy will have to be administered throughout the entire lifetime of the patients. It is therefore important, during therapy development, to test promising compounds over a long period of time and assess the effects at different time points during the course of the trial. During the Nb11 experiments, this had to be done by using different groups for every time point since the current methods of AGel analysis are end-stage [8, 9]. Not only does this greatly augment the amount of mice needed, it also makes it impossible to evaluate the drug effect and amyloid build-up in a continuous manner. In the hope of resolving this drawback, we set out to develop a nanobody-based imaging agent. The ultimate goal was to be able to visualize the AGel amyloid build-up in vivo in a non-invasive manner. This would facilitate evaluation of drug responses at different time points over the entire course of treatment in the same animal.

6.1. Labelling of nanobody through ^{99m}Tc linkage to His_6 tag

Thanks to their excellent stability, small size and single-chain nature, nanobodies represent an ideal antibody derived format for transformation into a radionuclide-based amyloid imaging agent. ^{99m}Tc was the radionuclide of choice being readily available and displaying a half-life long enough to allow good quality imaging, but short enough to minimize the overall radiation burden during the trial. Linking it to a nanobody is also a straightforward process. Simply equipping the nanobody with a N- or C-terminal His_6 tag allows chelation with ^{99m}Tc via the tricarbonyl method [48]. Furthermore, ^{99m}Tc is compatible with SPECT, the imaging modality most ideal for visualization in small laboratory animals used during research trials such as this.

FAF Nb1-3 were the prime candidates to be explored for their ability to serve as an imaging tool. When administered as in vivo imaging agents, FAF Nb1-3 are required to remain stable for some time in the complex environment of the blood and extracellular matrix. In a preliminary test phase, FAF Nb1-3 were therefore incubated in C57BL/6 mouse serum at 37°C and found to remain stable for up to 24 h without deterioration.

As a last test before the first in vivo trials, a test labelling was performed. Using instant thin-layer chromatography (ITLC) and reverse-phase high-performance liquid chromatography (RP-HPLC), the radiochemical purities were determined to be 99.7 ± 1.3%, 99.7 ± 0.9% and 98.3 ± 1.0% for FAF Nb1-3, respectively.

6.2. Specificity and background signal determination

One of the key aspects of a good imaging agent is the capability of specifically generating a high signal wherever its target is present without provoking a significant background signal. As discussed earlier, FAF Nb1-3 are capable of binding their target with great specificity in vitro. To test whether this remained true in vivo, a group of 9-month-old WT C57BL/6 mice were injected with ^{99m}Tc-FAF Nb1-3. Nanobody BcII10 against β-lactamase of Bacillus cereus was used as a negative control [49]. SPECT/CT images and dissection analysis revealed the classic high kidney and bladder uptake of renal-filtered small hydrophilic proteins of which nanobodies are a textbook example. All the other organs showed no significant high signal when comparing the FAF Nb1-3 with the BcII10 control. From these data, it can be concluded that the FAF Nb1-3 do not show any nonspecific binding when administered to mice (and they do not cross-react with mouse gelsolin either).

The experiment was repeated in 9-month-old AGel mice (**Figure 4C**). At this age, the animals show considerable gelsolin amyloid build-up in the muscle tissue. Both FAF Nb1 and 2 showed significant uptake in skeletal muscle, heart and diaphragm. In the AGel mouse model, these represent three out of the four tissues in which gelsolin amyloid builds up over time. The fourth, the skin, could not be identified with the FAF Nbs, although it is possible that this organ only becomes affected later in life. Overall, this experiment showed that FAF Nb1-2 are capable of specifically recognizing gelsolin amyloid build-up in the AGel model. FAF Nb3 on the contrary did not seem able to provoke a significant signal in the heart nor diaphragm.

The two experiments described above were used to calculate both a signal-to-noise and a signal-specificity score. The first is defined as the signals gained with FAF Nb1-3 in AGel mice muscle over the signal obtained in AGel mice liver. The latter is defined as the signal gained with FAF Nb1-3 in AGel mice over the signal gained with Nb BcII10 in AGel mice. On both characteristics, FAF Nb1 scored the best. Combined with the fact that it also has a slightly better affinity for the 8 kDa peptide (FAF Nb1: $3.8 \times 10^{-7} \pm 1.2 \times 10^{-8}$ M, FAF Nb2: Kd: $8.4 \times 10^{-7} \pm 4.7 \times 10^{-8}$ M and FAF Nb3: Kd: $6.6 \times 10^{-7} \pm 1.7 \times 10^{-7}$ M, determined by isothermal titration calorimetry), FAF Nb1 was appointed as the best candidate for further development as a AGel ^{99m}Tc-based imaging agent.

6.3. Qualitative and quantitative characteristics

The ultimate goal was to see whether the FAF Nbs could be implemented as imaging tools during the screening of potential AGel therapeutics. This of course means that not only do we want to qualitatively image the amyloid build-up, but we also want the rendered signal to hold quantitative information. Only then would it be possible to track the therapeutic effect in a longitudinal follow-up study.

The intervention study with the gelsolin Nb11-expressing mouse model presented an ideal opportunity to test ^{99m}Tc-FAF Nb1 for any quantitative properties. As stated above, by crossing the Nb11 expressing mice with the AGel mice, we were able to reduce AGel amyloid burden as detected by IHC. The experiment was repeated, but now, starting at the age of 3 months, the mice underwent a SPECT/CT scan with ^{99m}Tc-FAF Nb1 every two months. Two groups were analyzed with IHC: one at 9 months of age and another at 11 months.

In the SPECT/CT images, the signal coming from the heart and hind leg muscle was quantified using AMIDE software. The same size region of interest was used for every animal at every time point. No significant differences could be discerned in the heart tissue. This is not so surprising since IHC had revealed earlier that the heart only seems to be homogeneously affected from the age of 7–9 months onwards. Therefore, a good quantification is not possible before that time. In the muscle tissue, however, the SPECT/CT analysis revealed a significant difference at the age of 7 and 9 months. Why the same was not true at 11 months, further research will have to reveal.

At the end stages of 9 and 11 months, mice were dissected right after SPECT/CT imaging. Signal strengths were determined for hind leg muscle and the heart. The same pattern as with SPECT/CT analysis could be found, a difference at 9 months but not at 11 months. The same tissue also underwent IHC, which still is the golden standard when it comes to amyloid detection and quantification. The IHC analysis confirmed that gelsolin staining in the heart tissue is not yet homogenous so these samples were not quantified. The muscle on the other hand showed good overall staining. Hence, IHC confirmed the result obtained with SPECT/CT imaging and dissection analysis, a significant difference at the age of 9 months but no longer at 11 months.

7. Future prospects

7.1. Combined therapy

Gelsolin amyloidosis is caused by a point substitution in the GSN gene which has a destabilizing effect on the second gelsolin domain. As a result a cryptic, otherwise buried, furin cleavage site is exposed at the surface. The plasma isoform encounters furin along the secretory pathway in the trans-Golgi network, at which point it is cleaved, thereby releasing a 68 kDa C-terminal fragment. In its turn, this C68 fragment is processes by MT1-MMP–like proteases leading to the production of 8 and 5 kDa amyloidogenic fragments.

This two-step pathological process allows intervention at two very distinct levels. The furin section takes place intracellularly, inside the trans-Golgi network, a site which is still quite troublesome to target with non-small-compound therapeutics. The MT1-MMP section takes place in the extracellular matrix, a region easily accessible through injections.

Both routes were explored, and the results are described above. Although both approaches proved to hold a therapeutic potential, none of them completely solved the AGel pathogenesis. Therefore, the next logical step is to combine them in a single therapeutic format. Once again the single-domain nature of nanobodies came in handy. Using straightforward cloning techniques, FAF Nb1 was linked to the C terminus of Nb11 which contains a secretion signal. The linker between both nanobodies contains a MT1-MMP–sensitive linker. The idea behind the construct is that when expressed the bispecific nanobody will perform its PG* chaperone function in the trans-Golgi network. During secretion, the MT1-MMP–sensitive linker will lure MT1-MMP away from the already lower amount of C68. This process will also release FAF Nb1 from Nb11 in situ, making it available to chaperone C68 and further diminish the overall production of the 8 kDa amyloidogenic pathway (**Figure 5**).

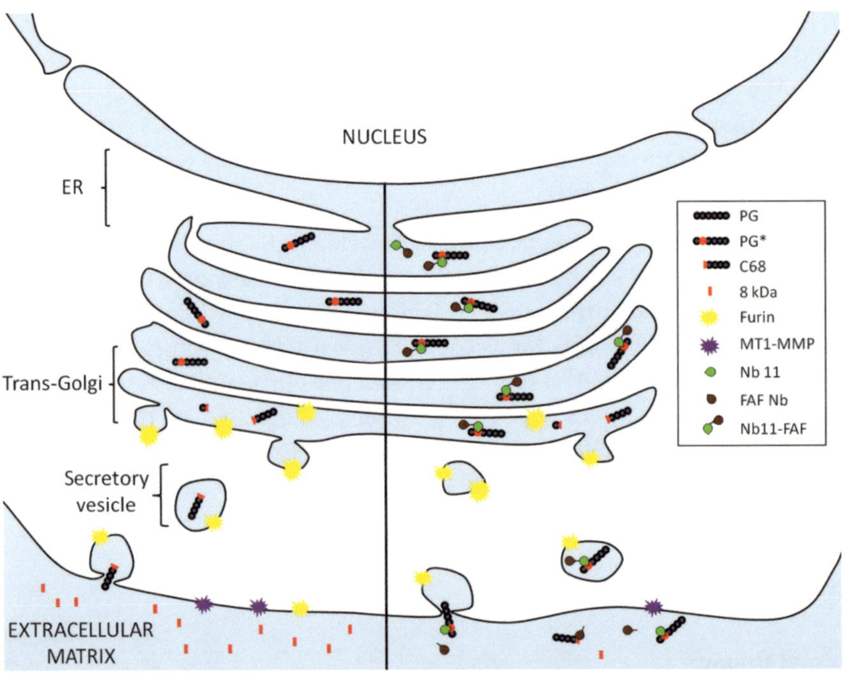

Figure 5. Envisioned molecular mechanism of the therapeutic bispecific Nb11-FAF1. The left-hand side depicts the pathological PG* processing with the formation of C68 in the trans-Golgi network and the 8 and 5 kDa amyloidogenic fragments in the extracellular matrix. On the right-hand side, the intervention with bispecific Nb11-FAF1 is shown. In the trans-Golgi network, the nanobody uses its Nb11 moiety to bind PG* and (partly) protect it from furin degradation. In the extracellular matrix, the MT1-MMP–sensitive linker between Nb11 and FAF1 serves as a decoy. At the same time, FAF Nb1 is released and is able to perform its C68 chaperoning effect, thereby further decreasing the overall formation of 8 and 5 kDa amyloidogenic fragments.

This hypothesis has already been tested in vitro. A combined Furin/MT1-MMP degradation assay was set up. Quantification of the amount of 8 kDa peptide showed Nb11-FAF1 outperformed both Nb11 and the individual FAF Nb1-3. Meaning that, in vitro, the double-hit approach shows a synergistic effect compared to the individual therapies.

For in vivo testing, a gene therapy approach could be chosen. Adeno-associated viruses (AAVs) are naturally occurring, non-pathogenic, replication-deficient viruses. They are capable of infecting non-dividing cells and reside in the nucleus under the form of episomal concatemers. This makes them ideal candidates to be used as gene therapy vectors. Their most important downside is the limited packaging capacity of about 5 kb [50]. Given its small size, this should not pose a problem for our Nb11-FAF1 application. Since AGel expression in the transgenic model is driven from muscle, a serotype with a muscle tropism would be preferential.

7.2. Beyond AGel

The studies performed with the AGel mouse model have shown that nanobodies are useful, potent therapeutics for both extra- and intracellular targets. They also highlighted that nanobodies can be used as an imaging tool in AGel, thereby facilitating the screening of potentially new therapeutic compounds. While AGel is an orphan disease, it should be emphasized that this strategy can be extrapolated to other amyloidogenic afflictions. The most infamous type of amyloidosis, Alzheimer's, actually has a quite similar pathogenesis; the sequential proteolysis of Alzheimer's precursor protein by β-secretase and γ-secretase results in the release of Aβ amyloidogenic peptides. Nanobodies against this β-secretase have already proven to be therapeutically active in a transgenic AD mouse model [43]. As already stated earlier, we believe that in the long run, it would prove more beneficial to target the APP instead of the secretases. Inhibiting a protease will most likely provoke unwanted side effects, whereas chaperoning the target, as in the AGel research discussed in this chapter, is more unlikely to do so.

Raising nanobodies against full length APP, s-APP β or Aβ, may result in nanobodies that bind near the β-secretase cleavage or docking site and that block the formation of s-APP β. A double-hit strategy as in the AGel case will most probably be more difficult to achieve. The gamma secretase is a multiunit integral membrane protein. It cleaves transmembrane passes. At the moment, there are no reports of nanobodies being able to integrate into the plasma membrane and remain functional. In addition, gamma secretase proteolysis also takes place in the non-pathogenic processing of APP. As the transmembrane part of C-terminal fragment-alpha and C-terminal fragment-beta is identical, even a chaperone-based intervention may provoke unwanted side effects.

Up until now, we have only discussed preventing the formation of amyloidogenic peptides. But directly targeting the amyloidogenic peptides, after their formation, also holds great therapeutic potential. The deposition of amyloid fibrils is the primary pathological feature of this group of afflictions. In recent years, however, scientific research towards the initial processes leads to fibrillation, implicated that the initial oligomeric aggregates may be the most toxic species in amyloid pathogenesis and mature fibrils may be far less pathogenic than previously thought [51, 52]. These new results hint to new therapeutic strategies. First, one could try to stimulate fibrillation, thus attempting to lower the half-life of small oligomeric aggregates. Secondly, one could try to remove the amyloidogenic peptides altogether as soon as they are formed. Most likely, the latter will prove to be the most rewarding in the long run. Because although evidence points at intermediate oligomeric species as highly toxic, the accumulation of amyloidogenic plaques would still impede normal homeostasis of the affected tissue from a certain point in time onwards.

FAF Nb1-3 are currently being tested for their ability to prevent 8 kDa AGel fibrillation. With transmission electron microscopy (TEM) and/or atomic-force microscopy (AFM), the differences in fibrillation could then be visualized in order to link reduced toxicity to a specific shift in amyloid oligomerization or fibril species.

Once more Alzheimer's researchers are also exploring this route. Studying the cytotoxic response of SH-SY5Y cells through LDL release, they found that oligomeric Aβ provoked a higher cytotoxic reaction compared to monomeric or fibrillar Aβ [53]. Next, the cells were incubated with oligomeric Aβ formed in the presence of anti-Aβ nanobodies. So far, two distinct nanobodies have been discovered, each binding a specific oligomeric species. Both are able to lower the intrinsic toxicity in SH-SY5Y cells. The first, Nb A4, does so by inhibiting further aggregation of its target. The second, Nb E1, acts in a different manner by binding to smaller Aβ species than Nb A4, thereby interfering earlier in the fibrillation process. Binding its target stabilizes the formation of small non-toxic low-n Aβ species.

It remains to be demonstrated if these approaches and beneficial effects can be translated in model organisms or even in patients, the current findings and results obtained with nanobodies in several amyloid diseases indicate that they could represent an instrument of choice in the diagnosis and/or treatment of these debilitating disorders.

Acknowledgements

This work was supported by the 'Stichting Alzheimer Onderzoek' (SAO-FRA Belgium), the Queen Elisabeth Medical Foundation (GSKE, Belgium) and the Amyloidosis Foundation (USA). A. Verhelle is supported by the Agency for Innovation by Science and Technology in Flanders.

Author details

Adriaan Verhelle and Jan Gettemans*

*Address all correspondence to: jan.gettemans@ugent.be

Department of Biochemistry, Faculty of Medicine and Health Sciences, Ghent University, Ghent, Belgium

http://dx.doi.org/10.5772/63981

References

[1] de la Chapelle A, Tolvanen R, Boysen G, Santavy J, Bleeker-Wagemakers L, Maury CP, et al. Gelsolin-derived familial amyloidosis caused by asparagine or tyrosine substitution for aspartic acid at residue 187. Nature Genetics. 1992;2(2):157–60.

[2] Sethi S, Theis JD, Quint P, Maierhofer W, Kurtin PJ, Dogan A, et al. Renal amyloidosis associated with a novel sequence variant of gelsolin. American Journal of Kidney Diseases: the Official Journal of the National Kidney Foundation. 2013;61(1):161–6.

[3] Efebera YA, Sturm A, Baack EC, Hofmeister CC, Satoskar A, Nadasdy T, et al. Novel gelsolin variant as the cause of nephrotic syndrome and renal amyloidosis in a large kindred. Amyloid: The International Journal of Experimental and Clinical Investigation: the Official Journal of the International Society of Amyloidosis. 2014;21(2):110–2.

[4] Burtnick LD, Urosev D, Irobi E, Narayan K, Robinson RC. Structure of the N-terminal half of gelsolin bound to actin: roles in severing, apoptosis and FAF. The EMBO Journal. 2004;23(14):2713–22.

[5] Chen CD, Huff ME, Matteson J, Page L, Phillips R, Kelly JW, et al. Furin initiates gelsolin familial amyloidosis in the Golgi through a defect in Ca(2+) stabilization. The EMBO Journal. 2001;20(22):6277–87.

[6] Robinson RC, Choe S, Burtnick LD. The disintegration of a molecule: the role of gelsolin in FAF, familial amyloidosis (Finnish type). Proceedings of the National Academy of Sciences of the United States of America. 2001;98(5):2117–8.

[7] Kiuru-Enari S, Haltia M. Hereditary gelsolin amyloidosis. Handbook of Clinical Neurology. 2013;115:659–81.

[8] Van Overbeke W, Verhelle A, Everaert I, Zwaenepoel O, Vandekerckhove J, Cuvelier C, et al. Chaperone nanobodies protect gelsolin against MT1-MMP degradation and alleviate amyloid burden in the gelsolin amyloidosis mouse model. Molecular Therapy: The Journal of the American Society of Gene Therapy. 2014;22(10):1768–78.

[9] Van Overbeke W, Wongsantichon J, Everaert I, Verhelle A, Zwaenepoel O, Loonchanta A, et al. An ER-directed gelsolin nanobody targets the first step in amyloid formation in a gelsolin amyloidosis mouse model. Human Molecular Genetics. 2015;24(9): 2492–507.

[10] Meretoja J. Familial systemic paramyloidosis with lattice dystrophy of the cornea, progressive cranial neuropathy, skin changes and various internal symptoms. A previously unrecognized heritable syndrome. Annals of Clinical Research. 1969;1(4): 314–24.

[11] Maury CP, Alli K, Baumann M. Finnish hereditary amyloidosis. Amino acid sequence homology between the amyloid fibril protein and human plasma gelsolin. FEBS Letters. 1990;260(1):85–7.

[12] Haltia M, Prelli F, Ghiso J, Kiuru S, Somer H, Palo J, et al. Amyloid protein in familial amyloidosis (Finnish type) is homologous to gelsolin, an actin-binding protein. Biochemical and Biophysical Research Communications. 1990;167(3):927–32.

[13] Kwiatkowski DJ. Functions of gelsolin: motility, signaling, apoptosis, cancer. Current Opinion in Cell Biology. 1999;11(1):103–8.

[14] Silacci P, Mazzolai L, Gauci C, Stergiopulos N, Yin HL, Hayoz D. Gelsolin superfamily proteins: key regulators of cellular functions. Cellular and Molecular Life Sciences: CMLS. 2004;61(19–20):2614–23.

[15] Khurana S, George SP. Regulation of cell structure and function by actin-binding proteins: villin's perspective. FEBS Letters. 2008;582(14):2128–39.

[16] Dominguez R, Holmes KC. Actin structure and function. Annual Review of Biophysics. 2011;40:169–86.

[17] McLaughlin PJ, Gooch JT, Mannherz HG, Weeds AG. Structure of gelsolin segment 1-actin complex and the mechanism of filament severing. Nature. 1993;364(6439):685–92.

[18] Burtnick LD, Koepf EK, Grimes J, Jones EY, Stuart DI, McLaughlin PJ, et al. The crystal structure of plasma gelsolin: implications for actin severing, capping, and nucleation. Cell. 1997;90(4):661–70.

[19] Yin HL, Albrecht JH, Fattoum A. Identification of gelsolin, a Ca2+-dependent regulatory protein of actin gel-sol transformation, and its intracellular distribution in a variety of cells and tissues. The Journal of Cell Biology. 1981;91(3 Pt 1):901–6.

[20] Vouyiouklis DA, Brophy PJ. A novel gelsolin isoform expressed by oligodendrocytes in the central nervous system. Journal of Neurochemistry. 1997;69(3):995–1005.

[21] Choe H, Burtnick LD, Mejillano M, Yin HL, Robinson RC, Choe S. The calcium activation of gelsolin: insights from the 3A structure of the G4-G6/actin complex. Journal of Molecular Biology. 2002;324(4):691–702.

[22] Bucki R, Levental I, Kulakowska A, Janmey PA. Plasma gelsolin: function, prognostic value, and potential therapeutic use. Current Protein & Peptide Science. 2008;9(6):541–51.

[23] Page LJ, Huff ME, Kelly JW, Balch WE. Ca^{2+} binding protects against gelsolin amyloidosis. Biochemical and Biophysical Research Communications. 2004;322(4):1105–10.

[24] Kangas H, Paunio T, Kalkkinen N, Jalanko A, Peltonen L. In vitro expression analysis shows that the secretory form of gelsolin is the sole source of amyloid in gelsolin-related amyloidosis. Human Molecular Genetics. 1996;5(9):1237–43.

[25] Creemers JW, Siezen RJ, Roebroek AJ, Ayoubi TA, Huylebroeck D, Van de Ven WJ. Modulation of furin-mediated proprotein processing activity by site-directed mutagenesis. The Journal of Biological Chemistry. 1993;268(29):21826–34.

[26] Molloy SS, Bresnahan PA, Leppla SH, Klimpel KR, Thomas G. Human furin is a calcium-dependent serine endoprotease that recognizes the sequence Arg-X-X-Arg and efficiently cleaves anthrax toxin protective antigen. The Journal of Biological Chemistry. 1992;267(23):16396–402.

[27] Molloy SS, Thomas L, VanSlyke JK, Stenberg PE, Thomas G. Intracellular trafficking and activation of the furin proprotein convertase: localization to the TGN and recycling from the cell surface. The EMBO Journal. 1994;13(1):18–33.

[28] Kangas H, Seidah NG, Paunio T. Role of proprotein convertases in the pathogenic processing of the amyloidosis-associated form of secretory gelsolin. Amyloid: The International Journal of Experimental and Clinical Investigation: the Official Journal of the International Society of Amyloidosis. 2002;9(2):83–7.

[29] Page LJ, Suk JY, Huff ME, Lim HJ, Venable J, Yates J, et al. Metalloendoprotease cleavage triggers gelsolin amyloidogenesis. The EMBO Journal. 2005;24(23):4124–32.

[30] Kiuru S. Familial amyloidosis of the Finnish type (FAF). A clinical study of 30 patients. Acta Neurologica Scandinavica. 1992;86(4):346–53.

[31] Pihlamaa T, Rautio J, Kiuru-Enari S, Suominen S. Gelsolin amyloidosis as a cause of early aging and progressive bilateral facial paralysis. Plastic and Reconstructive Surgery. 2011;127(6):2342–51.

[32] Page LJ, Suk JY, Bazhenova L, Fleming SM, Wood M, Jiang Y, et al. Secretion of amyloidogenic gelsolin progressively compromises protein homeostasis leading to the intracellular aggregation of proteins. Proceedings of the National Academy of Sciences of the United States of America. 2009;106(27):11125–30.

[33] Kohler G, Milstein C. Continuous cultures of fused cells secreting antibody of predefined specificity. Nature. 1975;256(5517):495–7.

[34] Beck A, Wurch T, Bailly C, Corvaia N. Strategies and challenges for the next generation of therapeutic antibodies. Nature Reviews Immunology. 2010;10(5):345–52.

[35] Hamers-Casterman C, Atarhouch T, Muyldermans S, Robinson G, Hamers C, Songa EB, et al. Naturally occurring antibodies devoid of light chains. Nature. 1993;363(6428): 446–8.

[36] Broisat A, Toczek J, Dumas LS, Ahmadi M, Bacot S, Perret P, et al. 99mTc-cAbVCAM1-5 imaging is a sensitive and reproducible tool for the detection of inflamed atherosclerotic lesions in mice. Journal of Nuclear Medicine: Official Publication, Society of Nuclear Medicine. 2014;55(10):1678–84.

[37] Put S, Schoonooghe S, Devoogdt N, Schurgers E, Avau A, Mitera T, et al. SPECT imaging of joint inflammation with Nanobodies targeting the macrophage mannose receptor in a mouse model for rheumatoid arthritis. Journal of Nuclear Medicine: Official Publication, Society of Nuclear Medicine. 2013;54(5):807–14.

[38] Vaneycken I, Devoogdt N, Van Gassen N, Vincke C, Xavier C, Wernery U, et al. Preclinical screening of anti-HER2 nanobodies for molecular imaging of breast cancer. FASEB Journal: Official Publication of the Federation of American Societies for Experimental Biology. 2011;25(7):2433–46.

[39] Dumoulin M, Last AM, Desmyter A, Decanniere K, Canet D, Larsson G, et al. A camelid antibody fragment inhibits the formation of amyloid fibrils by human lysozyme. Nature. 2003;424(6950):783–8.

[40] Pain C, Dumont J, Dumoulin M. Camelid single-domain antibody fragments: uses and prospects to investigate protein misfolding and aggregation, and to treat diseases associated with these phenomena. Biochimie. 2015;111:82–106.

[41] Domanska K, Vanderhaegen S, Srinivasan V, Pardon E, Dupeux F, Marquez JA, et al. Atomic structure of a nanobody-trapped domain-swapped dimer of an amyloidogenic beta2-microglobulin variant. Proceedings of the National Academy of Sciences of the United States of America. 2011;108(4):1314–9.

[42] Rasmussen SG, DeVree BT, Zou Y, Kruse AC, Chung KY, Kobilka TS, et al. Crystal structure of the beta2 adrenergic receptor-Gs protein complex. Nature. 2011;477(7366): 549–55.

[43] Dorresteijn B, Rotman M, Faber D, Schravesande R, Suidgeest E, van der Weerd L, et al. Camelid heavy chain only antibody fragment domain against beta-site of amyloid precursor protein cleaving enzyme 1 inhibits beta-secretase activity in vitro and in vivo. The FEBS Journal. 2015;282(18):3618–31.

[44] Vincke C, Loris R, Saerens D, Martinez-Rodriguez S, Muyldermans S, Conrath K. General strategy to humanize a camelid single-domain antibody and identification of a universal humanized nanobody scaffold. The Journal of Biological Chemistry. 2009;284(5):3273–84.

[45] Van Audenhove I, Debeuf N, Boucherie C, Gettemans J. Fascin actin bundling controls podosome turnover and disassembly while cortactin is involved in podosome assembly by its SH3 domain in THP-1 macrophages and dendritic cells. Biochimica et Biophysica Acta. 2015;1853(5):940–52.

[46] Bethuyne J, De Gieter S, Zwaenepoel O, Garcia-Pino A, Durinck K, Verhelle A, et al. A nanobody modulates the p53 transcriptional program without perturbing its functional architecture. Nucleic Acids Research. 2014;42(20):12928–38.

[47] Van den Abbeele A, De Clercq S, De Ganck A, De Corte V, Van Loo B, Soror SH, et al. A llama-derived gelsolin single-domain antibody blocks gelsolin-G-actin interaction. Cellular and Molecular Life Sciences: CMLS. 2010;67(9):1519–35.

[48] Xavier C, Devoogdt N, Hernot S, Vaneycken I, D'Huyvetter M, De Vos J, et al. Site-specific labeling of his-tagged Nanobodies with (9)(9)mTc: a practical guide. Methods in Molecular Biology. 2012;911:485–90.

http://dx.doi.org/10.5772/63981

[49] Conrath KE, Lauwereys M, Galleni M, Matagne A, Frere JM, Kinne J, et al. Beta-lactamase inhibitors derived from single-domain antibody fragments elicited in the camelidae. Antimicrobial Agents and Chemotherapy. 2001;45(10):2807–12.

[50] Wu Z, Yang H, Colosi P. Effect of genome size on AAV vector packaging. Molecular Therapy: the Journal of the American Society of Gene Therapy. 2010;18(1):80–6.

[51] Cecchi C, Stefani M. The amyloid-cell membrane system. The interplay between the biophysical features of oligomers/fibrils and cell membrane defines amyloid toxicity. Biophysical Chemistry. 2013;182:30–43.

[52] Bemporad F, Chiti F. Protein misfolded oligomers: experimental approaches, mechanism of formation, and structure-toxicity relationships. Chemistry & Biology. 2012;19(3):315–27.

[53] Kasturirangan S, Li L, Emadi S, Boddapati S, Schulz P, Sierks MR. Nanobody specific for oligomeric beta-amyloid stabilizes nontoxic form. Neurobiology of Aging. 2012;33(7):1320–8.